Contemporary Cardiology

Series Editor
Peter P. Toth, Ciccarone Center for the Prevention of Cardiovascular
Disease, Johns Hopkins University, Baltimore, MD, USA

For more than a decade, cardiologists and other clinicians have relied on the Contemporary Cardiology series to provide them with forefront medical references on all aspects of cardiology. Each title is carefully crafted by world-renown cardiologists who comprehensively cover the most important topics in this rapidly advancing field. With more than 75 titles in print covering everything from diabetes and cardiovascular disease to the management of acute coronary syndromes, the Contemporary Cardiology series has become the leading reference source for the practice of cardiac care.

Nathan D. Wong • Ezra A. Amsterdam
Peter P. Toth
Editors

ASPC Self-Assessment Program in Preventive Cardiology

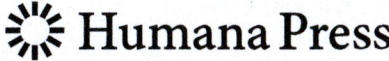

Editors
Nathan D. Wong
Heart Disease Prevention Program, Mary
and Steve Wen Cardiovascular Division
University of California, Irvine
School of Medicine
Irvine, CA, USA

Ezra A. Amsterdam
Division of Cardiovascular Medicine
University of California, Davis, School of
Medicine
Sacramento, CA, USA

Peter P. Toth
Division of Cardiology
Johns Hopkins School of Medicine and
Department of Family and Community
Medicine, University of Illinois
College of Medicine
Peoria, IL, USA

ISSN 2196-8969   ISSN 2196-8977   (electronic)
Contemporary Cardiology
ISBN 978-3-031-56237-2   ISBN 978-3-031-56238-9   (eBook)
https://doi.org/10.1007/978-3-031-56238-9

© The Editor(s) (if applicable) and The Author(s), under exclusive license to Springer Nature Switzerland AG 2024
This work is subject to copyright. All rights are solely and exclusively licensed by the Publisher, whether the whole or part of the material is concerned, specifically the rights of translation, reprinting, reuse of illustrations, recitation, broadcasting, reproduction on microfilms or in any other physical way, and transmission or information storage and retrieval, electronic adaptation, computer software, or by similar or dissimilar methodology now known or hereafter developed.
The use of general descriptive names, registered names, trademarks, service marks, etc. in this publication does not imply, even in the absence of a specific statement, that such names are exempt from the relevant protective laws and regulations and therefore free for general use.
The publisher, the authors and the editors are safe to assume that the advice and information in this book are believed to be true and accurate at the date of publication. Neither the publisher nor the authors or the editors give a warranty, expressed or implied, with respect to the material contained herein or for any errors or omissions that may have been made. The publisher remains neutral with regard to jurisdictional claims in published maps and institutional affiliations.

This Humana imprint is published by the registered company Springer Nature Switzerland AG
The registered company address is: Gewerbestrasse 11, 6330 Cham, Switzerland

Paper in this product is recyclable.

Preface

Over the past four decades, we have experienced explosive growth in our understanding of the prevention and treatment of cardiovascular diseases. With enhanced recommendations for lifestyle management as the foundation of cardiovascular disease prevention as well as the introduction of newer classes of antihypertensive agents, statins, lipid-modifying agents, antiplatelet drugs, anticoagulants, and anti-inflammatory agents, the prevention of cardiovascular disease and its progression has become a reality. Never before have we had such an astonishing impact on dyslipidemia, hypertension, insulin resistance, diabetes mellitus, obesity, atherosclerotic disease, heart failure, arrhythmias, and other cardiovascular diseases. Randomized prospective clinical trials have demonstrated the capacity of many therapeutic interventions to reduce risk of acute cardiovascular events, including myocardial infarction, stroke, atrial fibrillation, the need for revascularization, disability, and death, as well as all-cause mortality. Understandably, patients and their health care providers are now empowered to screen and characterize risk factor burden more aggressively, designing more comprehensive therapeutic approaches to both prevent and treat established disease in an evidence-based manner, utilizing highly efficacious drugs and lifestyle modifications.

The growing emphasis on, and need for, cardiovascular disease prevention is greater than ever. Populations around the world are aging. The young seek ways to prevent the clinical fate of their elders, and older individuals strive to maintain their health, aiming not only for a longer life but also for one of quality. Long-term health maintenance is also of interest to governments worldwide, as the cost of health care consumes an ever-increasing percentage of national budgets. Cardiovascular disease remains the number one cause for mortality worldwide and comes with considerable socioeconomic cost. The preventive cardiology specialist is uniquely positioned to make a significant global impact on cardiovascular diseases. It is clear that cardiovascular disease prevention is cost-effective and highly efficacious, resulting in substantially fewer premature deaths and disabilities.

The American Society of Preventive Cardiology (ASPC) and its members are committed to practicing state-of-the-art medicine in the prevention of cardiovascular disease. Preventive cardiology is emerging as a subspecialty of cardiology. The ASPC Self-Assessment Program (SAP) is intended to serve as an educational tool for clinicians to measure the adequacy of their current knowledge in the field of preventive cardiology. It is also intended to help guide further study and highlight some of the most important findings and recommendations from recent years. The questions contained with the SAP represent the entire spectrum of preventive cardiology and are based on clinical trials and established guidelines of care. All of the questions were written by members of the ASPC and their associates with expertise in their respective areas. Completion of the SAP is a component of a comprehensive program constructed by the ASPC to provide recognition of one's expertise in cardiovascular disease prevention. It is our sincere hope that clinician learners will find this resource of high educational value in their endeavors to provide excellent guidance and care in the prevention of cardiovascular disease.

Irvine, CA, USA   Nathan D. Wong
Sacramento, CA, USA   Ezra A. Amsterdam
Baltimore, MD, USA   Peter P. Toth

Contents

Questions 1
Answers 79
Index 255

Contributors

Matthew Allison Division of Preventive Medicine, University of California, San Diego School of Medicine, San Diego, CA, USA

Jaime Almandoz Division of Endocrinology, Department of Internal Medicine, University of Texas Southwestern, Dallas, TX, USA

Yousif Al-Saiegh Lankenau Medical Center, Wynnewood, PA, USA

Ezra A. Amsterdam Division of Cardiovascular Medicine, University of California, Davis, CA, USA

Alison Bailey Center for Heart, Lung and Vascular Health, Parkridge Health System, Chattanooga, TN, USA

Seth Baum Department of Integrated Medical Science, Florida Atlantic University, Boca Raton, FL, USA

Harold Bays Louisville Metabolic and Atherosclerosis Research Center, Louisville, KY, USA

Michael Blaha Division of Cardiology, Johns Hopkins University School of Medicine, Baltimore, MD, USA

Roger Blumenthal Division of Cardiology, Johns Hopkins University School of Medicine, Roger Blumenthal, MD, USA

William Boden Department of Medicine, Boston University School of Medicine, Boston, MA, USA

Matthew Budoff Division of Cardiology, Harbor-UCLA Medical Center, Torrance, CA, USA

Neal Dixit Division of Cardiovascular Medicine, University of California, Davis, CA, USA

Ramzi Dudum Department of General Internal Medicine, Stanford University School of Medicine, Stanford, CA, USA

Nada El Husseini Department of Cardiology, Duke University School of Medicine, Durham, NC, USA

Carter English Division of Cardiovascular Medicine, University of California, Davis, CA, USA

Keith Ferdinand Department of Medicine, Tulane University School of Medicine, New Orleans, LA, USA

Barry Franklin Department of Internal Medicine, Oakland University William Beaumont School of Medicine, Royal Oak, MI, USA

Charles German Department of Medicine, University of Chicago School of Medicine, Chicago, IL, USA

Dick Glassock Department of Medicine, Harbor-UCLA Medical Center, Torrance, CA, USA

Ty Gluckman Center for Cardiovascular Analytics, Research, and Data Science, Providence Heart Institute, Portland, OR, USA

Martha Gulati Department of Cardiology, Cedars-Sinai Medical Center, Los Angeles, CA, USA

Benjamin Hirsch Division of Infectious Diseases, Zucker School of Medicine, Manhasset, NY, USA

Adedapo Iluyomade Miami Heart and Vascular Institute, Miami, FL, USA

Carol Kirkpatrick Division of Cardiology, University of California, Irvine School of Medicine, Irvine, CA, USA

Arthur Klatsky Division of Research, Kaiser Permanente, Oakland, CA, USA

Stephen Kopecky Division of Cardiology, Mayo Clinic, Rochester, MN, USA

Anandita Kulkarni Department of Medicine, Texas A&M University College of Medicine, Bryan, TX, USA

Ryan Longmore Longmore Clinic, Portneuf Medical Center, Pocatello, ID, USA

Russel Luepker Division of Epidemiology and Community Health, University of Minnesota School of Public Health, Minneapolis, MN, USA

Shaista Malik Division of Cardiology, University of California, Irvine, School of Medicine, Irvine, CA, USA

David Maron Division of Cardiovascular Medicine, Stanford University School of Medicine, Stanford, CA, USA

Anurag Mehta Department of Cardiology, Virginia Commonwealth University, Tappahannock, VA, USA

Nehal Mehta Inflammation and Cardiometabolic Diseases, National Heart Lung and Blood Institute, Bethesda, MD, USA

Erin Michos Division of Cardiology, Johns Hopkins University School of Medicine, Baltimore, MD, USA

AnnMarie Navar Division of Cardiology, University of Texas Southwestern, Dallas, TX, USA

Adam Nelson Duke Clinical Research Institute, Duke University, Duram, NC, USA

Keith Norris Division of General Internal Medicine, University of California, Los Angeles School of Medicine, Los Angeles, CA, USA

Alex Razavi Division of Cardiology, Emory University School of Medicine, Atlanta, GA, USA

Fatima Rodriguez Division of Cardiovascular Medicine, Stanford University School of Medicine, Stanford, CA, USA

Ashish Sarraju Division of Cardiovascular Medicine, Stanford University School of Medicine, Stanford, CA, USA

Doug Schocken Department of Cardiology, Duke University School of Medicine, Durham, NC, USA

Geeta Sikand Division of Cardiology, University of California, Irvine School of Medicine, Irvine, CA, USA

Lance Sloan Texas Institute for Kidney and Endocrine Disorders, Lufkin, TX, USA

Laurence Sperling Division of Cardiology, Emory University School of Medicine, Atlanta, GA, USA

Neil Stone Division of Cardiology, Northwestern University, Chicago, IL, USA

Robert Superko Cholesterol, Genetics and Heart Disease Institute, Alameda, CA, USA

Peter P. Toth Division of Cardiology, Johns Hopkins School of Medicine and Department of Family and Community Medicine, University of Illinois College of Medicine, Peoria, IL, USA

Saqndhya Venugopal Division of Cardiovascular Medicine, University of California, Davis, CA, USA

Howard Weintraub Division of Cardiology, New York University, New York, NY, USA

Nathan D. Wong Heart Disease Prevention Program, Mary and Steve Wen Cardiovascular Division, University of California, Irvine School of Medicine, Irvine, CA, USA

Masood Younus Division of Cardiovascular Medicine, University of California, Davis, CA, USA

Questions

1. **Which of the following groups are adequately represented in cardiovascular clinical trials?**
   A. White men
   B. Black women
   C. Asian men
   D. Hispanic women

2. **Chronic venous disease**:
   A. Is associated with decreased morbidity
   B. Is associated with low BMI (body mass index)
   C. Is more common than peripheral arterial disease
   D. Is more common in men

3. A 48-year-old woman presents to clinic with progressive claudication symptoms over the last 3 years. She describes pain with ambulation and legs feeling "full," aching at night and not sleeping well. These symptoms are limiting her ability to function and causing decreased quality of life. Medical history is significant for hypertension, obesity, and 4 prior pregnancies.
   Exam: BP 120/64 mmHg, HR 75/min, BMI (body mass index) 31. She has a normal cardiac and respiratory exam. She has 2+/4 pulses in both lower extremities. There is 1+ lower extremity edema and dilated veins around the ankle bilaterally.
   Which one of the following tests is most likely to provide a diagnosis in this patient with suspected chronic venous disease (CVeD)?
   A. Ankle Brachial Index
   B. Nerve Conduction Study
   C. MRI of the lumbar spine
   D. Duplex scan of the veins

4. **Effective treatment options for chronic venous disease (CVeD) include which one of the following?**
   A. Clopidogrel
   B. Apixaban
   C. Arterial revascularization
   D. Weight loss

5. **A 57-year-old female with hypertension, hyperlipidemia, and obesity presents to your office for cardiovascular risk management. She is asymptomatic and denies family history of early ASCVD (arteriosclerotic cardiovascular risk) related events. She has three children and denies any history of pregnancy complications or other risk enhancing factors. LDL-cholesterol 146 mg/dL, triglycerides 167 mg/dL. She asks you if she needs medication. You calculate her 10-year ASCVD risk to be 8.5%.**
   What is the next best step in your management?
   A. Initiate moderate intensity statin
   B. Lifestyle modifications
   C. Obtain CT Calcium Score
   D. Initiate fenofibrate

6. **A 45-year-old male with Type 2 diabetes diagnosed 4 years prior presents to your office for management of hypertriglyceridemia. He currently takes fenofibrate 160 mg twice daily and aspirin 81 mg. His triglyceride level is 340 mg/dL on therapy.**
   What is the next best step in managing his hypertriglyceridemia?
   A. Addition of rosuvastatin 10 mg daily
   B. Increase fenofibrate dose
   C. Addition of icosapent ethyl
   D. Addition of niacin

7. **A 58-year-old female known to have Type 2 diabetes on oral hypoglycemics, history of gestational hypertension, mixed hyperlipidemia, obesity, and polycystic ovary syndrome presents to your office for management of cardiovascular risk. Recent CAC (coronary artery calcium score) 23 Agatson units, LDL cholesterol 66 mg/dL, triglycerides (TG) 163 mg/dL, HDL 41 mg/dL, hs-CRP 4.7 mg/L. She is currently on rosuvastatin 40 mg nightly and ezetimibe 20 mg daily. The addition of which pharmacotherapy is indicated to reduce her future risk of major adverse cardiovascular events?**
   A. Niacin
   B. PCSK-9
   C. silencing-RNA
   D. Icosapent ethyl

8. A 30-year-old male in generally good health presents to your office for management of dyslipidemia. He endorses a family history of father and brother (12 years old) with elevated cholesterol. His father experienced an acute myocardial infarction last year at age 54. The patient brings with him reports of laboratory evaluations obtained over the years. His most recent LDL-cholesterol is 168 mg/dL, and his peak LDL-cholesterol thus far has been 187 mg/dL. He is concerned about having a heart attack at a young age. What is the most appropriate next step in the management of this patient's future ASCVD risk?
   A. Calculate 10-year ASCVD risk using pooled cohort equation
   B. Initiate moderate intensity statin
   C. Lifestyle modifications
   D. Genetic testing

9. Among men over 40 years of age residing in the United States in the year 2000, which race/ethnic group had the highest prevalence of peripheral arterial disease (PAD)?
   A. African American
   B. American Indian
   C. Asian American
   D. Hispanic Americans
   E. Non-Hispanic Whites

10. Which of the following risk factors for peripheral arterial disease (PAD) is most often associated with artefactual elevations of ankle brachial index (ABI) values?
    A. Cigarette smoking
    B. Diabetes mellitus
    C. Hypertension
    D. Hyperlipidemia

11. Which one of the following pharmacologic agents should be prescribed to a patient with asymptomatic and uncomplicated peripheral arterial disease (PAD) to reduce the risk of future cardiovascular disease events?
    A. Aspirin
    B. Cilostazol
    C. Pentoxifylline
    D. Rivaroxaban

12. Among patients with symptomatic peripheral arterial disease (e.g., PAD with intermittent claudication), and compared to conservative management, early revascularization is associated with an increased risk for amputation.
    A. True
    B. False

13. A 52-year-old man with hypertension, Type 2 diabetes mellitus and obstructive sleep apnea presents for cardiovascular health optimization. Medications include amlodipine 5 mg daily and metformin 500 mg twice daily. There is no history of tobacco use, and he consumes two alcohol-containing beverages per week.
    Blood pressure is 120/80 mmHg, and heart rate is 75 beats/min. Height is 175 cm, and weight is 100 kg (BMI [body mass index] = 32.7 kg/m^2). Physical examination is unremarkable except for central obesity.
    What magnitude of weight loss would be beneficial to reduce his cardiovascular mortality?
    A. 3 kg
    B. ≥5%
    C. 7.5 kg
    D. 8 kg
    E. ≥10%

14. A 59-year-old female breast cancer survivor with Type 2 diabetes mellitus, mixed hyperlipidemia, hypertension, coronary artery disease, heart failure with preserved ejection fraction, and depression is referred by her oncologist for weight loss and health optimization.
    The patient has tried several low-calorie diets without any significant or durable weight loss. Physical activity is limited by arthralgia from aromatase inhibitor therapy. Current medications include: empagliflozin, atorvastatin, metoprolol succinate, lisinopril, low-dose aspirin, and bupropion. Blood pressure is 115/72 mmHg, and her heart rate is 70 beats/min. Height is 163 cm, and weight is 97 kg (BMI [body mass index] = 36.5 kg/m^2). Physical examination is unremarkable except for a left mastectomy scar.
    Laboratory results:
    Hemoglobin A1c = 6.8% (4.3–5.6%)
    CBC within normal limits; kidney and liver function tests within normal limits.
    Which anti-obesity medication is most appropriate for this patient?
    A. Semaglutide
    B. Phentermine
    C. Phentermine Topiramate ER
    D. Naltrexone Bupropion ER
    E. Metformin

15. A 65-year-old man with Type 2 diabetes, obstructive sleep apnea, hypertension, and hyperlipidemia presents for cardiovascular risk optimization. Type 2 diabetes was diagnosed 2 years ago at an annual health maintenance visit. Medications include metformin 1000 mg daily, atorvastatin 40 mg daily, and lisinopril 5 mg daily. His brother recently had a triple coronary artery bypass grafting, and the patient is concerned about his own risk for cardiovascular disease.

Blood pressure is 135/86 mmHg, and heart rate is 75 beats/min. Body mass index is 38 kg/m^2. Physical examination is remarkable for central adiposity with a palpable liver edge at the right costal margin.

Laboratory test results:
   Hemoglobin A1c = 9.0% (4.3–5.6%)
   Total cholesterol = 149 mg/dL (120–199 mg/dL)
   Triglycerides = 120 mg/dL (50–150 mg/dL)
   HDL cholesterol = 43 mg/dL (>39 mg/dL)
   LDL cholesterol = 67 mg/dL (<100 mg/dL)
   Non-HDL cholesterol = 106 mg/dL (95–160 mg/dL)
   Urine Microalbumin = 28 (<30)

Which one of the following is most likely to improve his cardiometabolic health and decrease his risk of future cardiovascular events?
A. Add empagliflozin 10 mg
B. Add liraglutide 0.6 mg
C. Roux-en-Y gastric bypass (RYBG)
D. Start insulin glargine
E. Start linagliptin

16. A 40-year-old Hispanic woman with nonalcoholic fatty liver disease, polycystic ovarian syndrome, and prediabetes presents for evaluation of shortness of breath on exertion. Her cardiovascular evaluation is unremarkable, and exercise testing suggests marked physical deconditioning. Her current BMI is 43 kg/m^2, and she would like to avoid bariatric surgery. Her fertility doctor has recommended 20% weight loss before she starts assisted fertility treatments.

Which one of the following medications is most likely to facilitate ≥20% weight loss?
A. Semaglutide
B. Empagliflozin
C. Liraglutide
D. Phentermine Topiramate ER
E. Tirzepatide

17. **A 59-year-old woman with exertional chest pain that occurs infrequently and is variably described by this patient, underwent a treadmill exercise test without imaging for assessment of this symptom. Select the best choice below.**
    A. Women should receive an imaging stress test rather than an electrocardiography (ECG) treadmill test without imaging because women have a high rate of false positive exercise ECGs.
    B. This patient's functional capacity on the treadmill test will provide an excellent estimation of her prognosis related to cardiovascular disease (CVD).
    C. The maximum heart rate x systolic blood pressure ("double product") achieved during exercise testing is an established indicator of prognosis in men.
    D. The percent positive predictive value of an exercise test is determined by the number of True-Positive results divided by the number of False-Positive results.
    E. Heart recovery (HRR) after an exercise test is not a useful method for estimating prognosis of CVD in women.

18. **A 40-year-old man was referred for a non-imaging exercise treadmill test as a screening method to detect coronary artery disease. The referral was occasioned by the patient's alarm over the recent myocardial infarction of a friend. The 40-year-old man has no family history of premature cardiovascular disease, and his arteriosclerotic cardiovascular disease risk score estimates that he has <1% probability of sustaining a cardiovascular event during the next 10 years. Select the best choice from the statements below.**
    A. Performance of a treadmill test is a useful addition to the evaluation of this 40-year-old man to screen for coronary artery disease.
    B. A stress imaging cardiac test (myocardial perfusion or echocardiography) is the preferred screening test for cardiovascular disease in this man.
    C. Family history of cardiovascular disease is one of the primary factors used in calculating an individual's arteriosclerotic cardiovascular disease (ASCVD) risk score to estimate future probability for fatal/nonfatal myocardial infarction or stroke.
    D. The Bruce exercise test protocol is characterized by modest increases in speed and grade of the successive stages of the test.
    E. The specificity (%) of an exercise test is based on the number of individuals with a normal test result divided by the number of all individuals without the condition tested for, multiplied by HMWS100, that is, number of True Negatives/(Number of True Negatives + False Positives) × 100.

19. **Select the one correct choice from the following statements regarding exercise testing.**
    A. The definition of 1 metabolic equivalent (MET), as used to estimate energy expenditure during exercise is: cc of oxygen expended per kilogram body weight per minute, that is, cc O_2/kg/min.
    B. The equation usually used to estimate an individual's predicted maximum exercise heart rate (220-age) is based on extensive exercise physiology studies.
    C. A fall of ≥20 mmHg in systolic BP during treadmill testing is associated with 3-V CAD or left main CAD in 95% of patients with this finding during exercise testing.
    D. ST segment elevation during a treadmill exercise test does not localize the myocardial region in which exercise has induced ischemia as reflected by this electrocardiographic finding.
    E. Ischemic ST segment depression during the post-exercise recovery phase of an exercise test is a false-positive result in the majority of individuals with this finding.

20. **Select the best single response to the following statements concerning exercise testing.**
    A. Bayes' theorem specifies that the accuracy of a test is determined by the sensitivity and specificity of the test.
    B. By convention, a treadmill exercise test in which the patient fails to reach at least 85% of age-predicted maximum heart rate with no ST depression is considered negative for ischemiA.
    C. Maximum functional capacity determined on a stress test is a less accurate indicator of prognosis than is exercise-induced ischemic ST segment depression.
    D. The Duke treadmill score (DTS) includes patient age and sex, minutes of treadmill exercise, millimeters of ST segment depression, and grade of exercise-induced chest pain.
    E. Studies have shown that individuals with an ischemic exercise ECG and excellent functional capacity (≥10 METs) have normal stress imaging tests and low prognostic risk.
    F. In a majority of patients with exercise-induced ischemic ST depression occurring initially during the recovery phase of an exercise test, this result is a false positive.

21. **The stagnation in preventable cardiovascular death rates among American adults over the past decade is associated with an increasing prevalence of all of the following risk factors except:**
    A. Smoking
    B. Diabetes mellitus
    C. Physical inactivity
    D. Obesity

22. **The American Heart Association has identified eight modifiable cardiovascular health factors and behaviors that are colloquially called Life's Essential 8. Which one of the following is an ideal cardiovascular health factor?**
    A. Systolic BP 120–139 or diastolic BP 80–89 mmHg
    B. Non-HDL-cholesterol <130 mg/dL
    C. Body mass index 25–29.9 kg/m^2
    D. 6–7 h of sleep

23. **The 2018 ACC/AHA/Multisociety cholesterol management guidelines recommend using risk-enhancing factors to improve personalization of cardiovascular risk assessment and better guide preventive pharmacotherapy use in primary prevention.**
    Which one of the following is not a risk-enhancing factor?
    A. Metabolic syndrome
    B. South Asian ancestry
    C. Ankle brachial index <1.0
    D. Family history of premature atherosclerotic cardiovascular disease

24. **Cardiac rehabilitation is a Class I guideline-recommended team-based approach for comprehensive secondary prevention of multiple cardiovascular disorders. Which of the following indications is not a Medicare covered guideline-recommended Class I indication for comprehensive cardiac rehabilitation or supervised exercise therapy (SET)?**
    A. Chronic heart failure with preserved ejection fraction
    B. Percutaneous coronary intervention
    C. Symptomatic peripheral artery disease
    D. Cardiac valve surgery

25. A 52-year-old woman presents to the office for follow up of Type 2 diabetes mellitus. She was diagnosed with diabetes 2 years ago and has tried lifestyle modifications. She is on the maximum daily dose of metformin and has no gastrointestinal complaints. She has a family history of Type 2 diabetes, hypertension, and coronary artery disease, and she has no history of pancreatitis. On examination, her blood pressure is 140/85 mmHg and pulse is 82/min; peripheral pulses are 2+ bilaterally without pedal edemA. Her BMI is 36 kg/m^2. Acanthosis nigricans is present on the neck and axilla. Monofilament test did not reveal any sensory loss in the lower extremities. The lungs are clear to auscultation. Normal S1 and S2 are heard, and no murmurs are present. Patient was found to have marked abdominal obesity.

Laboratory findings are as follows:
    Creatinine = 0.7 mg/dL
    Glucose = 150 mg/dL
    Alanine aminotransferase = 66 U/L
    Aspartate aminotransferase = 58 U/L
    Alkaline phosphatase = 80 U/L
    LDL Cholesterol = 145 mg/dL
    Triglycerides = 225 mg/dL
    Hemoglobin A1c = 8.7%
    Urine microalbumin/creatinine = 320 mg/g

Which one of the following measures is most likely to achieve a hemoglobin A1c goal of <6.5% person within 1 year in this patient?

A. Adding empagliflozin
B. Adding liraglutide
C. Continued intensive lifestyle changes
D. Adding tirzepatide
E. Starting insulin therapy

26. A 59-year-old African-American man presents to his cardiologist for a follow-up visit. He does not have any symptoms currently and is satisfied with his overall health. He runs about a mile daily and preforms strength training 2–3 times a week. He eats a healthy diet. He never smoked and drinks occasionally about 1–2 times a month. He is very compliant with his medications. He has a history of hypertension and was diagnosed with diabetes 1 year ago and is currently on the maximum daily dose of metformin without any gastrointestinal complaints. No history of pancreatitis. Family history includes diabetes, kidney disease, and coronary artery disease in his father and hypertension, hyperlipidemia, kidney disease, and stroke in his mother. His other medications are hydrochlorothiazide, losartan, rosuvastatin, multivitamins.

During this visit, his blood pressure is 118/76 mmHg and pulse is 68/min; peripheral pulses are 2+ bilaterally, with trace pedal edema. His BMI (body mass index) is 27 kg/m^2. Monofilament test did not reveal any sensory loss in the lower extremities. The lungs are clear to auscultation. Normal S1 and S2 are heard, and no murmurs are present. Apical impulse is felt in the fifth left intercostal space. Abdomen is soft and non-distended.

Laboratory findings are as follows:
- Sodium = 142 mEq/L
- Potassium = 4.0 mEq/L
- Bicarbonate = 24 mEq/L
- Blood urea nitrogen = 24 mg/dL
- Creatinine = 1.3 mg/dL
- Glucose = 140 mg/dL
- Alanine aminotransferase = 24 U/L
- Aspartate aminotransferase = 28 U/L
- Total Cholesterol = 140 mg/dL
- Triglycerides = 98 mg/dL
- HDL Cholesterol = 55 mg/dL
- VLDL Cholesterol = 20 mg/dL
- LDL Cholesterol = 65 mg/dL
- Hemoglobin A1c = 7.8%
- Urine microalbumin/creatinine = 320 mg/g

The patient's 10-year ASCVD (atherosclerotic cardiovascular disease) risk is 17.8%. Given his elevated cardiovascular risk and HbA1c, a shared decision to initiate cardiovascular risk lowering diabetes therapy was made.

According to the recent data, which one of the following is TRUE about use of cardiovascular risk lowering diabetes therapy by cardiologists?

A. 50% of all (GLP1-RA (glucagon-like peptide-1 receptor agonist) and SGLT2i (sodium-glucose cotransporter-2 Inhibitor) prescriptions are by cardiologists.

B. 25% of all GLP1-RA and SGLT2i prescriptions are by cardiologists.

C. 10% of all GLP1-RA and SGLT2i prescriptions are by cardiologists.

D. 5% of all GLP1-RA and SGLT2i prescriptions are by cardiologists.

E. <2.5% of all GLP1-RA and SGLT2i prescriptions are by cardiologists

27. A 38-year-old Caucasian man presents to the physician for complaints of gradual weight gain over the past few years. The patient works as an administrative assistant at an insurance company and spends most of his time at his desk. He lives a predominantly sedentary life and eats fast foods for lunch and precooked frozen foods for dinner along with 4–5 cans of fruit juices and sugared sodas daily. He started smoking in his late teens; he smoked about half a pack a day for 20 years and has not converted exclusively to electronic cigarettes. He also drinks a few beers on the weekends. He has a family history of Type 2 diabetes, hypertension, hyperlipidemia, and his father died of heart attack at the 49. His mother is alive with heart failure.

On examination, his blood pressure is 134/84 mmHg and pulse is 82/min; peripheral pulses are 2+ bilaterally. His BMI (body mass index) is 32 kg/m^2. There is no jugular venous distention. The lungs are clear to auscultation. Normal cardiac S1 and S2 are heard, and no murmurs are present. Cardiac apex is felt in the fifth left intercostal space. Patient was found to have abdominal obesity.

Laboratory findings are as follows:
    Glucose = 104 mg/dL
    Hemoglobin A1c = 5.7%
    Total Cholesterol = 250 mg/dL
    HDL Cholesterol = 55 mg/dL
    LDL Cholesterol = 115 mg/dL
    Triglycerides = 350 mg/dL

His electrolytes, renal function tests, liver function tests, and thyroid panel are normal.

In addition to intense lifestyle modification, which one of the following is the next best step in the overall evaluation and management of this patient?

A. Coronary artery calcium assessment
B. High intensity atorvastatin
C. Fenofibrate
D. Aspirin
E. No further intervention

28. A 54-year-old African-American woman presents to the office for follow up of elevated blood pressure noted during his routine annual visit 3 months ago. Her blood pressure was 142/88 mmHg during the initial visit. She works as a data analyst for a multinational bank and spends most of the time working from home at her desk. She mentions that her work has been stressful lately, which has been preventing her from engaging in any physical activity. She tries to eat healthy food except for occasional fried food 1–2 times a week. She has a family history of Type 2 diabetes, hypertension, hyperlipidemia, and obesity, but no history of premature cardiovascular disease was noted. She is a lifetime nonsmoker, drinks a glass of red wine nightly with dinner, and does not use any recreational drugs. The patient was started on low-dose hydrochlorothiazide and amlodipine.

She mentions that she has been sleeping well and she has been walking about 25 min about 5–6 times a week. She made changes to her diet including cutting down on salt and eating more vegetables and fruits. She lost about 4 lb in the past 3 months.

During this visit, her blood pressure is 126/78 mmHg and pulse is 78/min; peripheral pulses are 2+ bilaterally. Her BMI (body mass index) is 27 kg/m^2. There is no jugular venous distention. The lungs are clear to auscultation. Normal S1 and S2 are heard, and no murmurs are present. Cardiac apex is felt in the fifth left intercostal space. There is peripheral edemA. Abdomen in soft and nondistended.

Laboratory findings are as follows:
    Hemoglobin A1c = 5.3%
    Total Cholesterol = 220 mg/dL
    HDL Cholesterol = 45 mg/dL
    LDL Cholesterol = 108 mg/dL
    Triglycerides = 178 mg/dL

Her electrolytes, renal function tests, liver function tests, and thyroid panel are normal. Her 10-year ASCVD (atherosclerotic cardiovascular disease) risk is 5.8%.

On discussing statin therapy, the patient is hesitant to taking statins due to concern for side effects. A CAC scan was performed, and she was found to have a CAC (coronary artery calcium score) of 0. Given CAC score of zero, statin initiation was deferred with emphasis on intensive lifestyle changes and BP medication adherence.

Which one of the following is the most appropriate in the long-term management of this patient?

A. Repeat CAC scan every year
B. Repeat CAC scan in about 2–3 years
C. Repeat CAC scan in about 5 years
D. Repeat CAC scan in about 10 years
E. Do not repeat CAC scan

29. **You are seeing a 45-year-old male with no prior ASCVD (atherosclerotic cardiovascular disease) as a referral for primary ASCVD prevention. His primary care clinician estimated his 10-year ASCVD risk using the pooled cohort equations and found it to be 10%. The patient was recommended a statin but is reluctant to start it.**
    Which one of the following would be the best test to guide your risk discussion regarding statin therapy with this patient?
    A. No test is needed. Reassure the patient and remeasure his pooled cohort estimated risk in 5 years.
    B. Measure coronary artery calcium score.
    C. Measure Lp(a).
    D. Obtain ApoB measurement.

30. **You are seeing a 55-year-old woman for primary ASCVD (atherosclerotic cardiovascular disease) prevention recommendations. Which one of the following, if present in this patient, is a risk-enhancing factor that could guide clinician–patient risk discussions regarding preventive interventions?**
    A. Having a sister who suffered a heart attack at age 55 years.
    B. Premature menopause
    C. History of preeclampsia during her second pregnancy
    D. All of the above

31. **You are seeing a 60-year-old man with no past medical history in your cardiology cliniC. The patient is interested in getting your advice on how to lower his future risk of a heart attack or stroke. Which one of the following is recommended for primary ASCVD (atherosclerotic cardiovascular disease) prevention based on the 2018 AHA/ACC/Multisociety guidelines for primary prevention?**
    A. 75 min of moderate intensity exercise per week
    B. Increase intake of trans and polyunsaturated fatty acids
    C. Reducing the intake of processed red meats.
    D. Both B and C

32. **A 62-year-old female teacher presented to your cardiology clinic for advice on how to lower her future risk of ASCVD (atherosclerotic cardiovascular disease). She has diabetes that is well controlled on metformin but has no history of ASCVD. She is currently on atorvastatin 20 mg nightly for primary ASCVD prevention. Which one of the following, if present, would make you consider intensifying her statin therapy?**
    A. Diabetic Retinopathy
    B. ≥10-year duration of diabetes
    C. Elevated hsCRP (high sensitivity C reactive protein)
    D. Both A and B

33. **You are seeing a 65-year-old woman in your clinic for primary ASCVD (atherosclerotic cardiovascular disease) prevention. She has no history of diabetes. During her first clinic visit, you prescribed atorvastatin 20 mg nightly for primary ASCVD prevention after discussing her elevated ASCVD risk (10-year ASCVD risk was 20%). She comes back for a follow-up visit after being on atorvastatin for 2 months. Her lipid panel from the second visit showed that her LDL-C cholesterol was lower by 20%. In addition to maintaining a healthy lifestyle, what other recommendation would you give?**
    A. No change in therapy and remeasure LDL-cholesterol in 1 month
    B. Increasing atorvastatin to 40 mg nightly and remeasuring LDL-C in 3 months
    C. Start ezetimibe and remeasure LDL-C in 3 months
    D. Switch atorvastatin to rosuvastatin 10 mg nightly

34. **According to the 2018 AHA/ACC/Multisociety guideline on primary prevention, which of the following can be used to aid adults who use tobacco to maximize quit rates?**
    A. Nicotine patch
    B. Bupropion
    C. Varenicline
    D. All of the above

35. **You are seeing a 72-year-old man in your clinic for advice on primary ASCVD (atherosclerotic cardiovascular disease) prevention. He has an estimated 10-year ASCVD risk of >20%. A prior coronary artery calcium score obtained 5 years ago showed a score of 500 AU (Agatson units). He has been on low-dose aspirin for 10 years and has low bleeding risk. He is asking whether he should continue taking aspirin in light of the current primary ASCVD prevention recommendations.**
    Based on these recommendations, your response is:
    A. He should stop low-dose aspirin given the lack of benefit for primary ASCVD prevention.
    B. The physician should obtain another CAC (coronary artery calcium) measurement to guide treatment decision.
    C. The patient should consider continuing aspirin after a risk-benefit discussion.
    D. Aspirin is contraindicated in those >70 years of age.

36. A 55-year-old male truck driver is seeing you in clinic after measuring his blood pressure at home using his wife blood pressure machine and finding it to be 150/85 mmHg. You obtain two blood pressure readings which confirm that his blood pressure is elevated on two occasions. His estimated ASCVD (atherosclerotic cardiovascular disease) risk using pooled cohort equations was 7.5%. Which one of the following is the best next step for management of his blood pressure?
    A. The patient has elevated blood pressure and should be advised on non-pharmacological therapy alone.
    B. The patient has elevated blood pressure and should be advised to take non-pharmacological therapy plus BP-lowering medications.
    C. The patient has Stage 1 hypertension and should be advised to take non-pharmacological therapy alone since his estimated ASCVD risk is <10%.
    D. The patient has Stage 2 hypertension and should be advised on non-pharmacological therapy plus BP-lowering medications.

37. In patients who experience angina with moderate or strenuous exertional due to presumptive stable coronary artery disease (CAD), what should be the initial diagnostic approach to management?
    A. Obtain a careful history and perform a physical examination
    B. Perform a resting electrocardiogram (ECG)
    C. Undertake a noninvasive functional test (preferably with exercise, or with pharmacologic stress, if patient is unable to exercise) or an anatomic test (coronary computed tomography angiography)
    D. Proceed to invasive coronary angiography if a stenosis >50% is detected noninvasively
    E. A, B, C, and D

38. Among stable CAD (coronary artery disease) patients who have Canadian Cardiovascular Society (CCS) Class 1–2 angina and no diabetes in whom obstructive CAD ($\geq$70%) is diagnosed in one or two coronary arteries either by coronary computed tomography angiography (CCTA) or invasive coronary angiography, which one of the following constitutes the most appropriate initial management?
    A. Perform a functional test (e.g., exercise treadmill, stress myocardial perfusion imaging (MPI) scan, dobutamine stress echo, or CT-FFR, etC.) to assess the extent and severity of inducible myocardial ischemiA.
    B. Initiate guideline directed medical therapy (GDMT) alone including secondary prevention treatments targeted to blood pressure, lipids, and other cardiac risk factors including antianginal therapy
    C. Refer the patient for PCI + GDMT
    D. Refer the patient for CABG surgery
    E. A and B

39. **Which ONE of the following statements is true?**
    A. Treadmill exercise testing can help determine if patients' symptoms are consistent with angina pectoris.
    B. Cardiac magnet resonance imaging (CMR) in coronary artery disease (CAD) patients revealed superior diagnostic accuracy compared to myocardial perfusion imaging (MPI) [2, 3].
    C. Prognosis of patients with CCD is not related to extent and severity of wall motion abnormalities induced during stress echocardiography.
    D. Relief of angina by exercise ischemia-guided percutaneous coronary intervention (PCI) is not superior to medical therapy.
    E. Addition of clinical variables in an integrated score did not alter the risk estimate of a majority of patients evaluated by the Duke Treadmill Score (DTS).

40. **Which one of the following interventions is associated with a survival benefit?**
    A. Lipid-lowering therapy in patients with CCD, moderate to severe left ventricular dysfunction, and markedly elevated LDL cholesterol (>180 mg/dL)
    B. Beta blockers in patients with CCD and left ventricular diastolic dysfunction
    C. Coronary bypass graft (CABG) surgery plus medical therapy in the STICH trial in patients with CCD with ischemic cardiomyopathy and left ventricular dysfunction (ejection fraction ≑ 35%)
    D. Percutaneous coronary intervention (PCI) in patients with CCD, >70% stenosis of the left anterior descending coronary artery and normal left ventricular function
    E. PCI in patients with CCD, multi-vessel coronary artery disease (CAD) and normal left ventricular function

41. **Prediction of ASCVD (atherosclerotic cardiovascular disease) events with coronary artery calcium testing is?**
    A. Incremental to risk factors
    B. Superior to risk factors alone
    C. A robust predictor in women
    D. All of the above
    E. None of the above

42. **A 53-year-old asymptomatic male who is low risk based on risk assessment tools obtains a coronary calcium score due to concern of a family history of premature heart disease. His coronary artery calcium score is 156 (≥75th percentile for age, race, and gender). What is the next best recommended step for him?**
    A. Institute high intensity statin therapy
    B. Assess 10-year ASCVD (atherosclerotic cardiovascular disease) risk and number of risk factors to determine suitability for statin
    C. Perform coronary CT (computed tomography) angiography
    D. Perform nuclear stress test

43. A 58-year-old female with no cardiac symptoms is referred to your cliniC. She is concerned about the possibility of heart disease, as she heard that women after menopause are at increased risk, so she underwent a calcium scan. She is intermediate risk by the pooled risk calculator. Her calcium score is 0.
    Of the choices listed below, what is the one most appropriate next step?
    A. Add statin, given family history and concern of CHD (coronary heart disease)
    B. Reassure and continue lifestyle management for risk
    C. Recommend exercise treadmill testing
    D. Send for carotid intimal media thickness (IMT) assessment

44. Which of the following tests are most accurate to detect obstructive coronary artery disease?
    A. CCTA (coronary computed tomography angiography)
    B. Nuclear
    C. Stress Echocardiography
    D. Stress MRI (magnetic resonance imaging)
    E. Treadmill

45. According to the ACC/AHA 2018 Guidelines, coronary artery calcification imparts high risk status when the score is:
    A. Greater than zero
    B. 1–100
    C. ≥100
    D. ≥300
    E. Not recommended

46. The estimated radiation dose from a coronary artery calcium scan protocol will be approximately equal to:
    A. A chest X-ray
    B. Mammography
    C. 1 year of background radiation
    D. Nuclear scintigraphy

47. **A 32-year-old female with a past medical history of heterozygous familial hypercholesterolemia (HeFH) (genetically confirmed mutation in LDLR; low-density lipoprotein receptor) is seen in your office for further management. She has never received treatment for her cholesterol. She has a past medical history of pregnancy carried to term with infant at low birth weight. She is not on any contraception although she is not currently trying to conceive. She is a nonsmoker. The maternal side of her family has elevated cholesterol but no history of ischemic heart disease. Her blood pressure is 119/78. Today, her fasting lipid profile is TC (total cholesterol) 289 mg/dL, TG (triglycerides) 117 mg/dL, LDL (low-density lipoprotein cholesterol) 174 mg/dL, and HDL (high-density lipoprotein cholesterol) 92 mg/dL.**
    Considering this patient, which one of the following is FALSE?
    A. In addition to lifestyle intervention, statin therapy to reduce LDL-C by 50% is recommended based on her genetically determined HeFH.
    B. Women with HeFH are at increased risk for preterm delivery or of having infants with low birth weight or congenital malformations.
    C. If she starts a statin, she should be advised to use effective form of contraception and to stop her statin if trying to conceive or if pregnancy is discovered.
    D. A history of low-birth-weight infants has been shown to increase risk for atherosclerotic cardiovascular disease (ASCVD).

48. **A 71-year-old White female with history of hypothyroidism and recurrent SVT (supraventricular tachycardia) presents to establish cardiac care. She denies any symptoms suggestive of ischemic heart disease. Her untreated blood pressure is 113/67. Her fasting lipid profile is TC (total cholesterol) 212 mg/dL, TG (triglycerides) 106 mg/dL, LDL (low-density lipoprotein cholesterol) 151 mg/dL, and HDL (high-density lipoprotein cholesterol) 40 mg/dL. She has never smoked and has no history of diabetes. She is hesitant to start statin therapy. A coronary artery calcium (CAC) score is obtained and is zero.**
    Which statement is TRUE regarding the use of CAC score in this patient:
    A. She has an intermediate 10-year risk for ASCVD (atherosclerotic cardiovascular disease) based on the Pooled Cohort Equations (PCE), and despite her uncertainty and the CAC score, she should be initiated on moderate-intensity statin.
    B. The CAC score is reassuring in a nonsmoker and nondiabetic, and despite her intermediate 10-year risk for ASCVD by PCE, statin therapy may safely be withheld.
    C. The CAC score does not predict risk beyond traditional risk factors in women.
    D. If she were African American, a CAC score guided strategy to reclassify risk for ASCVD would not be cost-effective.

49. A 69-year-old male with past medical history significant for coronary artery disease complicated by myocardial infarction 1 year prior is admitted with unstable angina. He is found to have significant progression of atherosclerosis on invasive coronary angiogram that is treated with drug-eluting stent. He started on dual antiplatelet agent and his high-intensity statin, rosuvastatin 40 mg daily, is continued. He returns 2 weeks after this event. His blood pressure is well controlled, and he has no further ischemic symptoms. He has been adherent to dietary plan. His fasting lipid panel is TC (total cholesterol) 174 mg/dL, TG (triglycerides) 178 mg/dL, LDL-C (low-density lipoprotein cholesterol) 83 mg/dL, and HDL-C 55 mg/dL (high-density lipoprotein cholesterol).
    What is the next most appropriate therapeutic step?
    A. He is at very high risk for ASCVD (atherosclerotic cardiovascular disease). He should be continued on the high-intensity statin.
    B. He is at very high risk for ASCVD. A PCSK9i should be added to drug regimen.
    C. He is at very high risk for ASCVD. Ezetimibe should be added to drug regimen
    D. He is at very high risk for ASCVD. Due to moderate elevation in triglycerides, icosapent ethyl should be added to drug regimen.

50. A 60-year-old male with past medical history significant for hypertension is seen in a preventive cardiology clinic. His father died of an MI at the age of 52. He is eating a plant-based diet. He runs 3–5 miles most days of the week. He is extremely worried about his family history and would like to do everything possible to decrease his personal risk.
    Further workup reveals a blood pressure of 122/73 on medical management. He has a fasting lipid panel of TC (total cholesterol) 166 mg/dL, TG (triglycerides) 64 mg/dL, LDL (low-density lipoprotein cholesterol) 82 mg/dL, and HDL (high-density lipoprotein cholesterol) 71 mg/dL. His lipoprotein(a) is 154 nmol/L.
    Which one of the following statements is TRUE regarding his risk for a future atherosclerotic cardiovascular event?
    A. He is at borderline 10-year risk for ASCVD event based on the Pooled Cohort Equations, and therefore, lifestyle management alone is adequate.
    B. He is at borderline risk for 10-year ASCVD event based on the Pooled Cohort Equations, and therefore, statin therapy is not indicateD.
    C. It is reasonable to recommend statin therapy and lifestyle management after clinician–patient risk discussion given the high lifetime risk based on his family history and markedly elevated lipoprotein(a).

51. A 47-year-old man with a history of hypertension, hyperlipidemia, diabetes, and recent coronary stenting for myocardial infarction 2 months prior presents to establish care. Labs done the day of your visit demonstrate a total cholesterol of 141 mg/dL, LDL cholesterol of 62 mg/dL, HDL cholesterol of 48 mg/dL, and triglycerides of 155 mg/dL; hemoglobin A1C 5.5%. Relevant cardiovascular medications from discharge include rosuvastatin 40 mg daily, aspirin 81 mg daily, ticagrelor 90 mg twice daily, losartan 25 mg daily, metoprolol succinate 25 mg daily, and metformin 500 mg twice daily.
    What is the best next step in management?
    A. Repeat lipid panel in 4–12 weeks
    B. Add evolocumab 140 mg every 2 weeks
    C. Add icosapent ethyl 2 g twice daily
    D. Obtain a coronary artery calcium scan
    E. Obtain high-sensitivity C-reactive protein

52. A 23-year-old woman presents for a risk assessment given a family history of stroke (mother at the age of 56) and heart attack (maternal uncle at the age of 42). Lab tests are ordered.
    What result is most likely to impact the patient's future risk of atherosclerotic cardiovascular disease?
    A. Lipoprotein (a) = 109 mg/dL
    B. Apolipoprotein B100 = 117 mg/dL
    C. hsCRP = 1.9 mg/L
    D. Triglycerides = 162 mg/dL

53. A 67-year-old man without a clinical history of atherosclerotic cardiovascular disease and a history of statin intolerance presents for a second opinion of management strategies. He has tried atorvastatin, rosuvastatin, and pravastatin. His 10-year Pooled Cohort Equation risk is 16.2% and most recent lipid panel demonstrates: total cholesterol of 241 mg/dL, HDL-C (high-density lipoprotein cholesterol) of 48 mg/dL, LDL-C (low density lipoprotein cholesterol) of 176 mg/dL, and triglycerides of 87 mg/dL.
    After shared decision making, he is willing to try additional therapy for ASCVD risk reduction. What is the best next step in management?
    A. Start aspirin 81 mg daily
    B. Start pitavastatin 2 mg daily
    C. Start colchicine 0.6 mg dail
    D. Start ezetimibe 10 mg daily
    E. Start alirocumab 75 mg every 2 weeks

54. A 67-year-old man without a clinical history of atherosclerotic cardiovascular disease and a history of statin intolerance presents for a second opinion of management strategies. He has tried atorvastatin, rosuvastatin, and pravastatin. His 10-year Pooled Cohort Equation risk is 16.2% and most recent lipid panel demonstrates: total cholesterol of 241 mg/dL, HDL of 48 mg/dL, LDL of 176 mg/dL, and triglycerides of 87 mg/dL. Additional testing is ordered for the purposes of risk stratification.

    Which result best indicates it may be reasonable to delay additional medical therapy?
    A. Ankle-brachial index = 1.2
    B. Coronary artery calcium score = 0
    C. hsCRP (high sensitivity C reactive protein) = 1.7 mg/L
    D. Lipoprotein (a) = 33 mg/dL
    E. Carotid intima-media thickness <25 percentile

55. A 45-year-old Japanese man presents to your preventive cardiology clinic for a new patient assessment. He states he has had no cardiac history, although his father had an MI (myocardial infarction) at age 44. He currently smokes a half pack of cigarettes daily and has HTN (hypertension) and DM (diabetes mellitus) with a most recent blood pressure of 139/91 mmHg and HbA1C today of 8%. He is currently taking hydrochlorothiazide, amlodipine, metformin, and liraglutide. His lipid panel today is significant for total cholesterol of 214 mg/dL HDL (high-density lipoprotein cholesterol) 39 mg/dL, triglycerides 201 mg/dL, and LDL-C (low-density lipoprotein cholesterol) of 160 mg/dL. He is currently not taking a statin at this time.

    Which one of the following statements is true for initiating a statin in this patient?
    A. The patient should receive a coronary artery calcification (CAC) score before initiating high versus moderate-intensity statin.
    B. The patient should start a high-intensity statin.
    C. The ASCVD (arteriosclerotic cardiovascular disease) risk score risk score is very accurate in estimating 10-year cardiac risk for this individual.
    D. It may be best to start the patient on a low to moderate-intensity statin at this time.

56. Which of the following statements is true concerning the occurrence of atrial fibrillation in Black compared with White patients?
    A. Due to HTN (hypertension), the incidence of atrial fibrillation in Black is 0.20–0.50 times higher when compared with White patients, although Black have a lower odds of awareness.
    B. After adjusting for social determinants of health, Black are just as likely to receive novel oral anticoagulants and interventional therapies for atrial fibrillation as White patients.
    C. Although Black patients with atrial fibrillation have a lower incidence of atrial fibrillation than White patients, they also have a lower awareness and are less likely to receive anticoagulation therapy.
    D. None of the above are true.

57. Which of the following statements is true regarding uncontrolled HTN (hypertension) among US historically marginalized populations?
    A. Non-Hispanic Black patients have the highest uncontrolled rates of HTN when compared with all historically marginalized populations in the United States.
    B. Non-Hispanic Asian patients have the highest uncontrolled rates of HTN when compared with all historically marginalized populations of the United States.
    C. Hispanic or Latin populations have the highest uncontrolled rates of HTN when compared with other historically marginalized populations in the United States.
    D. White patients have the lowest number (in millions) of uncontrolled HTN when compared to all historically marginalized populations in the United States.

58. A 64-year-old self-identified non-Hispanic Asian woman with a past medical history of hypertension, anterior MI with PCI 6 months prior presents to your clinic. She is hesitant to take a high intensity statin since she was told this is not useful, and perhaps harmful, in East Asian patients. What is the most appropriate counseling prior to the initiation of therapy?
    A. Initiation of pitavastatin or other high-intensity statin while following closely for adverse effects
    B. Initiation ezetimibe and avoid statins
    C. Lifestyle modifications given more favorable lipid profile and metabolism in Asian patients
    D. Fish oil supplementation especially with higher prevalence of hypertriglyceridemia in Asian patients

59. A significant prevention target in atherosclerotic cardiovascular disease is the treatment of lipid disorders, as these lipid abnormalities, primarily elevated low-density lipoprotein, contribute to atherosclerotic plaque burden. Many studies have addressed findings that highlight racial and ethnic disparities in the diagnosis and treatment of hyperlipidemia. Which of these findings are false?
    A. Black patients tend to have similar or even more favorable lipid profiles when compared to the national average.
    B. There is little heterogeneity in risk within different racial and ethnic groups.
    C. In addition to higher cardiovascular disease outcomes, Black patients also may have consistently higher coronary artery calcium (CAC) scores than other racial and ethnic groups.
    D. Considerations of race and ethnicity are not impactful when providing or secondary prevention in all patients with lipid disorders.

60. Social determinants of health (i.e., adverse health behaviors, socioeconomic status [SES], and environmental factors) have a predominant effect on all chronic diseases, and systematically contribute to racial/ethnic disparities of cardiovascular disease health care and outcomes. Social determinants of health comprise what percentage of better health outcomes?
    A. 20%
    B. 40%
    C. 60%
    D. 80%

61. A 46-year-old non-Hispanic Black man presents with exertional fatigue and blood pressure 132/86 mmHg. He is unsure of any prior history of hypertension and has not been on antihypertensive medication. His echocardiogram demonstrated an ejection fraction of 35%. In consideration of his self-identified race and Stage 1 hypertension, a first step agent is chosen. As a first step agent, which may be most consistent with present evidence-based care?
    A. Lisinopril
    B. Losartan
    C. Amlodipine
    D. Atenolol

62. A tennis player's resting heart rate of 60 beats per minute (bpm) is increased to 120 bpm during a tennis match. Using the heart rate index equation, his estimated metabolic equivalent (MET) level at the heart rate of 120 bpm is?
    A. 5
    B. 7
    C. 9
    D. 11

63. The recent CARDIA study of 2100 Black and White men and women (38–50 years), with a mean follow-up of 10.8 years, reported that participants taking _____ steps/day had a 50–70% lower risk of mortality?
    A. ≥3000
    B. ≥5000
    C. ≥7000
    D. ≥10,000

64. For the primary and secondary prevention of ASCVD (arteriosclerotic cardiovascular disease), each 1-MET increase in cardiorespiratory fitness confers a ~ % decrease in mortality up to ~10 METs, beyond which the additional survival benefits largely plateau?
    A. 8
    B. 16
    C. 24
    D. 32

65. An increasing number of reports now suggest that potentially adverse cardiovascular manifestations may occur following high-volume, high-intensity long-term endurance training/competition. These adverse cardiovascular outcomes may include?
    A. Accelerated coronary artery calcification
    B. Myocardial fibrosis
    C. Atrial fibrillation
    D. All of the above

66. The defining features of all cardioprotective dietary patterns are:
    A. Plant centered, low in saturated fat, and dietary cholesterol
    B. Emphasize fruits, vegetables, whole grains, low-fat or fat-free dairy products, lean protein sources, legumes, pulses, nuts, seeds, and liquid vegetable oils.
    C. Low in red and processed meats, and low in refined grains, sugar sweetened foods and beverages.
    D. All of the above

67. The original Dietary Approaches to Stop Hypertension (DASH) dietary pattern, as well as the modified higher unsaturated fat DASH pattern, improved which of the following:
    A. Blood pressure
    B. Blood lipids
    C. ASCVD (atherosclerotic cardiovascular disease) risk
    D. All of the above

68. Patients with overweight or obesity improved blood pressure, delayed the onset of T2DM (Type 2 diabetes mellitus), improved glycemic control in T2D, prediabetes and metabolic syndrome, and improved lipid profile with a weight loss of _____%.
    A. 5–10% of initial weight
    B. 3–5% of initial weight
    C. 10–15% of initial weight
    D. 2–4% of initial weight

69. Current guidelines recommend consumption of viscous fiber and phytosterols to help reduce LDL-C (low density lipoprotein cholesterol) as adjunct therapy. What are the current amounts recommended by the National Lipid Association?
   A. 5–10 g viscous fiber and 5 g phytosterols
   B. 20–25 g viscous fiber and 2–3 g phytosterols
   C. 20–25 g viscous fiber and 5 g phytosterols
   D. 5–10 g viscous fiber and 2–3 g phytosterols

70. A 74-year-old male with a history of smoking and hypertension but no history of ASCVD asks if he should be taking aspirin to prevent a heart attack. Which of the following statements is true?
   A. He should be on aspirin given he has a history of smoking, making him high risk.
   B. A 10-year ASCVD (atherosclerotic cardiovascular disease) risk should be calculated to determine his candidacy for aspirin.
   C. He should not be given aspirin due to lack of net benefit.

71. A 55-year-old female with a history of obesity, diabetes mellitus, and hyperlipidemia but no history of ASCVD (atherosclerotic cardiovascular disease) presents to clinic asking if she should be on aspirin to prevent heart attack. She had a CAC (coronary artery calcium) score last year of 200 Agatston Units and is now on a statin.
   Which one of the following statements is true?
   A. There is no strong indication for primary prevention aspirin in any population.
   B. If there is no increased risk of bleeding, she should be offered low-dose aspirin to reduce her risk of future ASCVD.
   C. Her history of diabetes mellitus automatically qualifies her for aspirin, regardless of her CAC score or ASCVD risk.

72. Which one of the following have been shown to aid in smoking cessation?
   A. E-cigarettes
   B. Behavioral counseling
   C. Pharmacotherapy
   D. A, B, and C.
   E. B and C only

73. A 64-year-old male with a history of obesity, seizure disorder, depression, hyperlipidemia, and hypertension presents to clinic to discussion smoking cessation. Which one of the following medications should not be recommended to this patient?
   A. Varenicline
   B. Bupropion
   C. Nicotine patch
   D. A and B

74. A 35-year-old man with symptoms of congestive heart failure is seen for evaluation. He has a past history of diabetes and hypertension. A serum creatinine value 4 months ago was 1.9 mg/dL estimated GFR (glomerular filtration rate) = 57 mL/min/1.73 m²). Today, a serum creatinine was 2.0 mg/dL (estimated GFR = 54 mL/min/1.73 m²) and a urine specimen contained 190 mg of albumin per gram of creatinine.
    Which ONE of the following best describes the category of chronic kidney disease present in this patient?
    A. Category G2/A2
    B. Category G3A/A2
    C. Category G3B/A2
    D. Category G4/A2

75. Which ONE of the following cardiovascular diseases is MOST common among older patients with established CKD (chronic kidney disease), not on dialysis therapy?
    A. Congestive Heart Failure
    B. Atrial Fibrillation
    C. Ischemic Stroke
    D. Coronary Artery Disease

76. A 66-year-old woman has Category 3B/A3 CKD (chronic kidney disease) due to diabetes and hypertension. She has moderate congestive heart failure (AHA Class II) with a reduced ejection fraction (40%). Her serum potassium is 4.2 mmol/L, and her hemoglobin concentration is 10.1 g/dL.
    Which ONE of the following regimens would be MOST likely to improve her heart failure and slow the rate of progression of her CKD leading to better survival expectancy?
    A. Beta-blockers and subcutaneous insulin
    B. Oral chlorothiazide and metformin
    C. Oral renin-angiotensin system inhibitors and sodium glucose cotransporter 2 inhibitors
    D. Oral hydralazine and dipeptidyl–peptidase 4 inhibitors

77. A 55-year-old patient with Category 5 CKD (chronic kidney disease) has recently begun thrice weekly hemodialysis, carried out in the home. He has a history of diabetes and hypertension but has no symptoms of heart failure or coronary artery disease. He is on no hypolipidemic agents currently. His total serum cholesterol and LDL (low-density lipoprotein)-cholesterol are elevated at 220 mg/dL and 150 mg/dL, respectively. His fasting triglycerides are 200 mg/dL. His blood pressure pre-dialysis is 185/95 mmHg, and his hemoglobin A1c is 6.2%. His hemoglobin level is 10 g/dL.

Which ONE of the following agents should be prescribed to help prevent future development of symptomatic coronary artery disease.
- A. Simvastatin + Ezetimibe
- B. Atenolol
- C. Bezafibrate
- D. Losartan

78. Current guidelines give preference to direct-acting oral anticoagulants (DOACs) over warfarin for those with atrial fibrillation, unless there is:
- A. Moderate or severe aortic stenosis
- B. Moderate or severe aortic regurgitation
- C. Moderate or severe mitral stenosis
- D. Moderate or severe mitral regurgitation

79. Current guidelines recommend a higher INR (international normalized ratio) goal of 3.0 (range of 2.5–3.5) after mechanical aortic valve replacement (AVR) in those with each of the listed risk factors EXCEPT:
- A. Coronary artery disease
- B. Previous thromboembolism
- C. Hypercoagulable state
- D. Left ventricular systolic dysfunction

80. Current guidelines recommend use of dual antiplatelet therapy (aspirin and a $P2Y_{12}$ inhibitor) after percutaneous coronary intervention (PCI) with a drug-eluting stent (DES) among patients with stable ischemic heart disease (SIHD) for at least:
- A. 1 month
- B. 3 months
- C. 6 months
- D. 12 months

81. In general, periprocedural bridging of anticoagulation for those on a vitamin K antagonist (e.g., warfarin) is not routinely warranted. Among those at high thrombotic risk, bridging is also discouraged if the patient:
- A. Is on aspirin as well
- B. Is on a $P2Y_{12}$ inhibitor (e.g., clopidogrel) as well
- C. Is undergoing a low bleeding risk procedure
- D. Experienced a major bleed within the last 3 months

82. Bleeding in each of these locations constitutes a critical site bleed, *except*:
- A. Intracranial
- B. Gastric
- C. Intraarticular
- D. Pericardial

83. **The risk of developing coronary artery disease is lower among pre- and post-menopausal women compared to men of the same age.**
    A. True
    B. False

84. **All of the following have been established as independent female-specific risk enhancing factors for developing atherosclerotic cardiovascular disease, EXCEPT:**
    A. Gestational hypertension
    B. Gestational diabetes
    C. Preterm (<37 weeks) delivery
    D. Premature menopause
    E. Fertility therapy

85. **As per the 2018 ACC/AHA Cholesterol guidelines, which of the following condition is NOT a "risk enhancer" for developing atherosclerotic cardiovascular disease for women?**
    A. Metabolic Syndrome
    B. Pre-eclampsia
    C. Premature Menopause
    D. Hormonal Replacement Therapy
    E. Inflammatory diseases

86. **Which one answer is TRUE regarding the treatment of hypertension?**
    A. Nutritional interventions to lower blood pressure include lowering dietary intake of sodium, often achieved by substituting table salt with sea salt, which has more calcium and less sodium.
    B. Initial drug therapy with two first-line anti-hypertensive agents of different classes is recommended for adults with an average blood pressure >20/10 mmHg above their blood pressure target.
    C. Chlorthalidone is a "thiazide-like" diuretic with longer half-life than hydrochlorothiazide and is preferred over loop diuretics for treatment of heart failure.
    D. Angiotensin receptor blockers combined with direct renin inhibitors (i.e., aliskiren) provide additive blood pressure lowering and may mitigate potential hyperkalemia.
    E. Beta blockers have negative inotropic effects and should be avoided in patients with reduced ejection fraction, angina pectoris, cardiac dysrhythmias, and acute myocardial infarction.

87. **Which one answer is TRUE regarding the treatment of obesity?**
    A. In patients treated for obesity, semaglutide and liraglutide are examples of anti-obesity agents with cardiovascular disease (CVD) outcome trial support, and indicated use for reducing major adverse cardiac events (MACE) in patients with obesity.
    B. Semaglutide 2.4 mg oral per day is a glucagon-1 receptor (GLP-1) agonist indicated to reduce MACE in patients with Type 2 diabetes mellitus and reduce body weight to a clinically meaningful degree in patients with obesity.
    C. In patients with congestive cardiomyopathy and obesity, GLP-1 receptor agonists are preferred in patients with Type 2 diabetes mellitus because of their inhibition of renal tubular reabsorption and promotion of natriuresis.
    D. Tirzepatide is a unimolecular GLP-1 and glucose-dependent insulinotropic polypeptide (GIP) agonist that reduces glucose in patients with Type 2 diabetes mellitus and reduces body weight in patients with overweight or obesity.
    E. Phentermine is often described as the most commonly prescribed anti-obesity agent; in patients at high cardiovascular disease risk, phentermine has a neutral effect on major cardiovascular disease events (MACE).

88. **Which one answer is TRUE regarding cardiac imaging?**
    A. Cardiac diastolic function is best assessed by coronary computed tomography angiography.
    B. Cardiac microvascular dysfunction is best be evaluated by positron emission tomography and cardiac magnetic resonance.
    C. Cardiomyocyte injury is best evaluated by coronary artery calcium imaging and scoring.
    D. Myocardial macro- and microvascular perfusion is best evaluated by echocardiography.
    E. Cardiac microvascular perfusion is best evaluated by CCTA (coronary computerized tomography angiography) combined with computed tomography fractional flow reserve.

89. **Which one answer is TRUE about the sensitivity and specificity of cardiac imaging procedures?**
    A. Coronary computed tomography angiography (CCTA) has over 90% sensitivity for anatomically significant coronary artery disease
    B. Exercise stress electrography (treadmill) has over 90% sensitivity and specificity for functionally significant cardiovascular disease (CVD)
    C. Single-photon emission computed tomography (SPECT [single photon emission computed tomography]; e.g., technetium or thallium scan) has over 90% specificity for anatomically or functionally significant CVD
    D. Positron emission tomography (PET) and stress cardiac magnetic resonance (CMR) both have >80% sensitivity; but <70% specificity for functionally significant CVD
    E. Coronary calcium imaging/score has over 90% specificity for functionally significant cardiovascular disease CVD

90. **Which of the following statements are FALSE concerning alcoholic cardiomyopathy?**
    1. Has no diagnostic test, making it often difficult to distinguish from other types of dilated cardiomyopathy except by history of lifetime heavy alcohol drinking
    2. Probably has multiple potentiating cofactors, including genetic susceptibility, cardiotropic viruses and cobalt
    3. Is less often caused by beer drinking than by wine or liquor because beer has more nutrients and lower alcohol concentration than wine or liquor
    4. Is generally thought by experts to be due to chronic thiamine (Vitamin B1, co-carboxylase) deficiency
    5. May regress substantially with alcohol abstinence
        A. All of the above statements are false.
        B. None of the above statements are false.
        C. 1, 2, and 5 are false.
        D. 3 and 4 are false.
        E. 1, 2, and 3 are false.

91. **Holiday Heart Syndrome refers to which ONE of the following?**
    A. Supraventricular arrhythmias that occur with the ingestion of cold beer in patients who report a history of "brain freeze" headaches on Fourth of July
    B. Supraventricular arrhythmias that occur in the setting of syncope after a 10-km May Day marathon race
    C. Supraventricular arrhythmias that occur with the ingestion of leftover fermented cranberry sauce on Thanksgiving
    D. Supraventricular arrhythmias that are reversible and occur in the setting of acute consumption of heavy alcohol and meals on New Year's Eve

92. **Which one of these concepts of underreporting is FALSE?**
    A. Underreporting places some heavy drinkers spuriously into the light-moderate category, which affects threshold relationships of alcohol to adverse effects.
    B. Underreporting heavy drinkers who self-classified as light to moderate drinkers were identified via concurrent diagnoses associated with heavy alcohol intake like delirium tremens or alcoholic liver cirrhosis.
    C. Underreporting of alcohol intake only affects the individual person rather than outcome data or threshold relationships of harm.
    D. The sick quitter hypothesis refers to early studies that combined lifelong abstainers and past drinkers, who quit due to prior illness in one category.

93. **Which one of these definitions and statements about alcohol ingestion is FALSE?**
    A. The "Standard Drink" in the United States is defined as a 12 oz. (360 mL) of typical 5% US beer, 4 oz. (120 mL) of typical (13%) white or red table wine, and 1¼ oz. (a jigger) of 40% (80 proof) distilled spirits.
    B. The amount of alcohol in a standard drink in each beverage type is the same at approximately 14 g of alcohol.
    C. Much beer is sold in standard drink size, but wine and distilled spirits are more often poured to taste. This factor leads to greater underestimation of intake for people who drink spirits preponderantly.
    D. For all people over 21, consuming ≥2 drinks per day is considered heavy drinking.
    E. The pattern of drinking behavior is important, especially binge drinking.

94. **An elevated level of which ONE of the following biomarkers is an independent CVD risk factor and the most common monogenic cause of atherosclerotic CVD (cardiovascular disease)?**
    A. Lipoprotein(a) [Lp(a)]
    B. Brain natriuretic peptide (BNP)
    C. High-sensitivity c-reactive protein (hs-CRP)
    D. Estimated glomerular filtration rate (eGFR)
    E. Fasting blood glucose level

95. **The worldwide prevalence of elevated Lp(a) levels is estimated at approximately what percentage?**
    A. 5%
    B. 10%
    C. 15%
    D. 20%
    E. 30%

96. **In patients with the phenotype of familial hypercholesterolemia (FH), the absence of an identifiable genetic mutation for familial hypercholesterolemia excludes the diagnosis.**
    A. True
    B. False

97. **In patients with heterozygous familial hypercholesterolemia, statin treatment should be strongly considered beginning at the age of:**
    A. 2–4 years
    B. 8–10 years
    C. 18–20 years
    D. 30–35 years
    E. >40 years

98. **Nutraceutical options for addressing high blood pressure include all of the following, EXCEPT:**
    A. L-arginine
    B. Red yeast rice
    C. Beetroot
    D. Cocoa flavonoids

99. **Acupuncture has been shown to decrease frequency of angina and improve blood pressure. The following are proposed mechanisms for this effect**:
    A. Increased endogenous opioid production
    B. Direct vasodilation of arterioles
    C. Improved autonomic dysregulation, such as improved heart rate variability
    D. A and B
    E. A, B, and C
    F. A and C

100. **A 55-year-old male with diabetes mellitus is diagnosed with hyperlipidemia.**
    Integrative treatment modalities could include all of the following EXCEPT:
    A. Berberine
    B. Mediterranean diet
    C. Exercise program
    D. Chelation therapy

101. **The Dietary Approaches to Stop Hypertension (DASH) diet including low sodium, fruits, vegetables, and low-fat dairy has been shown to lower systolic blood pressure and diastolic blood pressure in the following amounts:**
    A. 10 mmHg for both
    B. 5 mmHg and 3 mmHg, respectively
    C. No impact

102. A 67-year-old man with no past medical history or current medications reports a 3-month history of chest discomfort while walking uphill. The discomfort resolves within a few minutes after he stops walking, and he is then able to resume walking without recurrent discomfort. His symptoms have never occurred at rest and has not been getting worse. Nuclear exercise stress testing reproduces his symptoms and demonstrates a large reversible inferior defect. Coronary CT (computerized tomography) angiography reveals a high-grade proximal stenosis of the right coronary artery. You start the patient on guideline-directed medical therapy that includes aspirin, high-intensity statin, a beta-blocker, and sublingual nitrate. Based on the results of the ISCHEMIA trial, which one of the following is the best next approach to this patient's management?
   A. Advise the patient to undergo PCI (percutaneous coronary intervention) of the right coronary stenosis to improve his chances of survival.
   B. Advise the patient that if his angina persists despite optimal medical therapy, PCI will improve his quality of life.
   C. Advise PCI to reduce his chances of having a heart attack.
   D. Advise the patient that his severity of ischemia portends a worse outcome without revascularization.

103. A 45-year-old Black woman is referred to you for management of hypertension. Her home blood pressure log shows an average systolic blood pressure of 133 mmHg over the last month. Based on a food frequency questionnaire, you determine that her diet includes high-sodium foods. She has a sedentary lifestyle. Her office blood pressure is 138/82 mmHg. Her BMI (body mass index) is 32 kg/m^2. She expresses a strong preference to avoid medications if possible. She has no history of cardiovascular disease, and her estimated 10-year risk for atherosclerotic cardiovascular disease (ASCVD) is <10%.
Which one of the following therapies should you initiate next?
   A. Pharmacologic therapy with an ACE (angiotensin converting enzyme) inhibitor or an angiotensin receptor blocker and have a repeat BP evaluation in 1 month
   B. Pharmacologic therapy with diuretic and have a repeat BP evaluation in 1 month
   C. Pharmacologic therapy with calcium channel blocker and have a repeat BP evaluation in 1 month
   D. Nonpharmacologic therapy and have a repeat BP evaluation within 3–6 months

104. **A 62-year-old woman with chronic kidney disease (eGFR 45 mL/min/m²) is referred to you because of a coronary artery calcium score of 837 Agatston units. The distribution of calcium is 0 in the left main, 380 in the left anterior descending, 111 in the circumflex, and 346 in the right coronary artery. She walks ~7000 steps daily and is asymptomatiC. She has hypertension that is well controlled, diabetes with recent HbA1c of 6.7% on dapagliflozin and metformin, and LDL-cholesterol of 152 mg/dL on 80 mg of atorvastatin and 10 mg of ezetimibe daily. Hypothyroidism, obstructive liver disease, and nephrotic syndrome had already been ruled out by the referring physician.**
    What should you recommend next?
    A. Refer for stress testing to rule out ischemia
    B. Refer for coronary CT angiography or invasive coronary angiography to rule out obstructive coronary artery disease
    C. Bempedoic acid 180 mg daily and repeat a lipid panel in 4–12 weeks
    D. A PCSK9 (proprotein convertase subtilisin/kexin type 9) inhibitor and repeat a lipid panel in 4–12 weeks

105. **A 58-year-old female patient reports to you that she has been having intermittent chest pain for the past 6 months. The pain is a central chest pressure that lasts for several minutes and occurs at rest, never with exertion, with no obvious precipitating causes. The symptoms have not been progressive. She has a remote history of smoking and a family history of coronary artery disease. She is on no medication. Her BMI (body mass index) is 27 kg/m². Blood pressure is 117/75 mmHg. ECG is normal. Non-fasting triglycerides are 191 mg/dL, and LDL-C (low-density lipoprotein cholesterol) is 123 mg/dL. You order a coronary CT (computerized tomography) angiogram and the result is mild 2-vessel atherosclerosis involving the left anterior descending and right coronary arteries, with no narrowing >25%. The coronary artery calcium score is 63.**
    What would you recommend next to this patient?
    A. Initiate at least moderate-intensity statin therapy.
    B. Order a stress test to rule out ischemia from obstructive coronary disease.
    C. Refer for invasive angiography to confirm the absence of obstructive coronary disease.
    D. Reassure the patient that her symptoms are not due to obstructive coronary disease and recommend that she return in 1 year.

106. **Which one of the following is TRUE about physical activity?**
   A. The ACC/AHA Guidelines recommend at least 600 min/week of moderate/vigorous activity for cardiovascular risk reduction.
   B. No cardiovascular benefit is seen with physical activity until one exceeds ≥150 min/week of moderate + vigorous physical activity.
   C. Greater fitness (METS) is associated with improved survival, even for older adults ≥70 years.
   D. Sedentary behavior does not confer any cardiovascular risk if individuals are physically active.
   E. Counseling about physical activity in clinic visits is not effective in improving physical activity behavior in patients.

107. **Which one of the following is TRUE about physical activity (PA)?**
   A. The PA guidelines from the Department of Health and Human Services additionally recommends muscle-strengthening activities on two or more days a week.
   B. Activity must be of vigorous intensity to achieve cardiovascular benefit.
   C. Moderate-intensity activity consists of activities at a workload of 6–9 METS.
   D. All adults should undergo medical screening by a health care provider before starting an exercise program.
   E. Trading sedentary time for light-intensity activity has no CV [cardiovascular] benefit.

108. **A 58-year-old South Asian woman with a history of polycystic ovary syndrome (PCOS), prior gestational diabetes, and early menopause at age 42 years of age is being seen for a preventive cardiology evaluation. She has mild hypertension treated with amlodipine 2.5 mg daily. She has a family history of premature coronary artery disease in her father. She does not currently have diabetes and does not smoke. Her treated systolic blood pressure is 128 mmHg. Her total cholesterol is 205 mg/dL, HDL-C (high-density lipoprotein) 36 mg/dL, TG (triglycerides) 185 mg/dL, and LDL-C (low-density lipoprotein cholesterol) of 132 mg/dL. She has no symptoms of cardiovascular disease.**
   Which one of the following is TRUE about her cardiovascular risk assessment?
   A. She is at low 10-year risk for atherosclerotic cardiovascular disease (ASCVD); thus, reassurance and lifestyle implementation is enough for now.
   B. She is at borderline ASCVD risk; a coronary artery calcium score may be reasonable to guide shared decision making about statin therapy.
   C. She is at high risk and should undergo cardiovascular stress testing for further risk stratification.
   D. She is at high lifetime risk, so low dose aspirin 81 mg daily is recommended for primary prevention.

109. **There are unique reproductive risk factors associated with elevated CVD [cardiovascular disease] risk in women.**
    All of the following have been associated with increased CVD risk in women, EXCEPT:
    A. Polycystic ovary syndrome
    B. Adverse pregnancy outcomes such as preeclampsia and gestational diabetes
    C. Early menopause before age 45
    D. Infertility
    E. Spontaneous pregnancy loss
    F. Menarche at age 12

110. **Which one of the following is TRUE about enrollment in cardiovascular clinical trials?**
    A. The proportion of women enrolled in CV [cardiovascular] clinical trials is lower in men, but this is explained by women being less likely to have coronary artery disease and thus not eligible for trial criteria.
    B. The proportion of Black adults in cardiometabolic clinical trials is low at 13%, but this is consistent with their proportion of the population based on US Census data.
    C. There is a correlation between the gender and racial/ethnic characteristics of study team investigators with proportion of enrollment of diverse individuals into trials.
    D. Most trial protocols for CV clinical trials do specify a target criterion for enrolling Black adults but fail to meet these targets.

111. **Which one of the following is TRUE regarding lipid management in women?**
    A. Women derive benefit from statin therapy in terms of reduction in major adverse cardiovascular events (MACE) in secondary prevention but not in primary prevention.
    B. Women develop ASCVD (atherosclerotic cardiovascular disease) approximately 10 years after men even in setting of familial hypercholesterolemia (FH), so treatment in FH can be delayed until after reproductive years.
    C. Statin therapy at prescribed doses is unlikely to be teratogenic, but further study is needed about statin use in pregnancy.
    D. Ezetimibe confers MACE risk reduction in both men and women, but a greater reduction in men.
    E. Evolocumab confers MACE risk reduction in both men and women, but a greater reduction in men.

112. A 58-year-old man with hypertension and diabetes, both reasonably well-controlled with medications, is already taking high-intensity statin therapy, but his fasting triglycerides remains at 310 mg/dL. Which one of the following is a reasonable next step in further reducing his risk of stroke?
    A. Add ezetimibe
    B. Add icosapent ethyl
    C. Add a PCSK9 inhibitor
    D. Switch to a PCSK9 inhibitor
    E. Switch to another high-intensity statin

113. A 62-year-old woman with diabetes presents to medical attention with 30 min of left-sided weakness and was diagnosed with a transient ischemic attack. Which one of the following is a recommended approach for the prevention of subsequent ischemic stroke in regard to her antithrombotic regimen?
    A. Start aspirin and clopidogrel for 21 days then aspirin monotherapy
    B. Start aspirin and clopidogrel to continue indefinitely
    C. Start ticagrelor
    D. Start apixaban

114. A 75-year-old woman with history of hyperlipidemia and a lacunar ischemic stroke 2 years ago presents for follow-up with her primary care physician. Her blood pressure in the office is 150 mmHg systolic and 95 mmHg diastolic. She reports that her systolic blood pressure at home is usually in the 150's and sometimes in the 160's. Which blood pressure goal should be recommended?
    A. Blood pressure of less than 150/90 mmHg
    B. Blood pressure of less than 140/90 mmHg
    C. Blood pressure of less than 140/80 mmHg
    D. Blood pressure of less than 130/80 mmHg

115. A 54-year-old man with history of hypertension, hyperlipidemia, and ischemic stroke with a body mass index (BMI) of 24.9 kg/m² presents for follow-up with his primary care physician. His blood pressure is overall well-controlled after being started on blood pressure medications, and his LDL is at goal with a high-intensity statin. He is asking about nutrition recommendations to prevent future strokes and cardiovascular events. Which one of the following dietary recommendations would be the most appropriate for him?
    A. Eliminate all salt from the diet and increase potassium intake
    B. Adopt a low-fat diet
    C. A Mediterranean and low-salt diet
    D. Restrict caloric intake to no more than 1400 cal

116. **Which one of the following patients should be considered for aspirin therapy for primary prevention of cardiovascular disease?**
    A. Person with Type 2 diabetes and 10-year risk of 6%
    B. 75-year-old person with well-controlled hypertension
    C. Person with 15% 10-year risk and atrial fibrillation on apixaban
    D. None of the above

117. **In a person at low risk of bleeding who is tolerating therapy, how long should dual antiplatelet therapy be continued after myocardial infarction?**
    A. 12 months
    B. 6 months
    C. 3 months
    D. 1 month
    E. Depends on whether PCI was performed

118. **In which patient populations is prasugrel recommended over clopidogrel?**
    A. Person with ACS (acute coronary syndrome) treated with coronary stent implantation
    B. Persons with ACS treated medically
    C. Persons with prior ischemic stroke
    D. Person with atrial fibrillation on warfarin

119. **Which one of the following is NOT a risk factor for bleeding on DAPT (dual antiplatelet) therapy?**
    A. Female sex
    B. Obesity
    C. Diabetes
    D. Chronic steroid use

120. **Mr. HH is a 55-year-old patient who is seeking care for the first time in 10 years at your clinic. He has no significant clinical history or concerns except that he was diagnosed with psoriasis 5 years ago and has since gained 25 lB. His psoriasis is not fully controlled by topical treatment therapy, and he has frequent flares. After laboratory assessment, you calculate his 10-year ASCVD (atherosclerotic cardiovascular disease) risk as borderline.**
    What would be an appropriate next step in managing his cardiovascular risk?
    A. Start a high intensity statin.
    B. Imaging guided therapy
    C. Counsel patient on exercise, hold statin therapy due to borderline risk, and repeat labs in 1 year.
    D. There is no need for further management; refer to dermatology and repeat 10-year ASCVD in 4 years.

121. In the Anti-inflammatory Therapy with Canakinumab for Atherosclerotic Disease (CANTOS) trial, patients on Canakinumab achieving levels of _____ had a 31% reduction in cardiovascular mortality compared to those treated with placebo.
    A. hs-CRP <2 mg/L and LDL-C <70 mg/dL
    B. Erythrocyte sedimentation rate (ESR) <12 mm/h and LDL-C <130 mg/dL
    C. ESR <12 mm/h and LDL-C <70 mg/dL
    D. hs-CRP <2 mg/L only

122. Results from CANTOS, utilizing canakinumab, and COLCOT, utilizing colchicine, suggest targeting residual inflammatory risk may be an important target for secondary CV event prevention. These two drugs share which common target in reducing inflammation?
    A. IL-1β reduction
    B. Microtubule assembly disruption
    C. NLRP3 inflammasome activation
    D. Absolute neutrophils and monocyte count reduction

123. The Justification for the Use of Statins in Prevention: An Intervention Trial Evaluating Rosuvastatin (JUPITER) study and subsequent analyses of the study evaluated the impact of statin therapy on inflammation, measured by hs-CRP (C-reactive protein), in those with low level of LDL-C (<130 mg/dL). Which of the following statements is FALSE regarding the study results?
    A. At 4 years, rosuvastatin was associated with a significant reduction in the levels of hs-CRP.
    B. Follow-up genetic determination analysis revealed statin-induced lipid reduction and statin-induced inflammation reduction share similar pathways.
    C. Statin associated reductions in LDL-C <70 mg/dL and hs-CRP <2 mg/L had a larger CV benefit than those reduction in LDL-C alone.
    D. High-dose statin therapy reduced by 50% the risk of myocardial infarction and stroke in those with low level of LDL-C but high hs-CRP ≥2 mg/L.

124. The primary analysis in the Therapy with Canakinumab for Atherosclerotic Disease Study (CANTOS) study found direct inhibition of IL-1β reduced recurrent rates of CV events compared to placebo. In secondary analysis, those who reached lower levels of this cytokine after treatment were also less likely to experience MACE (major adverse cardiac events).
    A. Tumor necrosis factor-α
    B. Interferon-γ
    C. Interleukin-1
    D. Interleukin-6

125. **A 51-year-old patient with severe psoriasis is referred by his PCP (primary care physician) to your cardiology office after a recent MI (myocardial infarction).**
    Which one of the following is FALSE about severe psoriasis and cardiovascular risk?
    A. Topical treatments and phototherapy have been shown to have cardioprotective in severe psoriasis.
    B. Patients with severe psoriasis have similar risk of major adverse cardiovascular events (MACE) as patients with Type 2 diabetes.
    C. Patients with severe psoriasis may benefit from early initiation of inflammation reducing biologic therapy.
    D. Current guidelines consider chronic inflammatory diseases a cardiovascular risk enhancing condition.

126. **A 54-year-old female with chronic kidney disease (CKD; estimated glomerular filtration rate [eGFR] of 50 mL/min/m², hypertension, dyslipidemia, and Type 2 diabetes mellitus (T2DM) attends your outpatient cliniC. She is otherwise well and presents for routine checkup. Blood pressure is 116/70 mmHg.**
    Her medications include aspirin 81 mg daily, perindopril/amlodipine 10/10 mg, metformin 1 g daily, sitagliptin 100 mg daily, and atorvastatin 40 mg daily.
    Investigations reveal an HbA1c of 6.8%, LDL 68 mg/dL, and urinary albumin to creatinine ratio (ACR) 250 mg/g.
    Which one of the following strategies is the next most important step to reducing her risk of adverse cardio-renal outcomes?
    A. Exchange sitagliptin 100 mg for empagliflozin 10 mg daily.
    B. Add insulin glargine 10 IU daily.
    C. Add ezetimibe 10 mg daily
    D. Add liraglutide 0.6 mg daily.

127. **A 52-year-old male attends your outpatient clinic following his recent admission to hospital for a myocardial infarction. He has been seeing you for stage 4 CKD (chronic kidney disease) (eGFR [estimated glomerular filtration rate] 21 mL/min/m²) for the last 4 years, which has been stable. His LDL-C after being on rosuvastatin 20 mg is 150 mg/dL.**
    What would be your next best step to lower LDL-C and reduce his risk of a recurrent event?
    A. Increase rosuvastatin to 40 mg
    B. Switch to atorvastatin 40 mg
    C. Add ezetimibe 10 mg
    D. Add evolocumab 420 mg monthly

128. **A 44-year-old female is referred to you for an opinion on reducing her cardiovascular risk. She has long-standing ESKD from reflux nephropathy and has now undergone cadaveric renal transplantation 6 months ago and has stable graft function.**
LDL-C is 160 mg/dL despite an attempt at dietary and lifestyle modification.
Blood pressure is 122/80 mmHg.
Medications include aspirin, mycophenolate, tacrolimus, perindopril, and amlodipine.
What is the next best appropriate management step of her elevated LDL-C?
   A. Re-attempt dietary and lifestyle modification, repeat in 6 months
   B. Ezetimibe 10 mg daily
   C. Atorvastatin 20 mg daily
   D. Alirocumab 75 mg fortnightly

129. **A primary care physician calls your office in the afternoon. A 62-year-old male patient of yours has attended there for routine blood tests and his eGFR (estimated glomerular filtration rate) has gone from 58 to 50 mL/min/m². Last month, you commenced him on empagliflozin 10 mg daily. According to the primary care physician, he is euvolemic and has a BP of 132/80 mmHg. Other medications include perindopril 5 mg daily.**
What is the next most appropriate course of action?
   A. Cease perindopril
   B. Cease empagliflozin
   C. Continue empagliflozin
   D. Repeat eGFR in 48 h

130. **Which one of the following in not an optimal approach to blood pressure control?**
   A. An appropriate sensitivity to, and an understanding of, demographic factors
   B. An appropriate sensitivity to, and an understanding of, sociocultural factors
   C. Smoking cessation in tobacco users
   D. Use of DASH diet or Mediterranean diet
   E. Daily walking and/or exercise at least once a week

131. **The most recent recommendations for the management of high blood pressure by the American College of Cardiology/American Heart Association include classifying the stage of hypertension. Stage 1 hypertension is a blood pressure level of:**
   A. 120–129/70–79 mmHg
   B. 120–129/80–89 mmHg
   C. 130–139/80–89 mmHg
   D. 140–149/90–99 mmHg

132. **For persons with blood pressure of ≥130/80 mmHg but <140/90 mmHg, pharmacologic therapy is recommended with lifestyle management if:**
    A. The estimated 10-year atherosclerotic cardiovascular disease risk is ≥2%
    B. The estimated 10-year atherosclerotic cardiovascular disease risk is ≥5%
    C. The estimated 10-year atherosclerotic cardiovascular disease risk is ≥10%
    D. The estimated 10-year atherosclerotic cardiovascular disease risk is ≥20%

133. **Patient-centered recommendations for blood pressure care include each of the following except:**
    A. Maintaining weight control and conducting regular physical activity
    B. Reduced dietary sodium intake and reduced dietary potassium intake
    C. Increased adherence to clinic visits and adherence to pharmacotherapy
    D. Practicing stress reduction techniques and smoking cessation in tobacco users

134. **Compared to cohort subjects with less adherence to healthy lifestyle habits, optimizing "Life's Simple 7" may reduce incident heart failure by?**
    A. 10%
    B. 20%
    C. 40%
    D. 60%

135. **In the management of Type 2 diabetes mellitus, which of the following has been shown to prevent the development of heart failure?**
    A. Glucagon like peptide-1 (GLP-1) agonists
    B. Sulfonylureas
    C. Metformin
    D. SGLT-2 inhibitors

136. **Which of the following diets has been shown to decrease incident heart failure?**
    A. DASH (Dietary Approaches to Stop Hypertension diet)
    B. Mediterranean Diet
    C. Triglyceride-rich diet
    D. Low-proportion plant-based diet

137. **Across all age groups, large randomized controlled clinical trials have shown that subjects who achieve control of their hypertension reduce new onset heart failure by how much?**
    A. 25%
    B. 36%
    C. 42%
    D. 50%

138. **In the Women's Health Study, which genetic polymorphism identified a group of women who had a twofold greater CVD (cardiovascular disease) event risk when randomized to placebo but a normal CVD event risk when randomized to aspirin?**
    A. *LDLR*
    B. *LPA*
    C. *LQST*
    D. *APOB*

139. **In 2007, the first common gene polymorphism that increases risk for CAD independent of traditional risk factors was identified. Which of the following polymorphisms was it?**
    A. *KIF6*
    B. *LPA*
    C. *9p21*
    D. *PITX2*

140. **Which one of the following is true?**
    A. African American patients have among the highest rates of ASCVD but may have better HDL (high density lipoprotein cholesterol) and TG (triglyceride) levels than Caucasian patients.
    B. South Asian patients may have increased Metabolic Syndrome due their increased BMI (body mass index).
    C. The increased ASCVD (atherosclerotic cardiovascular disease) risk in South Asian patients is characterized by impaired fibrinolysis and a 1-2X increased risk of MI (myocardial infarction) and CV (cardiovascular)death.
    D. African American patients tend to have lower levels of Lp(a) (lipoprotein (a)).

141. **All of the following are true EXCEPT:**
    A. Obesity can increase the risk of atrial fibrillation, and weight loss can reduce this risk.
    B. Obesity can increase the risk of CHF (congestive heart failure) especially HFpEF (heart failure with preserved ejection fraction).
    C. An elevated BMI (body mass index) predicts risk of an MI equally to waist-hip ratio.
    D. In 2017–2018, the age-adjusted prevalence of obesity was (BMI ≥ 30 kg/m^2) 40%.

142. **All of the following regarding atrial fibrillation are true except?**
    A. A large study published in 2021 showed that developing or maintaining metabolic syndrome were associated with increased risks of AF (atrial fibrillation).
    B. In the Legacy trial, weight loss of 10–15% allowed >45% of patients with AF to have no further episodes.
    C. Several studies have shown that very vigorous exercise (such as cross-country skiing) results in less AF.
    D. Alcohol consumption can reduce AF prevalence and CV (cardiovascular) mortality in a dose-dependent manner.

143. **All of the following regarding Lp(a) [lipoprotein(a)] are true except:**
    A. There has been suggestion that the risk of Lp(a) is significantly enhanced in the setting of increased levels of hs-CRP (C-reactive protein).
    B. Lp(a) appears to have equal impact on stroke risk as well as risk of MI (myocardial infarction).
    C. Based on data from the Copenhagen City Study, the risk of MI is tripled when levels of Lp(a) are ≥ four times the upper limits of normal.
    D. The risk of DVT (deep vein thrombosis) was reduced in both FOURIER and ODYSSEY in patients with Lp(a) > the median who were treated with a PCSK9i.

144. **For which of the following populations is use of the ASCVD (atherosclerotic cardiovascular disease) Pooled Cohort Risk Calculator not recommended?**
    A. Persons with diabetes
    B. Hispanic persons
    C. Persons with atherosclerotic cardiovascular disease
    D. All of the above

145. **Which of the following is the most appropriate next step for deciding on a treatment approach in someone with a 10-year calculated ASCVD risk (atherosclerotic cardiovascular disease) of 10%?**
    A. Lifestyle management only is indicated.
    B. Consideration of risk enhancing factors for deciding on the treatment decision
    C. Use of coronary calcium scores to decide the treatment decision
    D. Moderate-intensity statin therapy is indicated.

146. **In which one of the following cases should a calcium score of 0 not be used to withhold or delay statin therapy?**
    A. Persons with a 10-year risk of 10% or greater
    B. Persons with hypertension
    C. Persons with diabetes
    D. Persons of South Asian ancestry

147. **Which of the following is true regarding subclinical measures of cardiovascular disease?**
    A. Carotid ultrasound measures carotid intimal medial thickness and is recommended in the 2018 guidelines as an option for further risk stratification.
    B. An ankle brachial index of <1.0 is considered a risk-enhancing factor in the 2018 guidelines.
    C. Coronary artery calcium improves risk discrimination over standard risk factors more than carotid ultrasound or ankle brachial index.
    D. Coronary artery calcium screening is recommended for all intermediate risk persons to determine the appropriateness of statin therapy.

148. **Which of the following initial cardiovascular complications are most common in patients with diabetes?**
    A. Peripheral arterial disease
    B. Heart failure
    C. Myocardial infarction
    D. Stroke
    E. Stable Angina

149. **How often are diabetes patients typically at risk stratified, guideline specified target simultaneously for LDL-C, blood pressure, and HbA1c?**
    A. 60–70%
    B. 40–50%
    C. 10–20%
    D. Under 5%

150. **Approximately how much lower may cardiovascular disease event rates be from being at risk stratified target simultaneously for HbA1c, LDL-C, and blood pressure compared to NOT being at target for these risk factors?**
    A. 20%
    B. 35%
    C. 60%
    D. 80%

151. **A 61-year-old White male smoker with controlled hypertension and Type 2 diabetes, which was diagnosed 2 years ago, has been taking pravastatin 20 mg. His most recent total cholesterol is 180 mg/dL, HDL-C, 40 mg/dL, LDL is 99 mg/dL and triglycerides are 195 mg/dL. He has no history of heart failure or other cardiovascular disease. His hypertension is treated with an ACE inhibitor (current BP 120/80 mmHg), and his diabetes is diet controlled with a current HbA1c of 5.9%. What would be a reasonable next approach to optimize his cardiovascular risk?**
    A. His LDL-C is at reasonable levels for someone without known heart disease
    B. Add Icosapent ethyl
    C. Recommend changing to high intensity statin
    D. B and C are both appropriate
    E. Recommend adding PCSK9-i

152. **A 46-year-old patient with a past medical history of hypertension is seen during an outpatient cardiology visit. He is a second-generation immigrant from South India. He states that his father suffered a heart attack at age 61 and requests more information about his individual risk of future atherosclerotic cardiovascular events.**
    Which cardiovascular risk assessment tool is derived from, or prospectively validated in South Asian?
    A. Framingham Risk Score
    B. ASCVD risk calculator
    C. UKPDS
    D. WHO (World Health Organization) risk tables
    E. UK QRISK2

153. **A 59-year-old male presents to your office for routine follow up. He has a past medical history of obesity. He recently stopped consuming soda beverages and has started an exercise program. He is interested in learning more about modifiable and non-modifiable risk factors for ischemic heart disease.**
    Which ethnic/racial group carries the highest risk for ischemic heart disease and proportional mortality?
    A. Asian Indian
    B. Chinese
    C. Japanese
    D. Korean

154. **A 42-year-old male presents to your outpatient clinic. He has no medical history other than an appendectomy at age 14. He works as a software engineer, drinks two to three alcoholic beverages per week, and denies any recreational drug use. He has been smoking one pack of cigarettes daily for the past 11 years. He would like to hear more information about smoking cessation.**
Which statement regarding smoking is incorrect?
   A. Patients who are active smokers have a life expectancy that is up to 10 years shorter than nonsmokers.
   B. Smoking can affect multiple organ systems.
   C. Smoking is the leading cause of preventable death in the United States.
   D. Men are more likely to be smokers than women.
   E. Hispanic and Asian ethnic groups have a higher prevalence of smokers than other groups.

155. **A 33-year-old female has been referred to your outpatient clinic by her primary care doctor. She has been obese since the age of 14. Her review of systems is normal. Her vitals are within normal limits. Recent lab work revealed a hemoglobin A1c of 5.9% and she was consequently diagnosed with prediabetes. She is very concerned about this new diagnosis and is interested in losing weight. She has heard about the ketogenic diet and requests more information.**
Which statement about a ketogenic diet is incorrect?
   A. Ketogenic diet incorporates a very low carbohydrate diet which discourages processed and refined foods that have a high glycemic index.
   B. Increased consumption of monosaturated fats has been shown to increase LDL (low-density lipoprotein cholesterol) levels.
   C. Ketogenic diets may be effective in lowering triglycerides, blood pressure; postprandial glucose and insulin levels.
   D. Several long-term prospective clinical trials have shown a significant reduction in cardiovascular events in patients following a ketogenic diet for more than 12 months.
   E. Monosaturated fats are generally favored over saturated fats.

156. **A 43-year-old female presents to clinic for evaluation recently being diagnosed with Type 2 diabetes mellitus. She lives a sedentary lifestyle and wants to know what the best exercise regimen would be to reduce her hemoglobin A1C. Which of the following exercise modalities has been shown to be most effective in lowering hemoglobin A1c?**
   A. Aerobic training alone
   B. Resistance training alone
   C. Stretching
   D. Combination of aerobic exercise and resistance training
   E. Combination of aerobic training and stretching exercises

157. **A 64-year-old East Asian female with hypertension, pre-diabetes, and obesity presents to your clinic for preventive care. Using the pooled cohort equations, you calculate her ASCVD (atherosclerotic cardiovascular disease) 10-year risk to be intermediate: 7.9%. You want to further stratify her ASCVD risk. Which of the following is a risk-enhancing factor as outlined in the 2018 ACC/AHA Cholesterol Guidelines?**
    A. High-sensitivity C-reactive protein of 1.8 mg/L
    B. Southeast Asian ancestry
    C. Metabolic syndrome
    D. Family history of father suffering a heart attack at age 58

158. **A 55-year-old male with obesity, hypertension, and prediabetes has an ASCVD (atherosclerotic cardiovascular disease) risk score of 22% and is started on a moderate-intensity statin per the 2018 AHA/ACC Cholesterol Guidelines. On follow-up bloodwork, his hemoglobin A1c increases from 6.1% to 6.6%. What is the next best step in managing this patient?**
    A. Continue moderate-intensity statin therapy
    B. Switch the statin to ezetimibe
    C. Stop the moderate-intensity statin
    D. Repeat hemoglobin A1c in 3 months

159. **Which of the following dietary plans has *NOT* been shown to be heart-healthy in patients with Type 2 diabetes?**
    A. DASH (Dietary Approaches to Stop Hypertension)
    B. Mediterranean
    C. Low-fat
    D. Vegan/Vegetarian

160. **The most recent recommendations of the US Preventive Services Task Force (USPSTF) on the use of aspirin to prevent CVD (cardiovascular disease) includes all the following EXCEPT (select single best choice):**
    A. Recommends against aspirin use for prevention of a first heart attack or stroke in all individuals aged ≥60 years
    B. Recommends against aspirin use for prevention of a first heart attack or stroke in individuals aged ≥60 years with no clinical evidence or history of vascular disease
    C. Suggests low-dose aspirin for primary prevention of CVD in persons 40–59 years old with ≥10% 10-year risk for CVD
    D. Indicates that the adverse effects of aspirin may outweigh its benefits when used for primary prevention
    E. A variety of doses of aspirin has been used for primary prevention of CVD.

161. **Select the single choice that is NOT true regarding antiplatelet therapy to prevent CVD (cardiovascular disease)**
    A. Aspirin produces its antiplatelet effect by reversibly inhibiting platelet COX-1.
    B. Aspirin therapy improves patency of saphenous vein coronary bypass grafts.
    C. Aspirin reduces risk of vascular events in patients with stable angina, atrial fibrillation, and peripheral artery disease.
    D. Prasugrel is contraindicated in patients with prior stroke or TIA (transient ischemic attack) because of increased bleeding risk.
    E. In patients with an MI 1–3 years earlier, initiation of ticagrelor long term lowers subsequent CV death, MI (myocardial infarction), and stroke.

162. **Select the single correct choice regarding antiplatelet therapy.**
    A. In some patients, aspirin pseudoresistance may be related to poor adherence, delayed absorption, or drug interactions with aspirin.
    B. Oral thienopyridines inhibit platelet aggregation by reversibly blocking $P2Y_{12}$.
    C. The beneficial effects of aspirin plus clopidogrel in reducing vascular events are not greater than either drug alone in patients with acute coronary syndromes.
    D. The risk of bleeding is lower with prasugrel than with clopidogrel.
    E. Ticagrelor is less potent than clopidogrel in reducing vascular events in patients with acute coronary syndromes.

163. **Select the single correct choice regarding treatment with antiplatelet drug therapy.**
    A. The effects of ticagrelor and clopidogrel are equivalent in reducing vascular events in patients with non-STE (non-ST elevation) ACS.
    B. Enteric coating of aspirin delays achievement of therapeutic blood levels compared to regular aspirin.
    C. The frequency of administration with ticagrelor is once daily.
    D. Ticagrelor exerts its antiplatelet action by irreversible inhibition of the $P2Y_{12}$ platelet receptor.
    E. Bleeding rates with prasugrel are equivalent to those of clopidogrel.

164. **Coronary calcium scoring is most appropriate for use in patients with a 10-year ASCVD (atherosclerotic cardiovascular disease) risk of between:**
    A. $\geq 5\%$ and $<15\%$
    B. $\geq 10\%$ and $<20\%$
    C. $\geq 7.5\%$ and $<20\%$
    D. $\geq 2.5\%$ and $<15\%$

165. Per the 2018 American College of Cardiology/American Heart Association guideline on the management of blood cholesterol, in an intermediate risk patient with a calcium score of 0, statin therapy would still be recommended in patients with certain risk factors except for:
    A. Cigarette smoking
    B. LDL-C (low-density lipoprotein cholesterol) ≥150 mg/dL
    C. Diabetes mellitus
    D. Family history of premature coronary heart disease

166. Which cardiovascular risk assessment allows for the incorporation of a patient's calcium score in the estimation of their 10-year ASCVD (atherosclerotic cardiovascular disease) risk?
    A. ACC/AHA ASCVD risk calculator
    B. Framingham risk score
    C. MESA Multiethnic Study of Atherosclerosis) 10-year CHD risk score
    D. PREDICT CVD risk predictor

167. Which of the following coronary plaque characteristics observed by coronary CTA (computed tomography angiography) are most highly correlated with increased risk of future plaque rupture events:
    A. Calcified plaque with negative remodeling
    B. Mixed (calcified and noncalcified) plaque with positive remodeling
    C. Mixed (calcified and noncalcified) plaque with negative remodeling
    D. Noncalcified plaque with positive remodeling

168. **Non-alcoholic fatty liver disease (NAFLD) has become highly prevalent, affecting approximately 25% of the US population. The more severe form of fatty liver disease, nonalcoholic steatohepatitis (NASH), afflicts approximately 3–5% of the population. NASH predisposes to not only cirrhosis and hepatocellular carcinoma but a wide spectrum cardiovascular disease as well, including ASCVD, cardiomyopathy, and arrhythmias. The fatty liver diseases are a product of multiple metabolic, inflammatory, and fibrotic derangements. Type 2 diabetes mellitus, obesity, insulin resistance, hypertension, and dyslipidemias are the typical underlying comorbidities in patients with NAFLD and NASH. NASH is poised to become the leading cause for liver transplantation in the United States, soon to surpass hepatitis C infection. As a consequence of the burgeoning nature of this epidemic, in 2022 the American Association of Clinical Endocrinology (AACE) published a Clinical Practice Guideline for the Diagnosis and Management of Nonalcoholic Fatty Liver Disease in Primary Care and Endocrinology Clinical Settings Co-Sponsored by the American Association for the Study of Liver Diseases (AASLD). As all associated NAFLD comorbidities are also CV risk factors, and CV death is the leading cause of death among these patients, it is important for the CV prevention specialist to have enhanced understanding of this disease state. The following three questions pertain to NAFLD/NASH as discussed in the 2022 guidelines.**

1. NAFLD is the overarching term encompassing simple steatosis ($\geq 5\%$ liver fat), steatohepatitis, and cirrhosis in the absence of alcohol abuse or other secondary factors. NASH is defined as $\geq 5\%$ liver fat, with inflammation and hepatocyte injury (hepatocellular ballooning), with or without fibrosis. Though biopsy is imperfect, it remains the gold standard for diagnosis. Prior to biopsy, however, there are laboratory tests and imaging procedures that are helpful for determining which patients should be considered for biopsy. Concerning such tests, which of the following is false:

    A. FIB-4 is the preferred initial test to identify patients with fibrosis stages F2–F4.
    B. MRI-PDFF is the best imaging test to determine degree of fibrosis in NASH.
    C. VCTE is the optimal imaging test to assess NASH with advanced fibrosis.
    D. When treating patients with diabetes, clinicians should consider using FIB-4 to screen for advanced fibrosis even in the setting of normal liver enzymes.

2. **Although more than 50 drugs are in development, there is currently no FDA-approved medication for the treatment of NAFLD or NASH. There are, however, clear guidelines now that help clinicians support and treat these patients. Current recommendations include all of the following except:**
   A. Clinicians must manage persons with NAFLD for obesity, metabolic syndrome, prediabetes, Type 2 diabetes mellitus, dyslipidemia, hypertension, and CVD based on the current standards of care.
   B. Clinicians should recommend lifestyle changes in persons with excess adiposity and NAFLD with a goal of at least 5%, preferably ≥10%, weight loss, as more weight loss is often associated with greater liver histologic and cardiometabolic benefit, depending on individualized risk assessments.
   C. Clinicians must recommend participation in a structured weight loss program, when possible, tailored to the individual's lifestyle and personal preferences.
   D. Clinicians might consider treating diabetes with pioglitazone and/or GLP-1 RAs when there is an elevated probability of having NASH based on elevated plasma aminotransferase levels and noninvasive tests.
   E. Vitamin E is recommended for patients with NASH and T2D but not for patients without DM.
3. **The 2022 AACE Guidelines for the Diagnosis and Management of NAFLD present useful clinical algorithms for identifying and risk stratifying patients. Three high-risk groups for the development of NAFLD have been identified: (1) Pre-diabetes or diabetes, (2) Obesity and/or ≥2 cardiometabolic risks, (3) Hepatic steatosis on imaging or elevated transaminase ≥30 IU/L. When patients fall into any of these groups, they should undergo an assessment for NAFLD/NASH, the goal being to prevent downstream consequences of cirrhosis and CVD. Secondary causes of fatty liver should first be ruled out. A liver stiffness measure (LSM) test such as a VCTE should be performed in "intermediate risk" cases. Following FIB-4 and VCTE, which one of the following defines an intermediate risk individual?**
   A. FIB-4 <1.3 and LSM <8 kPa
   B. FIB-4 >2.67 and LMS <8 kPa
   C. FIB-4 1.3–2.67 and LMS 8–12 kPa
   D. FIB-4 1.3–2.67 and LMS >12 kPa

169. **Which one response is <u>TRUE</u> regarding the treatment of hypertension?**
   A. Nutritional interventions to lower blood pressure include lowering dietary intake of sodium, often achieved by substituting table salt with sea salt, which has more calcium and less sodium.
   B. Initial drug therapy with two first-line anti-hypertensive agents of different classes is recommended for adults with an average blood pressure >20/10 mmHg above their blood pressure target.
   C. Chlorthalidone is a "thiazide-like" diuretic with longer half-life than hydrochlorothiazide and is preferred over loop diuretics for treatment of heart failure.
   D. Angiotensin receptor blockers combined with direct renin inhibitors (i.e., aliskiren) provide additive blood pressure lowering and may mitigate potential hyperkalemia.
   E. Beta blockers have negative inotropic effects and should be avoided in patients with reduced ejection fraction, angina pectoris, cardiac dysrhythmias, and acute myocardial infarction.

170. **Which is <u>TRUE</u> regarding treatment of obesity?**
   A. In patients treated for obesity, semaglutide and liraglutide are examples of anti-obesity agents with cardiovascular disease (CVD) outcome trial support, and indicated use for reducing major adverse cardiac events (MACE) in patients with obesity
   B. Semaglutide 2.4 mg oral per day is a glucagon-1 receptor (GLP-1) agonist indicated to reduce MACE in patients with Type 2 diabetes mellitus and reduce body weight to a clinically meaningful degree in patients with obesity
   C. In patients with congestive cardiomyopathy and obesity, GLP-1 receptor agonists are preferred in patients with Type 2 diabetes mellitus because of their inhibition of renal tubular reabsorption and promotion of natriuresis.
   D. Tirzepatide is a unimolecular GLP-1 and glucose-dependent insulinotropic polypeptide (GIP) agonist that reduces glucose in patients with Type 2 diabetes mellitus and reduces body weight in patients with overweight or obesity
   E. Phentermine is often described as the most commonly prescribed anti-obesity agent; in patients at high cardiovascular disease risk, phentermine has a neutral effect on major cardiovascular disease events (MACE).

171. **Which statement is TRUE regarding cardiac imaging?**
    A. Cardiac diastolic function is best assessed by CCTA (coronary computed tomography angiography).
    B. Cardiac microvascular dysfunction is best be evaluated by positron emission tomography and cardiac magnetic resonance.
    C. Cardiomyocyte injury is best evaluated by coronary artery calcium imaging and scoring.
    D. Myocardial macro- and microvascular perfusion is best evaluated by echocardiography.
    E. Cardiac microvascular perfusion is best evaluated by CCTA combined with computed tomography fractional flow reserve.

172. **Which is TRUE about the sensitivity and specificity of cardiac imaging procedures?**
    A. Coronary computed tomography angiography (CCTA) has over 90% sensitivity for anatomically significant coronary artery disease.
    B. Exercise stress electrography (treadmill) has over 90% sensitivity and specificity for functionally significant cardiovascular disease (CVD).
    C. Single-photon emission computed tomography (SPECT; e.g., technetium or thallium scan) has over 90% specificity for anatomically or functionally significant CVD.
    D. Positron emission tomography (PET) and stress cardiac magnetic resonance (CMR) both have >80% sensitivity but <70% specificity for functionally significant CVD
    E. Coronary calcium imaging/score has over 90% specificity for functionally significant cardiovascular disease CVD.

173. **Which of the following is the recommended intensity of statin therapy to use in the treatment of a patient with Type 2 diabetes mellitus and a calculated 10-year ASCVD (atherosclerotic cardiovascular disease) risk score of 9.0% according to the 2022 ACC ECDP (Expert Consensus Decision Pathway)?**
    A. A moderate-intensity statin therapy
    B. A high-intensity statin therapy
    C. A high-intensity statin therapy only if diabetes-specific risk enhancers are present
    D. A low-intensity statin therapy

174. A 71-year-old gentleman with a history of an anterior wall myocardial infarction 2 years ago s/p percutaneous coronary intervention of the left anterior descending coronary artery and a prior stent to the left superficial femoral artery presents for management of dyslipidemia. He is currently on rosuvastatin 40 mg and ezetimibe 10 mg with an LDL-C (low-density lipoprotein-cholesterol) of 67 mg/dL. According to the 2022 ACC ECDP (Expert Consensus Decision Pathway), what is the recommended next step to optimize the treatment of his LDL-C?
    A. Switch to atorvastatin 80 mg
    B. Add a proprotein convertase subtilisin: kexin type 9 (PCSK9) inhibitor
    C. Continue current management
    D. Stop rosuvastatin and add bempedoic acid

175. A 52-year-old woman presents to your office requesting guidance on whether to start statin therapy. Her family history is notable for a father with a myocardial infarction at the age of 49 years. She is a nonsmoker; her HbA1c is 5.6%, LDL-C is 120 mg/dL, and calculated 10-year ASCVD (atherosclerotic cardiovascular disease) risk is 8.2%. No other risk-enhancing factors are present. She is evaluated for a coronary artery calcium score, which demonstrates a score of 0 Agatson units. Which of the following is recommended as the next step in management according to the 2022 ACC ECDP?
    A. Statin therapy is recommended.
    B. Repeat a coronary calcium score in 3–5 years is recommended.
    C. Routine follow up is recommended.

176. For a 50-year-old male with a 10-year ASCVD (atherosclerotic cardiovascular disease) risk estimate of 6.7%, which of the following would most significantly alter his risk category?
    A. Death of father by myocardial infarction at age 64
    B. HDL-C (high density lipoprotein-cholesterol) of 37 mg/dL
    C. Lp(a) [lipoprotein(a)] of 100 mg/dL (250 nmol/L)
    D. Fasting triglyceride level of 225 mg/dL
    E. All of the above are significant risk-enhancing factors

177. A 6-month-old newborn presents for a well-child visit. His mother, 31 years old, informs you that she recently had a lipid panel drawn on herself which was notable for a total cholesterol of 256 mg/dL and LDL (low-density lipoprotein cholesterol)) of 187 mg/dL. She asks what the best age would be to order lipid screening for her child. What is the best response?
    A. 2 years old
    B. 15 years old
    C. 21 years old
    D. 25 years old

178. The radiation exposure in a single computed tomography scan for coronary artery calcium scoring is nearest to the background radiation dose received by the average American in what time period?
    A. 4 days
    B. 4 weeks
    C. 4 months
    D. 4 years

179. A 56-year-old male patient with a history of severe hypertriglyceridemia and hypertension presents to clinic for follow-up. After initiation of atorvastatin 80 mg daily, his fasting triglycerides decreased from 623 to 509 mg/dL. His 10-year ASCVD (atherosclerotic cardiovascular disease) risk score is 9.7%. He also takes amlodipine. What is the best next step to reduce his risk of acute pancreatitis?
    A. Add gemfibrozil
    B. Initiate a very low-fat diet
    C. Switch amlodipine to hydrochlorothiazide
    D. Trial of a high carbohydrate diet

180. A 29-year-old male patient presents to clinic for a referral to evaluate for a significant family history of coronary artery disease in his father and paternal grandfather. Patient states his father was first diagnosed around 45 years old and died of a massive heart attack at 53 years old. He was told his father had an LDL-C (low-density lipoprotein-cholesterol) of 240 mg/dL when he was first diagnosed with high cholesterol. Patient has no findings of personal history of CAD (coronary artery disease), PAD (peripheral artery disease), and stroke with a benign physical exam. He has never had genetic testing nor anyone in his family for high cholesterol. Patients LDL-C (low-density lipoprotein-cholesterol) was 240 mg/dL. What is his likelihood of having familial hypercholesteremia?
    A. No Familial Hypercholesteremia
    B. Unlikely Familial Hypercholesteremia
    C. Possible Familial Hypercholesteremia
    D. Probable Familial Hypercholesteremia
    E. Definite Familial Hypercholesteremia

181. Which LDL-C (low-density lipoprotein-cholesterol) and TG (triglyceride) profile would be most effective for recommending icosapent ethyl 4 g daily in preventing of cardiovascular death?
    A. LDL-C 150 mg/dL, TG 200 mg/dL
    B. LDL-C 60 mg/dL, TG 200 mg/dL
    C. LDL-C 60 mg/dL TG 100 mg/dL
    D. LDL-C 150 mg/dL, TG 100 mg/dL

182. **If measured, lipoprotein(a) can be used as a risk factor to recalibrate which risk group of patients in the 10-year risk estimation by the Pooled Cohort Equation?**
    A. Low Risk (<5%) + Borderline risk (5–7.4%)
    B. Borderline risk (5–7.4%) + Intermediate (7.5–19.9%)
    C. Intermediate risk (7.5–19.9%) + High Risk (>20%)
    D. Low Risk + Borderline Risk + Intermediate Risk

183. **A non-ambulatory 64-year-old female with PMH history of CVA (cerebrovascular accident, i.e., stroke) with residual hemiparesis, Type 2 diabetes mellitus, and HTN (hypertension) has a PET/CT rubidium (positron emission tomography/computed tomography) myocardial perfusion scan for a preoperative evaluation for intermediate risk surgery. The results were a normal perfusion at rest/stress, LVEF (left ventricular ejection fraction) 55% at rest and 55% at stress, no wall motional abnormalities at rest/stress, and a CFR of 1.48. Patient does not remark of any symptoms of dyspnea or chest pain.**
    What is the patient patient's prognosis for major associated cardiac events? Should the patient proceed with intermediate risk surgery?
    A. Low Risk for annual MACE (major adverse cardiac events), more information is needed to proceed with surgery
    B. Low Risk for annual MACE, proceed with surgery
    C. Intermediate Risk for annual MACE, more information is needed to proceed with surgery
    D. Intermediate Risk for annual MACE, proceed with surgery
    E. High Risk for annual MACE, do not proceed with surgery

184. **What is the approximate lifetime prevalence of major depression disorder in the United States?**
    A. 10%
    B. 20%
    C. 30%
    D. 40%

185. **What is an appropriate approach for assessment of psychological factors in cardiology practice?**
    A. Schedule a separate consultation with a clinical psychologist
    B. Evaluation by the clinical cardiologist
    C. Administration of brief screening tools by front-line staff
    D. Arrange urgent psychiatric evaluation

186. **Which of the following clinical trials met their primary endpoint in showing the benefit of cognitive behavioral intervention on depression in reducing mortality?**
    A. Recurrent Coronary Prevention Project
    B. ENRICHD
    C. Montreal Heart Attack Readjustment Trial
    D. None of the above

187. **Which of the following is true regarding positive psychological factors and cardiovascular health?**
    A. Optimism is associated with reduced incident CVD (cardiovascular disease) and all-cause mortality.
    B. A high sense of purpose is associated with reduced CVD risk and all-cause mortality.
    C. Happiness and a more positive affect is associated with reduced incident of CHD.
    D. All of the above.

188. **65-year-old Caucasian male presents to Cardiology Clinic for regular follow up. His cardiac history is significant for chronic stable angina, hypertension, hyperlipidemia, obesity, and he has newly diagnosed Type 2 Diabetes. A coronary angiogram performed within the last 12 months showed non-obstructive coronary artery disease. A more recent exercise stress echocardiogram was negative for ischemia, but he reached limited functional aerobic capacity. He has no history of thromboembolic disease. During the office visit he reports decreased libido, erectile dysfunction, significant fatigue, and decreased muscle mass. No history of congenital anomalies or childhood infections. He is a nonsmoker. Family history is significant for premature coronary disease. For evaluation of decreased libido, testosterone levels were checked and showed total serum testosterone level 200 ng/dL on two morning samples (normal level is >300 ng/dL), with free testosterone 3 ng/dL (normal >3.5 ng/dL). LH and FSH were within normal range. PSA was normal. Patient inquiries about taking oral testosterone supplement to improve his sexual function. Which one of the following is the best advice to give to the patient?**
    A. Patient has primary hypogonadism. Testosterone therapy is indicated as it would improve his sexual function and it would not increase his risk of cardiovascular events.
    B. Testosterone therapy would improve his sexual function and also improve his functional aerobic capacity, but he could experience more exertional chest pain.
    C. Prescribe oral testosterone therapy for its cardioprotective effects.
    D. Testosterone will worsen his newly diagnosed Type 2 Diabetes.
    E. None of the above

189. Risk factors for cardiovascular disease are also recognized as risk factors for erectile dysfunction. Which of the following best describes the relationship between coronary disease and erectile dysfunction?
    A. Coronary artery disease is an early marker of erectile dysfunction.
    B. Although heart healthy lifestyle offers significant reduction in cardiovascular events, no incremental benefit of Mediterranean diet was demonstrated in improving erectile dysfunction.
    C. Erectile dysfunction presents 2–5 years earlier than coronary artery disease.
    D. Statins are not protective against progression of erectile dysfunction.

190. A 65-year-old obese female presents to your clinic for cardiovascular screening evaluation. She admits to poor dietary habits. Her calculated 10-year ASCVD (atherosclerotic cardiovascular disease) risk is 7%. You discuss with her the importance of regular exercise and healthy nutrition patterns. What is the major cardiovascular benefit of Mediterranean type of diet, especially the benefit of extra virgin olive oil compared to other oils such as canola, sunflower, and coconut oil?
    A. High anti-inflammatory properties
    B. Increase in HDL-C (high-density lipoprotein cholesterol)
    C. Decrease in LDL-C (low-density lipoprotein cholesterol)
    D. High mono-unsaturated fatty acids
    E. Improvement in blood pressure

191. A 50-year-old Caucasian man presents to your clinic for cardiovascular screening evaluation. He is obese, he also has borderline hypertension, and you calculate that his 10-year ASCVD risk is 8%. He has family history of premature heart disease. He is very motivated to improve his dietary habits and asks what the optimal amount of carbohydrates in his diet should be to reduce cardiovascular mortality. The lowest mortality is seen with carbohydrates in what % of total calories?
    A. 10–20%
    B. 20–30%
    C. 30–40%
    D. 40–50%
    E. 50–60%

192. The Agatston CAC (coronary artery calcium) score, per-lesion, is calculated as a function of which of the following?
    A. Mean calcium density factor multiplied by calcific plaque area
    B. Peak calcium density factor multiplied by calcific plaque area
    C. Calcium volume multiplied by calcific plaque area
    D. Calcium mass multiplied by calcific plaque area

193. **Which of the following best represents the most appropriate CAC (coronary artery calcium score) rescan intervals for asymptomatic primary prevention patients with an initial CAC score of 0?**
    A. <5% 10-year risk: *6–7 years*, 5–20% 10-year risk: *3–5 years*, ≥20% 10-year risk: *3 years*, Diabetes: *3 years*
    B. <5% 10-year risk: *8–9 years*, 5–20% 10-year risk: *5–7 years*, ≥20% 10-year risk: *4 years*, Diabetes: *4 years*
    C. <5% 10-year risk: *9–10 years*, 5–20% 10-year risk: *6–8 years*, ≥20% 10-year risk: *5 years*, Diabetes: *5 years*
    D. <5% 10-year risk: *10 years*, 5–20% 10-year risk: *7–9 years*, ≥20% 10-year risk: *6 years*, Diabetes: *6 years*

194. **Though metabolic syndrome and Type 2 diabetes are associated with an increased ASCVD risk, up to 40% of such patients may have absence of CAC (coronary artery calcium score) through middle age. Which of the following can help to most strongly predict the maintenance of long-term CAC = 0 over a 10-year period?**
    A. Normal fasting blood glucose
    B. Normal serum triglycerides
    C. Absence of extra-coronary atherosclerosis (e.g., thoracic aortic calcium, carotid plaque)
    D. Normal total cholesterol/HDL-cholesterol

195. **Which of the following statements is most accurate regarding CAC (coronary artery calcium score) burden and the demarcation between primary and secondary prevention risk?**
    A. CAC does not help to demarcate primary versus secondary prevention risk; demarcation and treatment decisions should strictly be limited to hard events (e.g., myocardial infarction, stroke).
    B. Individuals with CAC ≥1000 AU have an incident ASCVD (atherosclerotic cardiovascular disease) event risk similar to that of a stable secondary prevention population and should thus be treated as such.
    C. While individuals with moderate to severely increased CAC have a markedly elevated incident ASCVD risk, the increased incidence of myocardial infarction and stroke is only observed several decades later.
    D. While individuals with prevalent CAC have a markedly elevated ASCVD risk, there is no level of CAC burden in primary prevention patients that increases future risk to the level of that of secondary prevention patients.

196. A 41-year-old man is found to have a low-density lipoprotein cholesterol level of 192 mg/dL on a fasting lipid panel. His prior LDL-C was 196 mg/dL, which was measured 8 years prior during a health screening fair at his place of employment. He has no history of hypertension or diabetes. His father had a myocardial infarction at the age of 49 years. He has no cardiovascular symptoms. What is the next guideline-recommended step for the management of his hypercholesterolemia?
   A. Recommend a moderate-intensity statin
   B. Estimate his 10-year risk of atherosclerotic cardiovascular disease using the Pooled Cohort Equations to guide statin initiation decisions
   C. Measure a coronary artery calcium score and defer statin therapy if his score is zero
   D. Recommend a high-intensity statin

197. A 59-year-old woman presents for evaluation of hypercholesterolemia. She has a low-density lipoprotein cholesterol of 150 mg/dL. Her calculated 10-year risk of atherosclerotic cardiovascular disease (ASCVD) is 7.3% by the Pooled Cohort Equations (PCE). She has hypertension that is controlled on therapy. She exercises for 30 min daily. She is asymptomatic from a cardiovascular standpoint. She prefers to avoid statin therapy and opts for coronary artery calcium scoring after risk discussions. Her calcium score is 61. In addition to optimizing lifestyle measures, what is the next best recommended step regarding lipid management?
   A. Defer statin therapy and repeat coronary artery calcium scoring in 5 years.
   B. Consider initiating statin therapy.
   C. Defer statin therapy as her coronary calcium score is <100.
   D. Perform exercise stress testing since her coronary calcium score is greater than zero.

198. A 36-year-old man presents with hypercholesterolemia. He has no history of cardiovascular disease and no cardiovascular symptoms. His LDL-C is 168 mg/dL. His father had a myocardial infarction at the age of 54 years. He is normotensive and normoglycemic. His weight is normal. He plays soccer four times a week. He is working with a dietician and a personal trainer to improve his diet and exercise regimen. What is the next best guideline-recommended step regarding the management of hypercholesterolemia?
   A. Calculate his 10-year risk score by the Pooled Cohort Equations (PCE) to guide statin decisions
   B. Defer statin therapy until he turns 40
   C. Consider initiating statin therapy
   D. Recommend garlic supplements

199. **A 42-year-old South Asian woman presents for evaluation of hypercholesterolemia. Her low-density lipoprotein cholesterol (LDL-C) is 148 mg/dL. She has a history of asthma and preeclampsia. Her calculated 10-year risk of atherosclerotic disease by the Pooled Cohort Equations is 5.9%. She is asymptomatic. In addition to lifestyle optimization, what is the guideline-recommended next step for the management of hypercholesterolemia?**
    A. Consider initiating statin therapy
    B. Recommend against statin therapy because her 10-year risk is <7.5%
    C. Consider initiating statin therapy along with an exercise stress test to evaluate for "silent" ischemia
    D. Recommend against statin therapy because her 10-year risk is <20%

200. **Which one of the following statements is TRUE regarding studies on Renin Angiotensin System Inhibition (RASi) in patients with CKD (chronic kidney disease)?**
    A. RASi drugs can slow progression of CKD in all stages of CKD.
    B. RASi drugs reduce mortality in all stages of CKD.
    C. RASi drugs reduce proteinuria and BP in all stages of CKD.
    D. RASi are safe in patients with CKD unless they develop substantial hyperkalemiA.
    E. RASi reduces heart failure hospitalizations in all stages of CKD.

201. **The diagnosis of CKD (chronic kidney disease) requires which of the following for 3 months minimum:**
    A. GFR <60 mL/min/m^2
    B. Microalbumin greater than 30 in patients with a GFR of 60 mL/min/m^2 or greater any time of day.
    C. ACR (albumin to creatinine ratio) of 30 or greater preferably in the AM.
    D. A and/or C
    E. Both A and C are needed

202. **Sodium-glucose cotransporter-2 inhibitors (SGLT2i) have been shown to do all the following except:**
    A. Reduce kidney disease progression in CKD.
    B. Lower blood glucose in patients with Type 2 diabetes.
    C. Prevent diabetic ketoacidosis (DKA).
    D. Reduce acute kidney injury
    E. Reduce hospitalizations for heart failure regardless of ejection fraction.

203. **Individuals with anemia of kidney disease, with HgbA1c <10, have been shown to have:**
    A. Increased all cause and CV (cardiovascular) mortality
    B. Hospitalization and increased length of stay
    C. Major acute coronary events
    D. Chronic kidney disease progression
    E. All of the above

204. **Which one of the following metabolites produced by the gut microbiome exerts anti-inflammatory effects?**
   A. Trimethylamine
   B. Short chain fatty acids
   C. Histidine
   D. Lipopolysaccharide

205. **Specialized pro-resolving molecules induce each of the following effects except for:**
   A. Orderly macrophage efferocytosis
   B. Stimulate the production of lipoxins
   C. Stimulate the production of prostaglandins and leukotrienes
   D. Down-regulate endothelial cell adhesion molecules
   E. Increase expression of IL-10

206. **Which one of the following is incorrect concerning high sensitivity C-reactive protein?**
   A. It is a pentraxin molecule.
   B. It participates in the opsonization and phagocytosis of infectious agents via the classical complement pathway.
   C. It is valuable as a predictor of ASCVD (atherosclerotic cardiovascular disease) events and its use as a dual target with LDL-C (low-density lipoprotein cholesterol) provides incremental benefit in primary and secondary prevention trials of statins.
   D. It is causal in the pathway for atherosclerosis.
   E. When its value exceeds 2.0 mg/L, it can be used to adjust 10-year predicted risk higher when using standard risk calculators.

207. **Each of the following findings concerning the Canakinumab Anti-inflammatory Thrombosis Outcome Study (CANTOS) is true EXCEPT:**
   A. Outcomes reduction was dependent on both decreases in hsCRP (high sensitivity C reactive protein) and atherogenic lipoprotein burden in serum.
   B. There was no mortality benefit with Canakinumab in the trial as a whole.
   C. The incidence of neutropenia and death due to sepsis was increased in participants randomized to Canakinumab.
   D. Canakinumab reduced the incidence of lung cancer.
   E. Among participants with hsCRP <2.0 on treatment compared to those with hsCRP > 2.0, both all-cause and cardiovascular mortality were reduced by 31%.

208. Each of the following is true concerning lipoprotein-associated phospholipase A2 EXCEPT:
    A. It is a treatment target.
    B. It potentiates inflammation by hydrolyzing phospholipids into a lysophospholipid and an oxidized fatty acid.
    C. It is a risk marker highly predictive of CVD (cardiovascular disease) independent of other established risk factors.
    D. It is transported in serum by lipoproteins.
    E. It is produced locally by activated macrophages and foam cells.

209. Visceral adipose tissue that is insulin resistant is a potent source of inflammatory cytokines and interleukins (adipokines) that boosts risk for ASCVD (atherosclerotic cardiovascular disease). Each of the following biochemical changes are induced by insulin resistance in adipose tissue EXCEPT:
    A. Increased triglyceride hydrolysis by hormone sensitive lipase and release of free fatty acid
    B. Increased expression of c-Jun N-terminal kinase (JNK)
    C. Decreased production of TNF-α and retinol binding protein 4
    D. Decreased cell surface expression of glucose transport proteins

210. Resident macrophages within atherosclerotic plaques scavenge lipoproteins and can gradually form foam cells as excess intracellular cholesterol accumulates. If allowed to continue the excess cholesterol and oxysterols produced from cholesterol are toxic and lead to macrophage apoptosis. Foam cells are also detrimental because they are engines of inflammatory mediator expression. Which one of the following is NOT associated with protective macrophage cholesterol mobilization and externalization:
    A. Membrane cassette transport protein A1 (ABCA1)
    B. Membrane cassette transport protein G1 (ABCG1)
    C. Membrane cassette transport protein A5/A8 (ABCG5/8)
    D. Scavenger Receptor BI (SR-BI)
    E. Apoprotein E secretion (apo E)

211. Neutrophils are versatile and play key roles in host defense and inflammatory responses. Neutrophils contribute to inflammation and atherogenesis via all of the following EXCEPT for:
    A. Suicidal neutrophils can form neutrophil extracellular traps
    B. Secrete matrix metalloproteinases such as collagenase and elastase
    C. Secrete azurocidin and helicidin
    D. NLR3P inflammasome activation
    E. Inhibit alpha-defensins

212. A male patient has excessive daytime sleepiness, nonrefreshing sleep, and morning headaches. Which one of the following findings most strongly suggests further evaluation for the presence of sleep apnea?
    A. BMI (body mass index) of 27 kg/m^2
    B. Mallampati score of 2
    C. Presence of retrognathia
    D. Neck circumference of 15 in.

213. Mr. Jones is a 55-year-old obese man with metabolic syndrome, Type 2 diabetes mellitus, and coronary artery disease. His stress test is normal. Through dietary changes alone, his weight decreased from 122 to 112 kg, and his waist circumference decreased from 128 to 109 cm during a period of 8 months. Which one of the following is the best next step regarding his lifestyle-intervention plan?
    A. No change is recommended because the patient has already met appropriate weight-loss goals.
    B. Initiate brisk walking or jogging for 30 min three times/week.
    C. Initiate brisk walking or jogging for 30 min/day
    D. Participate in gardening for 20 min three times/week.

214. Which of the following statements regarding the epidemiology of metabolic syndrome is TRUE?
    A. The prevalence of metabolic syndrome is roughly the same among non-Hispanic White women and men.
    B. Metabolic syndrome is more prevalent among non-Hispanic Black men than non-Hispanic Black women.
    C. Metabolic syndrome is more prevalent among Mexican American men than Mexican American women.
    D. All of the above.

215. A patient states that she tends to overeat on weekends when socializing with friends. Her physician discusses ways to limit exposure to social cues that trigger her overeating. This type of behavior therapy is referred to as?
    A. Goal setting
    B. Self-monitoring
    C. Stimulus control
    D. Stimulus narrowing

216. A 67-year-old man with a history of hypertension, hyperlipidemia, diabetes, and known multivessel disease presents for persistent ongoing angina. He can walk two blocks before symptom onset and has relief with decreasing activity. A month prior, he could walk four blocks prior to symptom onset. SYNTAX score is 30. His current medications are rosuvastatin 40 mg daily, aspirin 81 mg daily, losartan 25 mg daily, metoprolol succinate 50 mg daily, and metformin 500 mg twice daily.
What is the one best next step in his management?
A. Add clopidogrel 75 mg daily
B. Proceed with percutaneous intervention
C. Increase metoprolol succinate to 100 mg daily
D. Refer for coronary artery bypass grafting
E. Add empagliflozin 10 mg daily

217. A 30-year-old female who was a former collegiate athlete presents for symptoms of chest pain with exertion that occurs 30 min into her exercise. She is not currently having symptoms. She has previously discussed with her PCP (primary care physician) where she underwent evaluation with a chest X-Ray (unremarkable), pulmonary function tests (no obstructive/restrictive deficit and normal lung volumes), and had a normal CBC (complete blood count), CMP, and proBNP. Her family history is notable for an older brother who is 5 years her senior with a CAC (coronary artery calcium) score of 10 and an Lp(a) [lipoprotein(a)] of 230 mg/dL.
What is the one best next step to establish a diagnosis?
A. Perform a coronary CT (computed tomography) angiogram
B. Perform a stress echocardiogram
C. Perform a coronary artery calcium score
D. Obtain a high-sensitivity troponin
E. Perform an exercise ECG (electrocardiographic) stress test

218. Which of the following is TRUE about physical activity?
A. The ACC/AHA Guidelines recommend at least 300 min/week of moderate/vigorous activity for cardiovascular risk reduction.
B. No cardiovascular benefit is seen with physical activity until one reaches ≥150 min/week of moderate + vigorous physical activity.
C. Greater fitness (METS) is associated with improved survival, even for older adults ≥70 years.
D. Sedentary behavior does not confer any cardiovascular risk if individuals are physically active.
E. Counseling about physical activity in clinic visits is not effective in improving physical activity behavior in patients

219. **Which one of the following is TRUE about physical activity?**
    A. The PA guidelines from the Department of Health and Human Services additionally recommends muscle-strengthening activities on 2 or more days a week.
    B. Activity must be of vigorous intensity to achieve cardiovascular benefit.
    C. Moderate-intensity activity consists of activities at a workload of 6–9 METS.
    D. All adults should undergo medical screening by a health care provider before starting an exercise program.
    E. Trading sedentary time for light-intensity activity has no CV (cardiovascular) benefit.

220. **The following glucagon-like receptor agonist is the most recently FDA-approved anti-obesity medication in this class:**
    A. Liraglutide
    B. Cagrilintide
    C. Semaglutide
    D. Tirzepitide
    E. Dulaglutide

221. **Which one is TRUE regarding humor, laughter and preventive cardiology:**
    A. Largely due to their comedy surroundings, stand-up comics have a reduced risk of cardiac and overall premature death.
    B. Humor does not improve capability to manage life stressors (i.e., coping).
    C. Humor does improve capability to manage life stressors (i.e., coping).
    D. Humor does not affect the immune system.
    E. Humor may favorably affect endothelial function (enhances vasodilation and blood flow).

222. **Lactic acidosis has been associated with which one of the following classes of medication?**
    A. Sulfonylureas (e.g., glipizide)
    B. Metformin
    C. SGLT-2 (e.g., empagliflozin)
    D. GLP1-RA (e.g., liraglutide)
    E. Thiazolidinedione (e.g., rosiglitazone)

223. **Increased risk for perineal infections have been associated with which one of the following?**
    A. GLP1-RA
    B. Long-acting insulin
    C. Thiazolidinediones
    D. SGLT-2

224. **Select the one statement that is TRUE:**
    A. Women have better outcomes than men after AMI (acute myocardial infarction).
    B. Women are equally likely as men to receive guideline directed medical therapies after AMI.
    C. Women with AMI are equally likely as men to have chest pain.
    D. Young women with AMI who sought care prior to AMI are equally likely to men to be told their chest pain may be heart-related.
    E. Women are adequately represented in FDA premarket approval of cardiovascular devices.

225. **Which one of the following is FALSE?**
    A. Women are more likely than men to have myocardial ischemia without coronary artery disease (INOCA) or myocardial infarction without obstructive coronary artery disease (MINOCA).
    B. Despite more INOCA/MINOCA, women have worse MACE and mortality than men.
    C. Young women (<55 years) have the lowest rates of improvements in CHD death rates compared with any other age or sex groups.
    D. High sensitivity troponin I improves the sensitivity for the diagnosis of AMI in both men and women.

226. **You are seeing a 56-year-old man for general evaluation who relates he has decreased libido and erectile function. You check total and free testosterone (T) levels. Which one of the following is generally accepted as "low T"?**
    A. Total T (TT) or Free T < Lower Limit of Normal
    B. TT <350 ng/dL (12 nmol/L)
    C. TT <300 ng/dL
    D. TT <200 ng/dL
    E. T Levels are not helpful in diagnosing Low T

227. **A 56-year-old man has TT (total testosterone) <300 ng/dL and after discussion, he opts to start testosterone replacement therapy (TRT). Which one of the following may improve with TRT?**
    A. Erectile dysfunction
    B. Libido
    C. Lean body mass
    D. Depressive symptoms
    E. All the above

228. Per AHA/ACC 2018 Cholesterol Guidelines, which of the following biomarkers are associated with increased ASCVD (atherosclerotic cardiovascular disease) risk?
    A. Apo B <130 mg/dL
    B. Lipoprotein(a) ≥50 mg/dL
    C. hs-CRP 1–2 mg/L
    D. Triglycerides 150–175 mg/dL
    E. Non-HDL-C 100–130 mg/dL

229. In a patient with diabetes and elevated triglycerides of 250 mg/dL, which one of the following biomarkers can be inaccurate?
    A. Direct LDL-C
    B. LDL-P
    C. Non-HDL-C
    D. Apo B
    E. LDL-C

230. The blood brain barrier blocks the entry of which of the following into the central nervous system?
    A. Low-density lipoprotein
    B. High-density lipoprotein
    C. Chylomicrons
    D. Very low-density lipoprotein
    E. All lipoproteins

231. Which one of the following studies definitively demonstrated that aggressive lipid-lowering is associated with increased risk for neurocognitive impairment?
    A. Heart Protection Study
    B. PROSPER Trial
    C. EBBINGHAUS Trial
    D. ODYSSEY Outcomes
    E. None of the above

232. Which one of the following statements about the Canakinumab Anti-inflammatory Thrombosis Outcome Study (CANTOS) is incorrect:
    A. This trial enrolled patients with history of a previous myocardial infarction.
    B. Patients enrolled needed to have elevated hs-CRP levels.
    C. hs-CRP levels decreased in those receiving canakinumab.
    D. LDL-C levels decreased by 20 mg/dL among those receiving canakinumab.
    E. Canakinumab use was associated with a reduction in major adverse cardiovascular events.

233. **Which one of the following about the Justification for the Use of Statins in Prevention: an Intervention Trial Evaluating Rosuvastatin (JUPITER) is correct:**
   A. JUPITER trial was performed in patients with a history of myocardial infarction.
   B. To be included in the trial, participants needed to have LDL-C levels of 160 mg/dL or lower.
   C. Rosuvastatin 20 mg per day was associated with a 25% relative risk reduction in the primary end point.
   D. Rosuvastatin 20 mg per day was associated with a reduction in both LDL-C (low-density lipoprotein cholesterol) and hs-CRP (high-sensitivity C-reactive protein) levels.
   E. To be included in the trial, participants needed to have hs-CRP levels of 3 mg/L or higher.

234. **Olive oil, considered to be a heart healthful food choice, contains substantial amounts of the following fats:**
   A. Monounsaturated fat
   B. Polyunsaturated fat
   C. Saturated fat
   D. All of the above
   E. Only A and B

235. **Which one of the following is FALSE?**
   A. In a recent study, the likelihood of an atrial fibrillation (AF) episode 4 h after alcohol ingestion increased from 3× to 4× after 1 or 2 drinks.
   B. Obstructive sleep apnea (OSA) increases the risk of AF post ablation but CPAP does not reduce the risk.
   C. CABANA showed a reduction in recurrent AF, but the overall outcome was not significantly improved.
   D. North American women were about 10× more likely to develop AF.
   E. There is no difference in mortality between paroxysmal AF and persistent AF.

236. **Which one of the following is FALSE?**
   A. Both low and very high BMI (body mass index) predispose to AF (atrial fibrillation).
   B. Over an 8-year follow-up, those with persistent metabolic syndrome had a 31% higher incidence of AF versus patients without metabolic syndrome.
   C. Both occasional exercise and very vigorous sustained exercise have the same impact on risk of AF.
   D. In a study of 5599 patients felt to not be a candidate for a VKA (vitamin K antagonist) with an average $CHADS_2$ (congestive heart failure, hypertension, age >75 (2 points), vascular disease. age 65×74, and female) of 2.1 had a significantly lower risk of stroke, with a non-significant increased risk of bleeding
   E. In the SPRINT Trial, the group assigned to more intensive BP reduction had a lower risk of AF.

237. Which one of the following therapies have NOT been shown to reduce cardiovascular mortality in patients with heart failure and reduced ejection fraction (HFrEF)?
   A. Angiotensin Receptor Neprilysin Inhibitors
   B. Beta blocker
   C. Mineralocorticoid receptor antagonist
   D. ACE (angiotensin converting enzyme) inhibitors
   E. Digoxin

238. Which one of the following therapies have been shown to reduce cardiovascular mortality in patients with heart failure and preserved ejection fraction (HFpEF)?
   A. Angiotensin Receptor Neprilysin Inhibitors
   B. Beta blockers
   C. Mineralocorticoid receptor antagonist
   D. None of the above
   E. All of the above

239. In stage 1 hypertension, medical therapy is started beyond non-pharmacological approaches when:
   A. Cardiovascular risk is ≥5%
   B. Cardiovascular risk is ≥7.5%
   C. Cardiovascular risk is ≥10%
   D. Cardiovascular risk is ≥20%

240. Initiation of antihypertensive drug therapy with stage 2 hypertension and an average BP more than 20/10 mmHg above their BP target is recommended:
   A. with 2 first-line agents of different antihypertensive classes
   B. as separate agents
   C. in a fixed-dose combination
   D. All of the above

241. Which one of the following is NOT associated with genetic variants etiologic for familial hypercholesterolemia:
   A. PCSK9
   B. Apoprotein B100
   C. Apoprotein CII
   D. LDL-RAP-1
   E. LDL receptor

242. Within the hepatocyte, PCSK9 does which one of the following:
   A. Enzymatically proteolyzes the LDL receptor (LDL-R)
   B. Serves as a chaperone molecule to shunt LDL-R into the lysosome
   C. Serves as a chaperone molecule to shuttle LDL-R to the golgi apparatus
   D. Dissociates the LDL-R from APO B
   E. Activates cholesterol 7-alpha-hydroxylase

243. **Which technique may be most effective to improve BP control and reduce disparities in hypertension goal attainment?**
    A. Multiple outpatient visits in the clinic setting
    B. The use of detailed recording of symptoms related to BP (blood pressure)
    C. Self-measured BP interventions
    D. Physician only based pharmacotherapy

244. **Which one of the following characteristics may affect evaluation of lipids in Black adults when compared to White adults or Hispanic/Latinx adults?**
    A. Lower level of HDL-C
    B. Higher level of triglycerides
    C. Higher severity of coronary artery calcium
    D. Equal responsiveness to statin dosage

245. **According to recent mortality rates attributed to CVD (cardiovascular disease) in the US between 1900 and 2018, the following trend has been noted:**
    A. Uptick in deaths attributable to CVD for non-Hispanic White, but not non-Hispanic Black individuals
    B. Small but insignificant decline in CVD deaths in all major racial/ethnic
    C. Plateau effect with CVD deaths essentially unchanged in all major racial/ethnic groups
    D. Lower CVD deaths projected in non-Hispanic White, but not in non-Hispanic Black individuals in 2020 and beyond

246. **Renal-artery stenting does not confer a significant benefit with respect to the prevention of clinical events when added to comprehensive, multifactorial medical therapy in people with atherosclerotic renal-artery stenosis and hypertension or chronic kidney disease.**
    A. False
    B. True
    C. In a fixed-dose combination
    D. All of the above

247. **Meta-analyses of randomized controlled trials suggest that the fall in blood pressure with treating OSA (obstructive sleep apnea) in hypertensive sleep apneic patients is approximately:**
    A. 10–15 mmHg
    B. 5–10 mmHg
    C. 0 mmHg
    D. 2–3 mmHg
    E. >15 mmHg

248. **Treating obstructive sleep apnea is proven to:**
    A. Prevent atrial fibrillation
    B. Reduce myocardial infarction
    C. Reduce sudden death
    D. All of the above
    E. None of the above

249. **A 55-year-old man with borderline dyslipidemia and a family history of premature CAD (coronary artery disease) presents for evaluation. He has no chest pain and exercises three times a week at the gym. He undergoes a coronary calcium scan which shows an Agatston score of 640. What do you recommend next?**
    A. Coronary CT angiography (CTA)
    B. Exercise treadmill testing (ETT)
    C. Carotid intima-media thickness (IMT) measurement
    D. No further testing

250. **A 67-year-old woman with Type 2 diabetes and hypertension undergoes a stress echocardiogram for evaluation of chest pain. She is able to perform 5 min (5 METS) of exercise before stopping due to chest pain. She has a normal resting ejection fraction but has a large anterior inducible wall motion abnormality with a decrement in her EF (ejection fraction) with exercise. What do you recommend next?**
    A. Invasive coronary angiography
    B. Coronary CT (computed tomographic) angiography
    C. Stress perfusion imaging
    D. No further testing

251. **For which one of the following should the Pooled Cohort Equation for estimating 10-year ASCVD (atherosclerotic cardiovascular disease) risk not be used?**
    A. Persons with LDL-C (low-density lipoprotein cholesterol) ≥190 mg/dL
    B. Persons with known ASCVD (atherosclerotic cardiovascular disease)
    C. Persons with diabetes
    D. Persons under age 40
    E. A and B
    F. A, B, and D
    G. All of the above

252. **What is an appropriate use of the coronary calcium score (CAC) based on the 2018 cholesterol management guideline?**
    A. For those at borderline or intermediate risk with a CAC score of 0, and without other risk enhancing factors, as well as without diabetes, heavy current cigarette smoking, or a strong family history of premature ASCVD, one can consider withholding or delaying statin therapy.
    B. For those with known ASCVD, the CAC score can help in deciding on the intensity of statin therapy.
    C. For those with diabetes, the CAC score can help in deciding whether to initiate statin therapy.
    D. All of the above.

253. **What proportion of patients hospitalized with an early-onset myocardial infarction harbor a monogenic familial hypercholesterolemia mutation?**
    A. 0.4%
    B. 1.7%
    C. 17%
    D. 25%
    E. 50%

254. **Among patients who inherit an increased risk for myocardial infarction on the basis of a high polygenic score, which one of the following have been associated with a significant decrease in risk?**
    A. None
    B. Adherence to a healthy lifestyle
    C. Statin therapy
    D. Both adherence to a healthy lifestyle and statin therapy
    E. Transitioning from traditional to e-cigarettes

255. **Absent contraindications, which patients should be given prasugrel or ticagrelor over clopidogrel in secondary prevention?**
    A. Acute MI treated medically
    B. Acute MI with stent implantation
    C. Drug eluting stent placement for stable angina
    D. High-risk primary prevention patients

256. **Recent clinical trials demonstrated statistically significant reductions in cardiovascular event risk from aspirin therapy in which group of patients?**
    A. Type 2 diabetes without prior cardiovascular disease
    B. High risk primary prevention patients based on 10-year risk score
    C. Older adults age 70+
    D. Patients with severely elevated CAC (coronary artery calcium) scores
    E. None of the above

Questions

257. **Among symptomatic patients with stable coronary artery disease (CAD) who receive optimal medical therapy (OMT) and therapeutic lifestyle intervention, the performance of PCI (percutaneous coronary intervention)/stenting to treat obstructive CAD:**
    A. reduces the composite of death or MI (myocardial infarction)
    B. reduces MI only
    C. improves short-term angina relief, but not long-term angina or quality of life
    D. may not improve even short-term angina/treadmill walking time when patients undergo a blinded treatment comparison
    E. B, C, and D
    F. C and D only

258. **Patients with symptomatic lower extremity peripheral artery disease are at high risk of:**
    A. Major adverse cardiovascular events including myocardial infarction and stroke
    B. Major adverse limb events including acute limb ischemia and amputation
    C. Functional limitation
    D. All-cause mortality
    E. All of the above

259. **Therapies that lower LDL-C in patients with lower extremity peripheral artery disease:**
    A. Reduce major adverse cardiovascular events
    B. Reduce major adverse limb events
    C. Reduce peripheral revascularizations
    D. Are under-utilized
    E. All of the above

260. **A 57-year-old female undergoes a coronary CTA to evaluate for rare episodes of brief chest discomfort. She has a high exercise capacity, and her symptoms are non-exertional. She is found to have a medium amount of mostly non-calcified atherosclerotic plaque resulting in minimal stenosis (<25%; CAD RADS 1) of multiple coronary segments, including the proximal and mid left anterior descending, the proximal and mid right coronary artery, and the left circumflex artery. She is not on any medical therapies. Her LDL-C is 122 mg/dL. Lp(a) is 62 mg/dL (normal <30 mg/dL). She is a nonsmoker.**
    Which one of the following would be the most important next step for reducing her risk of future cardiovascular events?
    A. Niacin
    B. Statin therapy
    C. PET MPI to evaluate for microvascular dysfunction
    D. Refer for genetic testing
    E. All of the above

261. **Which one of the following patients would be the most appropriate candidate for a coronary CT angiography?**
    A. A 62-year-old male with no known CAD who is presenting with typical chest pain
    B. A 62-year-old female with prior PCI to the LAD and RCA who is presenting with atypical chest pain
    C. A 48-year-old asymptomatic female with a family history of premature cardiovascular disease
    D. A 48-year-old male asymptomatic male with an elevated LDL-C who prefers to avoid statin therapy
    E. All of the above

262. **Chronic venous disease is:**
    A. Significantly more common than peripheral arterial disease
    B. Seen only in individuals with Type 2 diabetes and peripheral arterial disease
    C. Not associated with increased morbidity
    D. Not preventable or treatable

263. **Which one of the following is true for intermediate risk, asymptomatic, primary prevention patients?**
    A. CAC improves CVD risk discrimination beyond traditional risk factors.
    B. CAC provides better CVD risk discrimination compared to ankle-brachial index (ABI).
    C. The prevalence of CAC differs by ethnicity.
    D. Inflammation is important in the development of coronary artery calcification.
    E. All of the Above

264. **A 53-year-old woman with a history of diabetes mellitus, obesity, and hypertension presents to establish care after her primary care physician performed a nuclear perfusion scan for symptoms of exertional dyspnea. The nuclear perfusion scan demonstrated a severe defect. Current medications include aspirin 81 mg daily, rosuvastatin 40 mg daily, metoprolol succinate 100 mg daily and semaglutide 1.7 mg weekly. Since initiation of metoprolol therapy, her symptoms have improved and only occur after walking three blocks. Her vital signs during the clinic visit are as follows: afebrile, heart rate 52 beats/min, and blood pressure 113/64 mmHg.**
    What is the best next step in her management?
    A. Add clopidogrel 75 mg daily
    B. Add rivaroxaban 2.5 mg twice daily
    C. Obtain a coronary CT angiogram
    D. Increase metoprolol succinate to 200 mg daily
    E. Obtain a coronary artery calcium scan

Questions 77

265. A 53-year-old woman with a history of diabetes mellitus, obesity and hypertension presents to establish care after her primary care physician for persistent symptoms of exertional chest pain. Three months prior, she had undergone invasive coronary angiography that had demonstrated obstructive mid left anterior descending coronary artery disease. Her current cardiovascular medicines include: aspirin 81 mg daily, rosuvastatin 40 mg daily, ezetimibe 10 mg daily, metoprolol succinate 100 mg daily amlodipine 5 mg daily, isosorbide mononitrate 60 mg daily. Her vital signs during the clinic visit are as follows: Afebrile, heart rate 52 beats/min, and blood pressure 103/64.
    What is the best next step in management?
    A. Add clopidogrel 75 mg daily
    B. Add rivaroxaban 2.5 mg twice daily
    C. Perform angioplasty and stent placement along mid LAD
    D. Increase metoprolol succinate to 200 mg daily
    E. Add ranolazine 500 mg twice daily

266. A 53-year-old woman with a history of Type 2 diabetes mellitus, obesity, and hypertension presents to establish care. Recently, a coronary artery calcium score was performed and found a total Agatston score of 435 with calcifications in all epicardial vessels. Labs from 1 month prior demonstrate a hemoglobin A1C of 6.8% and a total cholesterol of 175 mg/dL, triglycerides of 40 mg/dL, HDL-C of 89 mg/dL, and LDL-C of 76 mg/dL. Her current medications include aspirin 81 mg daily, atorvastatin 40 mg daily, sitagliptin 100 mg daily, and metformin 1000 mg twice daily.
    What is the best next step in management?
    A. Start ezetimibe 10 mg daily
    B. Start empagliflozin 10 mg daily
    C. Start alirocumab 75 mg twice weekly
    D. A and B
    E. All of the above

267. A 53-year-old woman with a history of Type 2 diabetes mellitus, obesity (BMI 33.9), and hypertension presents to establish care. Recently, a coronary artery calcium score was performed and found a total Agatston score of 435 with calcifications in all epicardial vessels. Labs from 1 month prior demonstrate a hemoglobin A1C of 7.8% and a total cholesterol of 175 mg/dL, triglycerides of 40 mg/dL, HDL-C of 89 mg/dL, and LDL-C of 76 mg/dL. Her current medications include aspirin 81 mg daily, atorvastatin 40 mg daily, sitagliptin 100 mg daily, and metformin 1000 mg twice daily.
    What is the best next step in management?
    A. Start ezetimibe 10 mg daily
    B. Start tirzepatide 2.5 mg weekly with planned uptitration
    C. Start alirocumab 75 mg twice weekly
    D. A and B
    E. All of the above

Answers

1. Correct Answer: A

Rationale
A recent ASPC Clinical Practice Statement reviewed the demographics of individuals enrolled in cardiovascular clinical trials including both prevention and treatment. While racial and ethnic minority groups account for 36% of the population of the United States, individuals from these groups are considerably less likely to be enrolled in clinical trials, and the percentages vary by disease state. Likewise, women remain much less likely than men to enroll in trials.

Reference
1. Michos ED, Reddy TK, Gulati M, et al. Improving the enrollment of women and racially/ethnically diverse populations in cardiovascular clinical trials: an ASPC clinical practice statement. Am J Prev Cardiol. 2021;8:100250. PMID: 34485967.

2. Correct Answer: C

Rationale
More than 25 million people in the United States have some form of chronic venous disease (CVeD). The prevalence of CVeD is 10 times that of peripheral arterial disease and is underdiagnosed and undertreated. There are multiple established risk factors for CVeD including older age, female sex, family history, prolonged standing, and obesity. CVeD is a major source of morbidity, and most admissions are for venous ulcers. The direct cost of treating venous disease in the United States is $3 billion annually.

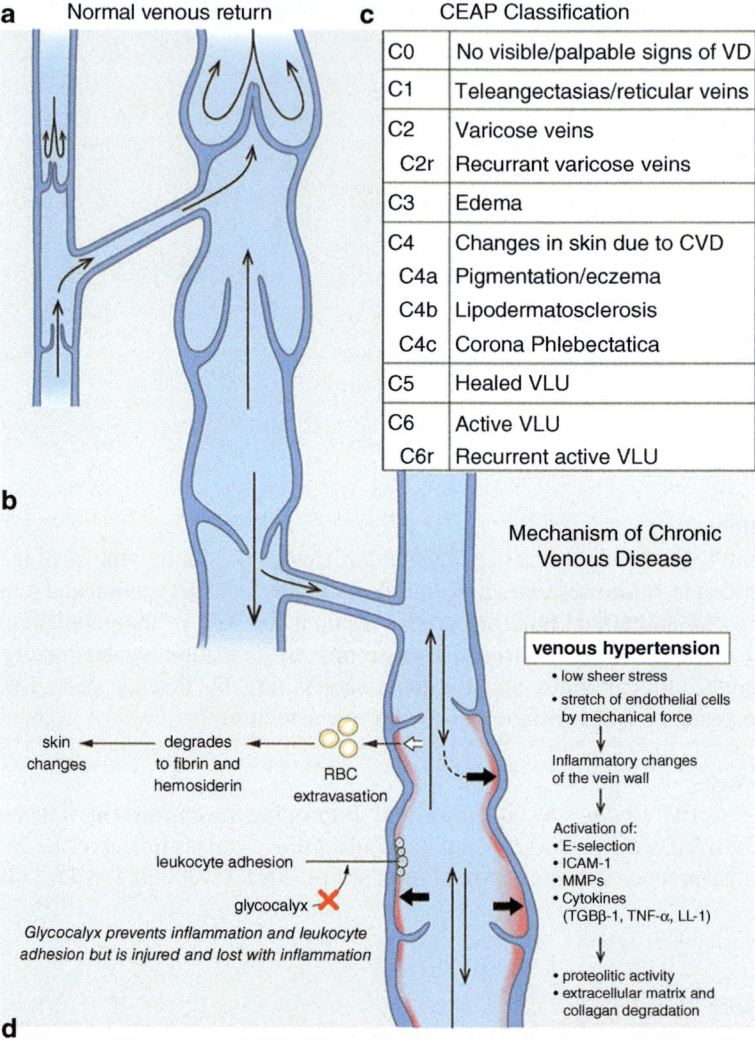

Chronic venous disease. (**a**) Normal venous return occurs through a system of superficial, perforating, and deep (intermuscular) veins propelled by the pressure gradient derived from muscle contraction and a network of bicuspid venous valves to prevent retrograde blood flow. During proper functioning, the pressure within the thin-walled veins remains relatively low ($\approx$20–30 mmHg). (**b**) Chronic venous disease occurs in the setting of prolonged venous hypertension arising from multiple factors including degenerate venous valves, weakened muscle contraction, and proximal obstruction. Rather than the standard flow of blood from the superficial to the deep veins, incompetent valves allow for blood to flow back into the superficial veins or pool in the deep vein increasing their local pressure. Over time, the increased volume and pressures in the veins incites endothelial dysfunction including loss of the protective glycocalyx and venous wall inflammation resulting in adverse extracellular matrix remodeling. This is further exacerbated by RBC extravasation and leukocyte adhesion. Further, support for these mechanistic changes within the venous wall has been derived from gene expression studies comparing healthy and diseased veins. (**c**) Clinical-Etiology-Anatomy-Pathophysiology (CEAP) classification system for patients with chronic venous disorders. (**d**) Summary table of genetic abnormalities (and when appropriate their associated genetic syndrome) that have been associated with varicose vein formation. (Figure and legend reproduced with permission from Baylis RA, Smith NL, Klarin D, Fukaya E. Epidemiology and Genetics of Venous Thromboembolism and Chronic Venous Disease. Circ Res. 2021 Jun 11;128(12):1988–2002)

References
1. McArdle M, Hernandez-Vila EA. Management of chronic venous disease. Tex Heart Inst J. 2017;44(5):347–9. PMID: 29259507.
2. Baylis RA, Smith NL, Klarin D, Fukaya E. Epidemiology and genetics of venous thromboembolism and chronic venous disease. Circ Res. 2021;128(12): 1988–2002. PMID: 34110897.

3. **Correct Answer: D**

Rationale

Duplex scanning is recommended as the first diagnostic test for all patients with suspected CVeD. It is safe, noninvasive, and cost-effective. Ankle-brachial indexes (ABIs) are unlikely to be helpful as the patient has no signs of arterial disease. Nerve conduction studies and MRI of the lumbar spine are used for the evaluation of a suspected neuropathic disorder.

Risk factors for CVeD are related to conditions that lead to venous dilation or other disruption of basic vein structure. These include older age, family history, female sex, pregnancy, obesity, occupations performed while standing, high-impact physical activity, and comorbid conditions such as deep vein thrombosis (DVT), superficial thrombophlebitis, and obstructive sleep apnea.

Dilated veins around the ankle is called corona phlebectatica and, importantly, is considered by many venous authorities to be an early sign of advanced venous disease and associated with an increased risk of developing a venous ulcer.

References
1. Gloviczki P, Comerota AJ, Dalsing MC, et al. Society for Vascular Surgery; American Venous Forum. The care of patients with varicose veins and associated chronic venous diseases: clinical practice guidelines of the Society for Vascular Surgery and the American Venous Forum. J Vasc Surg. 2011;53(5 Suppl):2S–48S.
2. Lurie F, Passman M, Meisner M, et al. The 2020 update of the CEAP classification system and reporting standards. J Vasc Surg Venous Lymphat Disord. 2020;8(3):342–52.

4. **Correct Answer: D**

Rationale
The first line therapy for CVeD is weight loss, exercise, and elevation and compression of the legs. Antiplatelet and/or anticoagulant therapy is not recommended in the management of these disorders prior to invasive interventions. Arterial revascularization has no role in the therapy of CVeD.

Reference
1. Gloviczki P, Comerota AJ, Dalsing MC, et al. Society for Vascular Surgery; American Venous Forum. The care of patients with varicose veins and associated chronic venous diseases: clinical practice guidelines of the Society for Vascular Surgery and the American Venous Forum. J Vasc Surg. 2011;53(5 Suppl):2S–48S.

5. **Correct Answer: C**

Rationale
Based on the atherosclerotic cardiovascular disease (ASCVD) risk estimator, the patient's risk for a vascular event is ≥ 7.5–20% (intermediate risk). Risk discussion: use moderate-intensity statins and increase to high-intensity with risk enhancers. There is the option for CAC (coronary artery calcium) to risk stratify if there is uncertainty about risk after consideration of risk enhancing factors. If CAC = 0, one can avoid statins and repeat CAC in the future (5–10 years), the exceptions being high-risk conditions such as diabetes, family history of premature CHD (coronary heart disease), and smoking. If CAC 1–100, it is reasonable to initiate moderate-intensity statin for persons ≥ 55 years. If CAC ≥ 100 or 75th percentile or higher, consider high intensity statin.

For persons at intermediate predicted risk ($\geq 7.5\%$ to $<20\%$) by the ASCVD risk estimator or borderline (5% to <7.5%) predicted risk, CAC helps refine risk assessment. CAC can re-classify risk upward (particularly when score is ≥ 100 or ≥ 75th age/sex/race percentile) or downward (if CAC = 0), which is not uncommon, particularly in men <50 and women <60 years. In MESA (Multi-Ethnic Study of Atherosclerosis), the CAC was strongly associated with 10-year ASCVD risk in a graded fashion across age, sex, and race/ethnic groups, and independent of traditional risk factors.

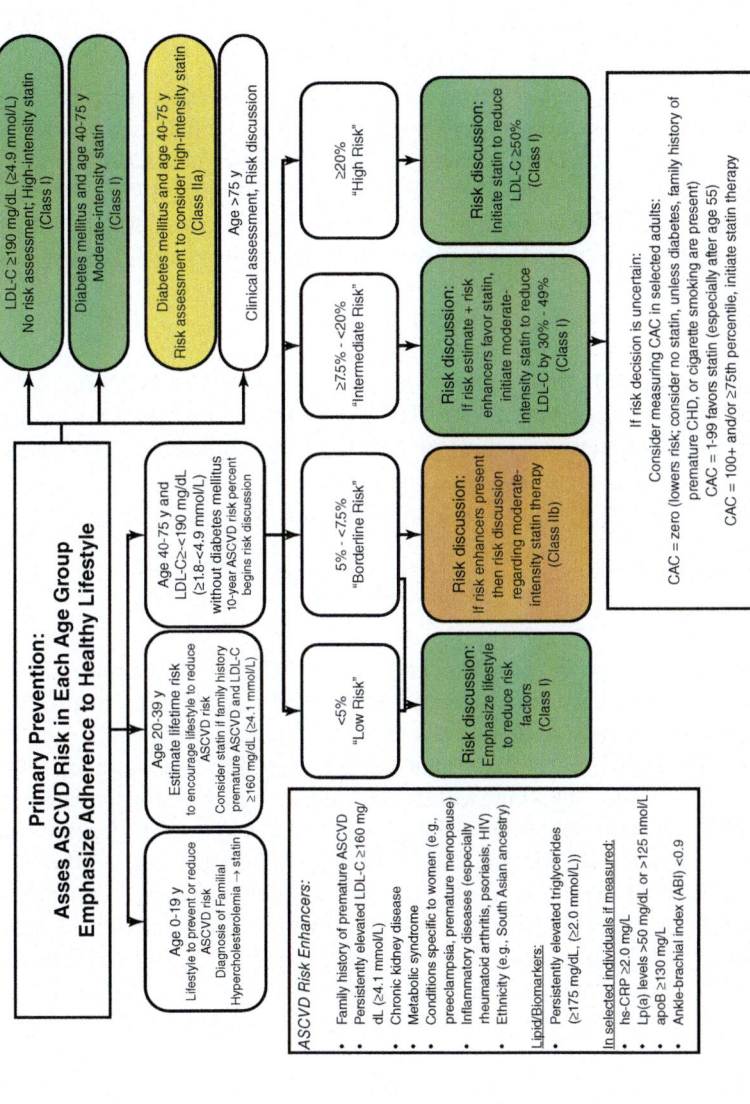

ABI ankle-brachial index, *apoB* apolipoprotein B, *ASCVD* atherosclerotic cardiovascular disease, *CAC* coronary artery calcium, *CHD* coronary heart disease, *HIV* human immunodeficiency virus, *hs-CRP* high-sensitivity C-reactive protein, *LDL-C* low-density lipoprotein cholesterol, *Lp(a)* lipoprotein (a). (Reproduced with permission from Arnett D, Blumenthal R, Albert M, et al. 2019 ACC/AHA Guideline on the Primary Prevention of Cardiovascular Disease. *J Am Coll Cardiol.* 2019 Sep, 74 (10) e177–e232)

Reference
1. Arnett D, Blumenthal R, Albert M, et al. 2019 ACC/AHA guideline on the primary prevention of cardiovascular disease. J Am Coll Cardiol. 2019;74(10):e177–232.

6. **Correct Answer: A**

Rationale
In adults with diabetes mellitus (DM) and aged 40–75, a moderate-intensity statin is recommended regardless of risk, and a high-intensity statin is reasonable for those with multiple ASCVD risk factors. The 2018 AHA/ACC/Multisociety Guideline identifies moderate hypertriglyceridemia (triglycerides ≥175 mg/dL) as a "risk-enhancing factor" to be considered in the clinician–patient risk discussion, the presence of which favors the initiation or intensification of statin therapy as a first step.

Reference
1. Grundy SM, Stone NJ, Bailey AL, et al. 2018 AHA/ACC/AACVPR/AAPA/ABC/ACPM/ADA/ AGS/APhA/ASPC/NLA/PCNA guideline on the management of blood cholesterol: a report of the American College of Cardiology/American Heart Association task force on clinical practice guidelines. J Am Coll Cardiol. 2019;73:e285–350.

7. **Correct Answer: D**

Rationale
For patients 45 years of age or older with clinical ASCVD (arteriosclerotic cardiovascular disease), or 50 years or older with diabetes mellitus requiring medication and >1 additional risk factor (additional risk factors include the following, based on the entry criteria in REDUCE-IT: age [men ≥55, women ≥65 years of age], cigarette smoker or stopped smoking within 3 months, hypertension [treated or untreated], high-density lipoprotein [HDL]-cholesterol <40 mg/dL for men or <50 mg/dL for women, hs-CRP [high sensitivity C-reactive protein] >3.0 mg/L, renal dysfunction with creatinine clearance >30 and <60 mL/min, retinopathy, microalbuminuria or macroalbuminuria, ABI <0.9 without symptoms of intermittent claudication, with fasting TG 135–499 mg/dL on high-intensity or maximally tolerated statin, with or without ezetimibe), treatment with icosapent ethyl is recommended for ASCVD risk reduction; evidence rating: (Class I, level BR).

Reference
1. Orringer CE, Jacobson TA, Maki KC. National Lipid Association Scientific Statement on the use of icosapent ethyl in statin-treated patients with elevated triglycerides and high or very-high ASCVD risk. J Clin Lipidol. 2019;13(6):860–72.

8. Correct Answer: B

Rationale
Current guidelines recommend a moderate intensity statin in a young adult aged 20–39 years reporting a positive premature family history of ASCVD and with an LDL-C ≥160 mg/dL.

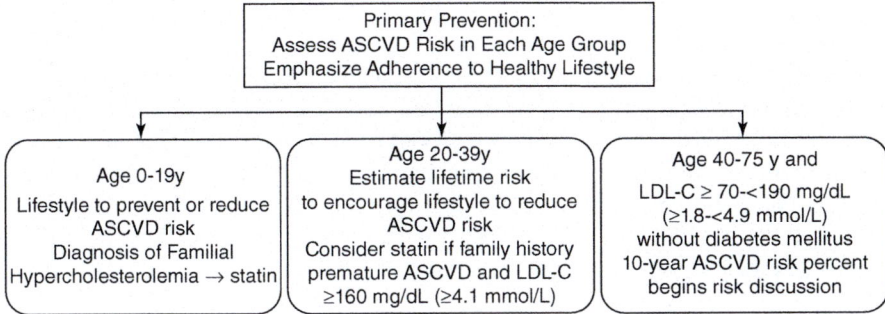

Reference
1. Grundy SM, Stone NJ, Bailey AL, et al. 2018 AHA/ACC/AACVPR/AAPA/ABC/ACPM/ADA/ AGS/APhA/ASPC/NLA/PCNA guideline on the management of blood cholesterol: a report of the American College of Cardiology/American Heart Association task force on clinical practice guidelines. J Am Coll Cardiol. 2019;73:e285–350.

9. Correct Answer: A

Rationale
In an analysis of data from seven different cohort studies in the United States and using a definition that included the ABI and lower extremity revascularizations, African–Americans were found to have the highest prevalence of peripheral arterial disease (PAD) compared to the other four groups listed above.

Reference
1. Allison MA, Ho E, Denenberg JO, et al. Ethnic specific prevalence of PAD in the United States. Am J Prev Med. 2007;32:328–33.

10. Correct Answer: B

Rationale
Diabetes mellitus, and the resulting insulin resistance, glycolates, and other biologic mechanisms, can lead to medial artery calcification, especially in the infrageniculate arteries to include the anterior and posterior tibial arteries. The medial artery calcification increases the "stiffness" of the artery, thereby requiring a higher pressure to collapse the arterial lumen. This results in a higher systolic blood pressure (SBP) reading in the ankle arteries and an elevated ABI, potentially despite significant luminal atherosclerotic disease.

References
1. Jeffcoate WJ, Rasmussen LM, Hofbauer LC, Game FL. Medial artery calcification in diabetes and its relationship to neuropathy. Diabetologia. 2009;52:2478–88.
2. Chistiakov D. Mechanisms of medial arterial calcification in diabetes. Curr Phar Des. 2014;20:5870–83.

11. Correct Answer: A

Rationale
A single antiplatelet agent (e.g., aspirin) is recommended to reduce the major cardiovascular events in patients with PAD. Cilostazol is recommended to improve pain-free walking distance in patients with PAD and associated intermittent claudication. Pentoxifylline has been assessed in patients with PAD and intermittent claudication but is currently not recommended for them. Rivaroxaban with aspirin is recommended for patients with coronary artery disease comorbid with PAD to reduce major cardiovascular events.

References
1. Gerhard-Herman MD, Gornik HL, Barrett C, et al. 2016 AHA/ACC guideline on the management of patients with lower extremity peripheral artery disease: executive summary. Vasc Med. 2017;22(3):NP1–43.
2. Bedenis R, Stewart M, Cleanthis M, et al. Cilostazol for intermittent claudication. Cochrane Database Syst Rev. 2014;2014(10):CD003748.
3. Salhiyyah K, Forster R, Senanayake E, et al. Pentoxifylline for intermittent claudication. Cochrane Database Syst Rev. 2015;9(9):CD005262.

12. Correct Answer: A

Rationale
Prior studies have shown that patients should be medically optimized prior to undergoing a lower extremity revascularization procedure.

Reference
1. Golledge J, Moxon JV, Rowbotham S, et al. Risk of major amputation in patients with intermittent claudication undergoing early revascularization. Br J Surg. 2018;105(6):699–708.

13. Correct Answer: E

Rationale
The Look AHEAD trial was a randomized controlled trial comparing an Intensive Lifestyle Intervention (ILI) to a Diabetes Support and Education (DSE) in people with overweight, obesity, and Type 2 diabetes. Initial results suggested a differential effect on weight loss and fitness between the two groups, and there was no effect on cardiovascular outcomes; however, in a post hoc analysis of those who lost 10% or more body weight, there is a 20% reduction in cardiovascular mortality and 21% reduction in major adverse cardiovascular events (MACE).

Reference
1. Look AHEAD Research Group; Gregg EW, Jakicic JM, Blackburn G, et al. Association of the magnitude of weight loss and changes in physical fitness with long-term cardiovascular disease outcomes in overweight or obese people with type 2 diabetes: a post-hoc analysis of the Look AHEAD randomised clinical trial. Lancet Diabetes Endocrinol. 2016;4(11):913–21.

14. Correct Answer: A

Rationale
Anti-obesity medications are indicated for treating adults with a BMI ≥30 kg/m^2 or those with a BMI ≥27 kg/m^2 with a weight-related comorbidity. There are many considerations on choosing anti-obesity medications, including contraindications, comorbidities, cues, combinations, cost/coverage. Semaglutide (answer A) is a glucagon-like receptor-1 agonist that is approved for treating obesity and Type 2 diabetes. The average weight loss at 68 weeks in a clinical trial was 14.9% versus 2.4% with placebo, and 69.1% achieved ≥10% weight loss, and third of subjects achieved 20% weight loss. In addition, semaglutide treatment reduces waist circumference, systolic blood pressure, and glycemia. In the SUSTAIN-6 trial, in participants with Type 2 diabetes who were at high cardiovascular risk, the rate of cardiovascular death, nonfatal myocardial infarction, or nonfatal stroke was significantly lower among patients receiving semaglutide than among those receiving placebo. This patient has known cardiovascular disease and hypertension so phentermine alone (answer B) or in combination as Phentermine Topiramate ER (answer C) would not be an ideal. In addition, the patient is already on bupropion for depression and adding Naltrexone Bupropion ER (answer D), a combination medication, is not correct. Metformin (answer E) is not an FDA-approved for obesity treatment.

References
1. Wilding JPH, Batterham RL, Calanna S, et al. STEP 1 Study Group. Once-weekly semaglutide in adults with overweight or obesity. N Engl J Med. 2021;384(11):989–1002.
2. Marso SP, Bain SC, Consoli A, et al. SUSTAIN-6 Investigators. Semaglutide and cardiovascular outcomes in patients with type 2 diabetes. N Engl J Med. 2016;375(19):1834–44.

15. Correct Answer: C

Rationale
This patient has uncontrolled Type 2 diabetes on metformin monotherapy. While the addition of empagliflozin or liraglutide will improve glycemia, body weight, and cardiovascular risk (CV) risk, RYGB is most likely to get his diabetes under control, treat obesity-related comorbidities (hypertension, OSA, etc.), and decrease his future risk of cardiovascular events. Insulin glargine will improve glucose but will likely contribute to weight gain and does not lower CV. Linagliptin is weight neutral and will not control his diabetes or CV risk to the same extent as RYGB.

Reference

1. Aminian A, Wilson R, Zajichek A, et al. Cardiovascular outcomes in patients with type 2 diabetes and obesity: comparison of gastric bypass, sleeve gastrectomy, and usual care. Diabetes Care. 2021;44(11):2552–63.

16. Correct Answer: E

Rationale

Tirzepatide is a GLP-1/GIP dual receptor agonist that was shown in the SURMOUNT-1 trial to achieve ≥20% weight loss in 57% of participants taking 15 mg once weekly. It appears to be superior to semaglutide, liraglutide, and phentermine topiramate ER in helping to achieve this magnitude of weight loss. Empagliflozin is not an approved anti-obesity medication and is not associated with this magnitude of weight reduction.

Reference

1. Frías JP, Davies MJ, Rosenstock J, et al. SURPASS-2 Investigators. Tirzepatide versus semaglutide once weekly in patients with type 2 diabetes. N Engl J Med. 2021;385(6):503–15.

17. Correct Answer: B

Rationale

A. Incorrect

ECG exercise testing is appropriate to assess potential cardiac symptoms in women if a woman has (1) adequate functional capacity (by history or data) and (2) a normal baseline electrocardiogram. The 2014 Consensus Statement of the American Heart Association includes the following recommendations: low-risk patient: no test or exercise electrocardiography (EECG); low-intermediate or intermediate risk: EECG; intermediate-high risk, stress imaging test. The misconception that EECG testing is fraught with false positives in women is a result of early correlative studies between coronary angiography and exercise ECG testing in which premenopausal, relatively young women comprised a large proportion of the subjects. Based on Bayes' theorem that the predictive accuracy of a test is a function of the sensitivity and specificity of the test and the prevalence of the disease (e.g., coronary artery disease [CAD]) in the population being tested), a high rate of false positives for CAD resulted because of the low prevalence of CAD in relatively young women in these studies. Additionally, evidence suggestive of a false positive exercise test for CAD is afforded by the following characteristics of the test in women (and men): high functional capacity, absence of exercise-induced symptoms, excellent heart rate recovery, only minimally positive ST segment criteria for ischemia (1.0-mm horizontal ST depression, and rapid reversal of ST depression post-exercise (≤30 s).

References
1. Levinson JM, Aspry K, Amsterdam EA. Improving the positive predictive value of exercise testing in women for coronary artery disease. Am J Cardiol. 2012;110:1619–22.
2. Mieres J, Gulati M, Bairey Merz N, et al. Role of noninvasive testing in the clinical evaluation of women with suspected ischemic heart disease. A consensus statement from the American Heart Association. Circulation. 2014;130:350–79.

B. Correct

Maximum functional capacity is one of the most valuable prognostic indicators for cardiovascular disease in symptomatic or asymptomatic women and men.

References
1. Blair SN, Kohl HW, Paffenbarger RS, et al. Physical fitness and all-cause mortality. A prospective study of healthy men and women. JAMA. 1989;262:2395–401.
2. Bhat A, Desai A, Amsterdam EA. Usefulness of high functional capacity in patients with exercise-induced ST-depression to predict a negative result on exercise echocardiography and low prognostic risk. Am J Cardiol. 2008;10:1541–3.
3. Beri N, Dang P, Bhat A, et al. Usefulness of excellent functional capacity in men and women with ischemic exercise electrocardiography to predict a negative stress imaging test and very low late mortality. Am J Cardiol. 2019;124:661–5.
4. Bourque JM, Beller GA. Value of exercise stress electrocardiography for risk stratification in patients with suspected or known coronary artery disease in the era of advanced imaging technologies. JACC Cardiovasc Imaging. 2015;8:1309–21.

C. Incorrect

Although the double product is closely related, in relative terms, to myocardial oxygen demand and coronary blood flow, there have been no large, prospective trials to investigate the utility of the double product for estimating prognosis in women or men.

References
1. Nelson RR, Gobel FL, Jorgensen CR, et al. Hemodynamic predictors of myocardial oxygen consumption during static and dynamic exercise. Circulation. 1974;50:1179–89.
2. Amsterdam EA, Price J, Berman D, et al. Exercise testing in the indirect assessment of myocardial oxygen consumption: application for evaluation of mechanisms and therapy of angina pectoris. In: Amsterdam EA, DeMaria A, Wilmore JH, editors. Exercise in health and disease. New York: LeJacq; 1997. p. 218–33.

D. Incorrect

The positive predictive value (percent) of an exercise test is determined by dividing the number of True Positive results by the total number of Positive results (True Positives + False Positives) and multiplying the resulting fraction by 100.

References
1. Fletcher GF, Balady GI, Amsterdam EA, et al. Exercise standards for testing and training: a statement for healthcare professionals from the American Heart Association. Circulation. 2001;104:1694–740.
2. Fletcher GF, Ades PA, Kligfield, et al. Exercise standards for testing and training. A scientific statement from the American Heart Association. Circulation. 2013;128:873–934.

E. Incorrect

Heart rate recovery is a potent and independent predictor of risk for estimating cardiovascular prognosis in women and men.

References
1. Cole CR, Blackstone EH, Pashkow EJ, et al. Heart recovery immediately after exercise as a predictor of mortality. NEJM. 1999;341:1351–7.
2. Lauer MS. Heart rate recovery. Coming back full circle to the baroreceptor reflex. Circ Res. 2016;119:582–3.

18. Correct Answer: E

Rationale
A. Incorrect

"Screening" of very low-risk individuals for CAD by stress testing is not recommended because of the high rate of false positives that results in very low-risk persons as well as the potential for unnecessary additional tests and expense.

References
1. Fletcher GF, Balady GI, Amsterdam EA, et al. Exercise standards for testing and training: a statement for healthcare professionals from the American Heart Association. Circulation. 2001;104:1694–740.
2. Fletcher GF, Ades PA, Kligfield P, et al. Exercise standards for testing and training. A scientific statement from the American Heart Association. Circulation. 2013;128:873–934.
3. Franklin BA, Berra K, Lavie CJ. Should I have an exercise stress test? JAMA Cardiol. 2016;9:1084.
4. Lauer M, Froelicher VF, Williams M, et al. Exercise testing in asymptomatic adults: a statement for professionals from the American Heart Association. Circulation. 2005;112:771–6.

Answers

B. Incorrect

See response above in (A).

C. Incorrect

Family history is not one of the major factors utilized to determine the risk for future fatal/nonfatal MI or stroke. The major factors are age, race, sex, blood pressure, total and high-density serum cholesterol level, cigarette smoking, and diabetes. Family history is one of the multiple "enhancing risk factors" that can be considered to refine the arteriosclerotic cardiovascular disease risk score.

References
1. Goff DC Jr, Lloyd-Jones DM, Bennett G, et al. American College of Cardiology/American Heart Association task force on practice guidelines. 2013 ACC/AHA guideline on the assessment of cardiovascular risk: a report of the American College of Cardiology/American Heart Association task force on practice guidelines. Circulation. 2014;129(25 Suppl 2):S49–73.
2. Agarwala A, Liu J, Ballantyne C, et al. The use of risk enhancing factors to personalize ASCVD risk assessment: evidence and recommendations from the 2018 AHA/ACC multi-society cholesterol guidelines. Curr Cardiovasc Rep. 2019;13:8.

D. Incorrect

The Bruce exercise test protocol comprises relatively large increases in speed and grade for the successive stages of the test. To provide a more gradual increase in intensity, two additional 3-min stages of relatively modest speed and grade (1.7 mph, 0 grade, and 1.7 mph, 5% grade) are added prior to the initial portion of the standard Bruce protocol.

References
1. Fletcher GF, Balady GI, Amsterdam EA, et al. Exercise standards for testing and training: a statement for healthcare professionals from the American Heart Association. Circulation. 2001;104:1694–740.
2. Fletcher GF, Ades PA, Kligfield P, et al. Exercise standards for testing and training. A scientific statement from the American Heart Association. Circulation. 2013;128:873–934.

E. Correct

Specificity is as defined in the question. True positive results and false negative results do not have a role in the calculation of specificity. This parameter relates only to individuals who do not have the abnormality tested for (true negatives and false positives).

References

1. Fletcher GF, Balady GI, Amsterdam EA, et al. Exercise standards for testing and training: a statement for healthcare professionals from the American Heart Association. Circulation. 2001;104:1694–740.
2. Fletcher GF, Ades PA, Kligfield P, et al. Exercise standards for testing and training. A scientific statement from the American Heart Association. Circulation. 2013;128:873–934.

19. Correct Answer: A

Rationale

A. Correct

    The statement in (a) above is correct. Additionally, METs are multiples of basal oxygen consumption. 1 MET = basal oxygen consumption, 5 METs reflect a light workload, and 10 METs indicate high exercise capacity.

References

1. Fletcher GF, Balady GI, Amsterdam EA, et al. Exercise standards for testing and training: a statement for healthcare professionals from the American Heart Association. Circulation. 2001;104:1694–740.
2. Fletcher GF, Ades PA, Kligfield P, et al. Exercise standards for testing and training. A scientific statement from the American Heart Association. Circulation. 2013;128:873–934.

B. Incorrect

    There are no large studies validating the formula 220-age = age-predicted maximum heart rate, although the use of this formula is conventional and widespread. If this formula is used to plot maximum heart rate vs. age for multiple patients, the result is a scattergram. The formula overestimates maximum heart rate in some subjects and underestimates it others, thereby resulting in a considerable number of erroneous estimates for this variable. One authority regards this formula as "relatively useless for clinical purposes." More accurate assessment of exercise capacity is based on nomograms of healthy individuals which provide a continuum of average exercise capacity in healthy individuals based on age and sex.

References

1. Morris CK, Myers J, Froelicher VF. Nomogram based on metabolic equivalents and age for assessing aerobic capacity in men. JACC. 1993;22:175–82.
2. Gulati M, Black HR, Shaw LJ. The prognostic value of a nomogram for exercise capacity in women. NEJM. 2005; 353:468–75.
3. Froelicher VF, Quaglietti S. Handbook of exercise testing. Boston: Little, Brown and Co. p. 88.

C. Incorrect

This finding on an exercise treadmill test has been associated with three-vessel CAD or left main coronary disease in ≥50% (not >95%) of patients. Although this finding has been an important one during the history of exercise testing, exercise-induced hypotension (decrease of ≥20 mmHg) has multiple causes in addition to severe coronary disease, including cardiomyopathy, obstructive valvular disease, frailty, and technical factors marring accurate blood pressure measurement. Additionally, this finding should always be interpreted in terms of the pretest probability of cardiovascular disease.

References
1. Thomson PD, Keleman MH. Hypotension accompanying the onset of exertional angina. Circulation. 1975;52:28–32.
2. Dubach P, Froelicher VF, Klein J, et al. Exercise-induced hypotension in a male population. Criteria, causes, and prognosis. Circulation. 1988;78:1380–7.

D. Incorrect

Exercise-induced ST segment elevation does localize the myocardial region and coronary artery related to this phenomenon.

References
1. Takahashi N, Gail E, Fan D, et al. ST segment elevation during recovery phase of an exercise test. Am J Med. 2020;133:1287–90.
2. Walters D, Chaitman B, Bourassa M, et al. Clinical and angiographic correlates to exercise-induced ST-segment elevation. Increased detection with multiple ECG leads. Circulation. 1980;61:286–96.
3. Bruce R, Fisher L. Unusual prognostic significance of exercise-induced ST elevation in coronary patients. J Electrocardiol. 1987;20:84–8.

E. Incorrect

Whether occurring during the active or recovery phases of an exercise test, ST depression has the same clinical significance. About 15% of exercise-induced ischemic ST depression occurs initially during the recovery phase of an exercise test.

References
1. Fletcher GF, Balady GI, Amsterdam EA, et al. Exercise standards for testing and training: a statement for healthcare professionals from the American Heart Association. Circulation. 2001;104:1694–740.
2. Fletcher GF, Ades PA, Kligfield P, et al. Exercise standards for testing and training. A scientific statement from the American Heart Association. Circulation. 2013;128:873–934.

20. Correct Answer: D

Rationale

A. Incorrect

Bayes' theorem specifies that the accuracy of a test is determined by the sensitivity and specificity of the test and the pretest probability of the disease in the subject being tested or the prevalence of the disease in the population undergoing testing. Bayesian analysis demonstrates the importance of the latter factor.

References
1. Laslett L, Mason DT, Amsterdam EA. Management of the asymptomatic patient with an abnormal exercise ECG. JAMA, 1984;252:1744–6.
2. Epstein SE. Implications of probability analysis on the strategy used for noninvasive detection of coronary artery disease: role of single or combined use of exercise electrocardiographic testing, radionuclide cineangiography and myocardial perfusion imaging. Am J Cardiol. 1980;46:491–9.

B. Incorrect

Functional capacity is considered the single most reliable indicator of prognosis.

References
1. Ahmed HM, Al-Mallah MH, McEvoy JW, et al. Maximal exercise testing variables and 10-year survival: fitness risk score derivation from the FIT project. Mayo Clinic Proc. 2015;90:346–55.
2. Myers J, Prakash M, Froelicher VF, et al. Exercise testing and mortality among men referred for exercise testing. NEJM. 2002;346:793–801.

C. Incorrect

The Duke treadmill score includes minutes of treadmill exercise, millimeters of ST segment depression, and grade of exercise-induced chest pain; among its limitations are absence of patient age and sex.

References
1. Fletcher GF, Balady GI, Amsterdam EA, et al. Exercise standards for testing and training: a statement for healthcare professionals from the American Heart Association. Circulation 2001;104:1694–740.
2. Fletcher GF, Ades PA, Kligfield P, et al. Exercise standards for testing and training. A scientific statement From the American Heart Association. Circulation. 2013;128:873–934.

D. Correct

The statement is correct. Multiple studies have shown that patients with excellent functional capacity and an ischemic ST segment response on exercise testing have low probability of CAD and low prognostic risk.

References
1. Bhat A, Desai A, Amsterdam EA. Usefulness of high functional capacity in patients with exercise-induced ST depression to predict a negative result on exercise echocardiography and low prognostic risk. Am J Cardiol. 2008;10:1541–3.
2. Beri N, Dang P, Bhat A, et al. Usefulness of excellent functional capacity in men and women with ischemic exercise electrocardiography to predict a negative stress imaging test and very low late mortality. Am J Cardiol. 2019;124:661–5.
3. Bourque JM, Beller GA. Value of exercise stress electrocardiography for risk stratification in patients with suspected or known coronary artery disease in the era of advanced imaging technologies. JACC Cardiovasc Imaging. 2015;8:1309–21.

E. Incorrect

The clinical significance of this finding does not differ whether it occurs initially during active or recovery phase of an exercise test.

References
1. Mark DB, Hlatky MA, Harrell FE Jr, et al. Exercise treadmill score for predicting prognosis in coronary artery disease. Ann Intern Med. 1987;106:793–800.
2. Fletcher GF, Balady GI, Amsterdam EA, et al. Exercise standards for testing and training: a statement for healthcare professionals from the American Heart Association. Circulation 2001;104:1694–740.
3. Fletcher GF, Ades PA, Kligfield P, et al. Exercise standards for testing and training. A scientific statement from the American Heart Association. Circulation. 2013;128:873–934.

21. Correct Answer: A

Rationale
According to NHIS data, the age-adjusted rates of smoking among adults have declined from 51% in 1965 to 15.6% in 2018 for males and from 34% in 1965 to 12.0% in 2018 for females. In contrast, the rates of diabetes mellitus, physical inactivity, and obesity have increased in the past two decades and are associated with stagnation in rate of preventable cardiovascular deaths among American adults.

References
1. Creamer MR. Tobacco product use and cessation indicators among adults—United States, 2018. MMWR Morb Mortal Wkly Rep. 2019;68.
2. Tsao CW, Aday AW, Almarzooq ZI, et al. Heart disease and stroke statistics—2022 update: a report from the American Heart Association. Circulation. 2022;145(8):e153–639.

22. Correct Answer: B

Rationale

The Goals and Metrics Committee of the Strategic Planning Task Force of the American Heart Association developed objective definitions for "ideal," "intermediate," and "poor" cardiovascular health based on seven modifiable cardiovascular risk factors that have been colloquially termed Life's Essential 8. They consist of blood pressure, non-HDL- cholesterol, fasting blood glucose, smoking, physical activity, body mass index, sleep, and healthy diet, with each scored on a scale of 0–100 points, with 100 being ideal. A non-HDL-C of <130 mg/dL is the only of the options provided above that would score 100 points.

Reference

1. Lloyd-Jones DM, Allen NB, Anderson CAM, et al. American Heart Association. Life's essential 8: updating and enhancing the American Heart Association's construct of cardiovascular health: a presidential advisory from the American Heart Association. Circulation. 2022;146(5):e18–43.

23. Correct Answer: C

Rationale

Ankle brachial index (ABI) is a commonly used test used to diagnose PAD. The ABI cut-off for diagnosing PAD is less than 0.9, and it is associated with an increased cardiovascular risk. The 2018 Multisociety Cholesterol Management Guideline has recognized ABI <0.9 as a risk enhancing factor along with the remaining options listed above. The full list of risk enhancing factors is provided below.

Risk-enhancing factors in the 2018 ACC/AHA Cholesterol Guideline:

1. Family history of premature ASCVD (males <55 years; females <65 years)
2. Primary hypercholesterolemia (LDL-C 160–189 mg/dL; non-HDL-C 190–219 mg/dL)
3. Metabolic syndrome (three of the following: increased waist circumference, elevated triglycerides ≥150 mg/dL, elevated glucose, low HDL-C)
4. Chronic kidney disease
5. Chronic inflammatory conditions
6. History of premature menopause (before 40 years) and history of pregnancy-associated conditions (i.e., preeclampsia)
7. High-risk ethnicities (i.e., South Asian ancestry)
8. Elevated biomarkers (high-sensitivity C-reactive protein ≥2 mg/L; lipoprotein (a) ≥50 mg/dL or ≥125 nmol/L; apo B ≥130 mg/dL)
9. Ankle-brachial index <0.9

Abbreviations: *ASCVD* atherosclerotic cardiovascular disease, *LDL-C* low-density lipoprotein cholesterol, *HDL-C* high-density lipoprotein cholesterol, *apoB* apolipoprotein B

References
1. Aboyans V, Criqui MH, Abraham P, et al. American Heart Association Council on Peripheral Vascular D, Council on E, Prevention, Council on Clinical C, Council on Cardiovascular N, Council on Cardiovascular R, Intervention, Council on Cardiovascular S, and Anesthesia. Measurement and interpretation of the ankle-brachial index: a scientific statement from the American Heart Association. Circulation. 2012;126(24):2890–909.
2. Grundy SM, Stone NJ, Bailey AL, et al. 2018 AHA/ACC/AACVPR/AAPA/ABC/ACPM/ADA/AGS/APhA/ASPC/NLA/PCNA guideline on the management of blood cholesterol: executive summary: a report of the American College of Cardiology/American Heart Association task force on clinical practice guidelines. J Am Coll Cardiol. 2019;73(24):3168–209.

24. Correct Answer: A

Rationale

Cardiac rehabilitation (CR) is an integral component in the care of patients with cardiovascular disease, but CR services are highly underutilized in clinical practice. Current guidelines provide Class IA recommendation for utilizing CR in patients with myocardial infarction, percutaneous coronary intervention, coronary artery bypass graft surgery, chronic stable heart failure with reduced ejection fraction, stable angina, cardiac transplantation, symptomatic peripheral arterial disease (SET), and cardiac valve surgery. Heart failure with preserved ejection fraction (HFpEF) is increasing in prevalence with the aging population, is associated with high morbidity and mortality, and continues to be refractory to most pharmacotherapies. Current evidence suggests that exercise training improves quality of life in patients with HFpEF and expanding CR indication for these patients may help improve patient outcomes.

References
1. Thomas RJ, Beatty AL, Beckie TM, et al. Home-based cardiac rehabilitation: a scientific statement from the American Association of Cardiovascular and Pulmonary Rehabilitation, the American Heart Association, and the American College of Cardiology. Circulation. 2019;140(1):e69–89.
2. Pandey A, Parashar A, Kumbhani DJ, et al. Exercise training in patients with heart failure and preserved ejection fraction. Circ Heart Fail. 2015;8(1):33–40.

25. Correct Answer: D

Rationale

Tirzepatide is a novel incretin-based drug with agonistic activity to both glucagon-like peptide-1 (GLP-1) and glucose-dependent insulinotropic polypeptide (GIP). As such, it has been referred to as a "twin-cretin." Tirzepatide's GIP activation appears to be synergistic to GLP-1 receptor activation allowing for greater weight loss and HbA1c reduction than GLP1-RA alone, although gastrointestinal side effects are also increased. Like other GLP1-RAs, Tirzepatide has pleiotropic effects resulting in improvement in blood pressure, lipid profile, and body weight. In meta-analysis, GLP1-RAs appears to improve albuminuria and slow eGFR decline. Tirzepatide decreases HbA1c by 2–2.5% which is substantially higher when compared to other medications such as empagliflozin and liraglutide which reduce the HbA1c by 0.5–1% and 1–1.5%, respectively. Moreover, insulin therapy is associated with about 2% reduction in HbA1c but causes weight gain which is not ideal in our patient, in addition to increased hypoglycemic side effects without cardiovascular risk reduction.

References
1. Rosenstock J, Wysham C, Frías JP, et al. Efficacy and safety of a novel dual GIP and GLP-1 receptor agonist tirzepatide in patients with type 2 diabetes (SURPASS-1): a double-blind, randomised, phase 3 trial. Lancet. 2021;398(10295):143–55.
2. Frías JP, Davies MJ, Rosenstock J, et al. SURPASS-2 Investigators. Tirzepatide versus semaglutide once weekly in patients with type 2 diabetes. N Engl J Med. 2021;385(6):503–15.
3. Ludvik B, Giorgino F, Jódar E, et al. Once-weekly tirzepatide versus once-daily insulin degludec as add-on to metformin with or without SGLT2 inhibitors in patients with type 2 diabetes (SURPASS-3): a randomised, open-label, parallel-group, phase 3 trial. Lancet. 2021;398(10300):583–98.
4. Del Prato S, Kahn SE, Pavo I, et al. SURPASS-4 Investigators. Tirzepatide versus insulin glargine in type 2 diabetes and increased cardiovascular risk (SURPASS-4): a randomised, open-label, parallel-group, multicentre, phase 3 trial. Lancet. 2021;398(10313):1811–24.
5. Shaman AM, Bain SC, Bakris GL, et al. Effect of the glucagon-like peptide-1 receptor agonists semaglutide and liraglutide on kidney outcomes in patients with type 2 diabetes: pooled analysis of SUSTAIN 6 and LEADER. Circulation. 2022;145(8):575–85.

26. Correct Answer: E

Rationale
As of 2020, though the monthly prescriptions of GLP1-RA and SGLT2i by cardiologist increased by 12-fold and 4-fold, respectively, in the past 6 years, they only account for 0.4% of all GLP1-RA and 1.5% of all SGLT2i prescriptions. Potential barriers to cardiologist usage of these medication include (a) perceived specialty boundaries: management of diabetes is beyond traditional cardiology purview and cardiologists may avoid overlap of diabetes care with endocrinology/PCP colleagues, (b) lack of clinician familiarity with the evidence base, (c) discomfort with the routine use of injectable medications, and (d) preference to avoid management of side effects. Dedicated interdisciplinary "Cardiometabolic Clinics" staffed by cardiologists that focus on the management of all aspects of cardiometabolic disease promise to overcome many of these traditional barriers.

References
1. Adhikari R, Jha K, Dardari Z, et al. National trends in use of sodium-glucose cotransporter-2 inhibitors and glucagon-like peptide-1 receptor agonists by cardiologists and other specialties, 2015 to 2020. J Am Heart Assoc. 2022;11(9):e023811.
2. Reiter-Brennan C, Cainzos-Achirica M, Soroosh G, et al. Cardiometabolic medicine—the US perspective on a new subspecialty. Cardiovasc Endocrinol Metab. 2020;9(3):70–80.

27. Correct Answer: A

Rationale
Individuals with cardiovascular risk factors such as smoking history, dyslipidemia, and family history of CAD develop CAC 3–4 years earlier when compared with those without these risk factors. In addition, presence of diabetes and multiple risk factors was associated with development of CAC 6–8 years earlier when compared to those without any risk factors. In the past, CAC was difficult to interpret in patients under the age of 45 because population-based reference values were unavailable. However, reference values are now available for white and black patients aged 33–45 (www.cac-tools.com). Approximately 15% of White males were noted to have CAC >0 by the age of 35 years. In this patient with multiple risk factors, but with LDL near the population average, CAC assessment should be considered for early risk stratification and initiation of pharmacotherapy if CAC >0. A moderate intensity statin could be considered without risk stratification, but current guidelines would not recommend routine statin initiation in this patient's scenario; in this case, a CAC score could guide early statin initiation including selection of statin intensity versus exclusive emphasis on lifestyle. Fibrates have not been associated with cardiovascular benefit and should not be routinely used when triglycerides are below 500 mg/dL. Without knowledge of this patient's burden of subclinical atherosclerosis, an aspirin should not be recommended here and may cause more harm than benefit. The National Lipid Association recommends an aspirin only when CAC >100, and there are no bleeding risk factors.

References
1. Javaid A, Dardari ZA, Mitchell JD, et al. Distribution of coronary artery calcium by age, sex, and race among patients 30–45 years old. J Am Coll Cardiol. 2022;79(19):1873–86.
2. Dzaye O, Razavi AC, Dardari ZA, et al. Modeling the recommended age for initiating coronary artery calcium testing among at-risk young adults. J Am Coll Cardiol. 2021;78(16):1573–83.
3. Orringer CE, Blaha MJ, Blankstein R, et al. The National Lipid Association scientific statement on coronary artery calcium scoring to guide preventive strategies for ASCVD risk reduction. J Clin Lipidol. 2021;15(1):33–60.

28. Correct Answer: C

Rationale

This patient is in the borderline risk group, with a 10-year risk of ASCVD of 6%. She was found to have a CAC score of 0, which is a strong "negative risk marker" for developing ASCVD in near term. Her lone risk factor is hypertension, which is very well controlled. Based on recent data and guidelines from the National Lipid Association, among borderline to intermediate risk patients, there is about a 20–25% change of developing a positive CAC score in about 5 years after the initial scan with CAC score of zero. A repeat CAC scan can be helpful to readdress the potential need for statin or other preventive pharmacotherapy like aspirin.

Summary Look-up Table for Individualized Risk Estimation And Appropriate Timing Of CAC Rescans

Risk Group	Recommended Rescan Interval
Low-risk (<5% 10-yr risk)	6–7 yrs
Borderline to Intermediate risk (5–20% 10-yr risk)	3–5 yrs
High risk (>20% 10-yr risk)	3 yrs
Diabetes	3 yrs

Look-up table for individualized risk estimation and appropriate timing of CAC rescans. CAC = coronary artery calcium

References

1. Dzaye O, Dardari ZA, Cainzos-Achirica M, et al. Warranty period of a calcium score of zero: comprehensive analysis from MESA. JACC Cardiovasc Imaging. 2021;14(5):990–1002.
2. Dzaye O, Dardari ZA, Cainzos-Achirica M, et al. Incidence of new coronary calcification: time to conversion from CAC = 0. J Am Coll Cardiol. 2020;75(13):1610–3.
3. Orringer CE, Blaha MJ, Blankstein R, et al. The National Lipid Association scientific statement on coronary artery calcium scoring to guide preventive strategies for ASCVD risk reduction. J Clin Lipidol. 2021;15(1):33–60.

Answers

29. Correct Answer: A

Rationale

Measure CAC score. In adults at intermediate risk (≥7.5% to <20% 10-year risk) for ASCVD as measured by the pooled cohort equations in whom uncertainty about their calculate risk exists, the 2018 AHA/ACC/Multisociety guideline recommends the use of additional risk-enhancing factors selectively measuring a CAC score to guide decisions regarding preventive interventions. CAC measurement is reliable in reclassifying ASCVD risk and has superior discrimination and risk reclassification properties compared with other tests such as Lp(a) or measuring ApoB.

Reference
1. Arnett DK, Blumenthal RS, Albert MA, et al. 2019 ACC/AHA guideline on the primary prevention of cardiovascular disease: a report of the American College of Cardiology/American Heart Association task force on clinical practice guidelines. Circulation. 2019;140(11):e596–646.

30. Correct Answer: D

Rationale

All of the above. Estimating ASCVD risk using the pooled cohort equations (PCE) remains the foundation for primary prevention risk discussion and interventions. However, the PCE estimates may underestimate risk in certain subgroups. The 2018 AHA/ACC/Multisociety guideline on primary prevention recommends considering the presence of additional risk-enhancing factors to help guide decisions regarding pharmacologic interventions. These factors are shown in box 1. Preeclampsia is a pregnancy-specific condition resulting in hypertension and possibly organ dysfunction. It is important to know that recognizing prior history of estimating ASCVD risk using the PCE remains the foundation for primary prevention risk discussion and interventions. However, the PCE estimates may underestimate risk in certain subgroups. The 2018 AHA/ACC/Multisociety guideline on primary prevention recommends considering the presence of additional risk-enhancing factors to help guide decisions regarding pharmacologic interventions. These factors are shown in the box below. Preeclampsia is a pregnancy-specific condition resulting in hypertension and possibly organ dysfunction. It is important to recognize prior history of preeclampsia, since it is associated with a twofold increase in ASCVD risk and a fourfold increase in the risk of heart failure. Similarly, early menopause is associated with a twofold increase in the risk of CHD and stroke.

ASCVD Risk Enhancers:
- Family history of premature ASCVD
- Persistently elevated LDL-C≥160 mg/dL (≥4.1 mmol/L)
- Chronic kidney disease
- Metabolic syndrome
- Conditions specific to women (e.g., preeclampsia, premature menopause)
- Inflammatory diseases (especially rheumatoid arthritis, psoriasis, HIV)
- Ethnicity (e.g., South Asian ancestry)

Lipid/Biomarkers:
- Persistently elevated triglycerides (≥175 mg/dL, (≥2.0 mmol/L))

In selected individuals if measured:
- hs-CRP ≥2.0 mg/L
- Lp(a) levels > 50 mg/dL or >125 nmol/L
- apoB ≥130 mg/dL
- Ankle-brachinal index (ABI) <0.9

Based on Grundy et al. Circulation. 2019 Jun 18;139(25):e1082–e1143

References
1. Wu P, Haththotuwa R, Kwok CS, et al. Preeclampsia and future cardiovascular health: a systematic review and meta-analysis. Circ Cardiovasc Qual Outcomes. 2017;10(2):e003497.
2. Wellons M, Ouyang P, Schreiner PJ, et al. Early menopause predicts future coronary heart disease and stroke: the Multi-Ethnic Study of Atherosclerosis. Menopause. 2012;19(10):1081–7.
3. Grundy SM, Stone NJ, Bailey AL, et al. 2018 AHA/ACC/AACVPR/AAPA/ABC/ ACPM/ADA/AGS/APhA/ASPC/NLA/PCNA guideline on the management of blood cholesterol: a report of the American College of Cardiology/American Heart Association task force on clinical practice guidelines. Circulation. 2019;139(25):e1082–143.

Answers

31. Correct Answer: C

Rationale
Reducing the intake of processed red meats. Adopting a healthy lifestyle is the cornerstone of primary prevention. This includes exercise, healthy dietary patterns, weight loss, and smoking cessation. Adults should engage in at least 150 min per week of moderate-intensity exercise or at least 75 min per week of high-intensity exercise. Decreasing sedentary behavior is helpful to reduce ASCVD risk. A healthy diet emphasizing vegetables, fruits, legumes, nuts, whole grains, and fish is highly recommended. While individuals are encouraged to substitute saturated fat with polyunsaturated fat in their diet, trans fats should be avoided to reduce ASCVD risk. Individuals should also minimize the intake of red meat or processed meat (e.g., bacon, salami, and hot dogs). In a study of US healthcare professionals, compared to consuming plant protein, consuming processed red meat was associated with a 34% higher all-cause mortality rate and 39% higher CVD-mortality rate.

References
1. Arnett DK, Blumenthal RS, Albert MA, et al. 2019 ACC/AHA guideline on the primary prevention of cardiovascular disease: a report of the American College of Cardiology/American Heart Association task force on clinical practice guidelines. Circulation. 2019;140(11):e596–646.
2. Song M, Fung TT, Hu FB, et al. Association of animal and plant protein intake with all-cause and cause-specific mortality. JAMA Intern Med. 2016;176(10):1453–63.

32. Correct Answer: D

Rationale
Both A and B. Patients with diabetes are at elevated risk for ASCVD. Therefore, all patients >40 years of age with diabetes should strongly consider being on a moderate-intensity statin. In the presence of multiple ASCVD risk factors, it is reasonable to prescribe high-intensity statin therapy aiming to reduce LDL-cholesterol by ≥50% (Class IIa recommendations). Independent of the traditional ASCVD risk factors, the presence of diabetes-specific risk enhancers should promptly consider prescribing high-intensity statins. These diabetes specific risk enhancers include long duration (>10 years for Type 2 diabetes mellitus and >20 years for Type 1 diabetes mellitus) albuminuria > 30-mg albumin/mg creatinine, eGFR <60 mL/min/1.73 m^2, retinopathy, neuropathy, or ankle brachial index <0.9.

Reference
1. Grundy SM, Stone NJ, Bailey AL, et al. 2018 AHA/ACC/AACVPR/AAPA/ABC/ACPM/ADA/ AGS/APhA/ASPC/NLA/PCNA guideline on the management of blood cholesterol: a report of the American College of Cardiology/American Heart Association task force on clinical practice guidelines. Circulation. 2019;139(25):e1082–143.

33. Correct Answer: B

Rationale

Increasing atorvastatin to 40 mg nightly and remeasuring LDL-C in 3 months. In adults without diabetes between 40 and 75 years, estimating 10-year ASCVD risk is the starting point of the ASCVD risk discussion. Based on the 10-year ASCVD risk, patients can have low (<5%), borderline risk (5% to <7.5%), intermediate (≥7.5% to <20%), or high (>20%) estimated risk. Estimating the patient's ASCVD risk guides prevention interventions.

The patient in this question has high ASCVD risk and, therefore, initiating statin therapy to reduce LDL-C ≥50% is strongly recommended (Class I). Her current regimen reduced her LDL-C by 20% and, therefore, needs to be intensified. Increasing her atorvastatin dose to at least 40 mg, emphasizing the importance of taking the statin daily, and rechecking her cholesterol in 3 months would be the correct answer. Adding ezetimibe should be considered in patients who are on maximally tolerated statin doses who did not achieve the desired LDL-C reduction. Since the dose of atorvastatin can be increased, adding ezetimibe would not be the best next step. Switching to rosuvastatin 10 mg may lower LDL-C a little more than atorvastatin 20 mg. However, this switch is unlikely to achieve a 50% reduction from baseline. Sometimes, patients with a high Lp(a) (lipoprotein a) do not get the anticipated amount of LDL-cholesterol reduction since the apoB (apolipoprotein B) associated with an elevated Lp(a) does not go down with statin therapy.

Reference

1. Arnett DK, Blumenthal RS, Albert MA, et al. 2019 ACC/AHA guideline on the primary prevention of cardiovascular disease: a report of the American College of Cardiology/American Heart Association task force on clinical practice guidelines. Circulation. 2019;140(11):e596–646.

34. Correct Answer: D

Rationale

All of the above. Tobacco use is the most important modifiable cause of ASCVD. Adults who use tobacco should be firmly advised to quit. The 2018 AHA/ACC/Multisociety guideline on primary prevention recommends a combination of behavioral interventions and pharmacotherapy to improve quit rates. There are seven FDA approved pharmacotherapies including several forms of nicotine replacement therapy (such as nicotine patches) and other medications (such as Bupropion and Varenicline).

Reference

1. Arnett DK, Blumenthal RS, Albert MA, et al. 2019 ACC/AHA guideline on the primary prevention of cardiovascular disease: a report of the American College of Cardiology/American Heart Association task force on clinical practice guidelines. Circulation. 2019;140(11):e596–646.

35. Correct Answer: C

Rationale
The patient should consider aspirin after a risk-benefit discussion. According to the 2018 AHA/ACC/multisociety guideline on primary prevention, aspirin should not be routinely administered for primary prevention of ASCVD among adults >70 years of age or adults at any age who are at increased risk of bleeding. However, aspirin may be considered for primary prevention among adults between 40 and 70 years of age not at increased bleeding risk in selected circumstances. Physicians should consider discussing the benefit of prophylactic aspirin in adults >70 of age who have significant ASCVD risk factors such as significant elevation in CAC score or are unable to achieve lipid or glucose targets.

This patient is at elevated ASCVD risk and has significant CAC. Given his low bleeding risk, it is reasonable to continue his low-dose aspirin at this point. Given his elevated CAC, there is no utility of remeasuring CAC in his case.

Reference
1. Arnett DK, Blumenthal RS, Albert MA, et al. 2019 ACC/AHA guideline on the primary prevention of cardiovascular disease: a report of the American College of Cardiology/American Heart Association task force on clinical practice guidelines. Circulation. 2019;140(11):e596–646.

36. Correct Answer: D

Rationale
The patient should be advised on non-pharmacologic therapy plus BP-lowering medications. According to the 2017 Hypertension Clinical Practice Guidelines, hypertension in adults is defined as a systolic blood pressure ≥130 mmHg or diastolic blood pressure ≥80 mmHg. Those with elevated BP measurements (120–129 <80 mmHg) or those with hypertension, non-pharmacological therapies such as a DASH (Dietary Approaches to Stop Hypertension) dietary pattern, weight loss, and exercise should be recommended regardless of estimated 10-year ASCVD risk.

In adults with stage, I hypertension (defined as BP of 130–139/80–89 mmHg) with a 10-year ASCVD risk estimate of <10% non-pharmacological therapy would be the initial step in management. However, in patients with stage 1 hypertension who also have an estimated 10-year ASCVD risk of ≥10%, starting a BP-lowering medication in addition to non-pharmacological therapy is recommended (Class I). All patients with Stage 2 hypertension (defined as BP ≥140/90) should be recommended non-pharmacological therapy and started on a BP-lowering medication.

The patient in this question has Stage 2 hypertension; therefore, both non-pharmacological therapies and BP-lowering medication should be recommended.

Reference
1. Whelton PK, Carey RM, Aronow WS, et al. 2017 ACC/AHA/AAPA/ABC/ACPM/AGS/APhA/ASH/ASPC/NMA/PCNA guideline for the prevention, detection, evaluation, and management of high blood pressure in adults: a report of the American College of Cardiology/American Heart Association task force on clinical practice guidelines. Circulation. 2018;138(17):e484–594.

37. Correct Answer: E

Rationale
This is supported both by the 2014 ACC/AHA stable ischemic angina guidelines and the 2019 ESC chronic coronary syndromes guidelines.

References
1. Fihn SD, Blankenship JC, Alexander KP, et al. 2014 ACC/AHA/AATS/PCNA/SCAI/STS focused update of the guideline for the diagnosis and management of patients with stable ischemic heart disease: a report of the American College of Cardiology/American Heart Association task force on practice guidelines, and the American Association for Thoracic Surgery, Preventive Cardiovascular Nurses Association, Society for Cardiovascular Angiography and Interventions, and Society of Thoracic Surgeons. Circulation. 2014;130(19):1749–67.
2. Knuuti J, Wijns W, Saraste A, et al. ESC Scientific Document Group. 2019 ESC guidelines for the diagnosis and management of chronic coronary syndromes. Eur Heart J. 2020;41(3):407–77.

38. Correct Answer: D

Rationale
This is supported both by the 2014 ACC/AHA stable ischemic angina guidelines and the 2019 ESC chronic coronary syndromes guidelines.

References
1. Fihn SD, Blankenship JC, Alexander KP, et al. 2014 ACC/AHA/AATS/PCNA/SCAI/STS focused update of the guideline for the diagnosis and management of patients with stable ischemic heart disease: a report of the American College of Cardiology/American Heart Association task force on practice guidelines, and the American Association for Thoracic Surgery, Preventive Cardiovascular Nurses Association, Society for Cardiovascular Angiography and Interventions, and Society of Thoracic Surgeons. Circulation. 2014;130(19):1749–67.
2. Knuuti J, Wijns W, Saraste A, et al. ESC Scientific Document Group. 2019 ESC Guidelines for the diagnosis and management of chronic coronary syndromes. Eur Heart J. 2020;41(3):407–77.

39. Correct Answer: A

Rationale

Treadmill exercise testing can help determine if patients' symptoms are consistent with angina. B is False as CMR and MPI have comparable accuracy for evaluating CAD. C is false as Prognosis is related to wall motion abnormalities induced during stress echocardiography. D is false as relief of angina is better by exercise ischemia-guided PCI than by medical therapy. E is false as the addition of clinical variables to the DTS reclassified a majority of patients from low-risk DTS to intermediate or high risk.

References
1. Ho PM, Rumsfeld JS, Peterson PN, et al. Chest pain on exercise treadmill test predicts future cardiac hospitalizations. Clin Cardiol. 2007;30:505–10.
2. Schwitter J, Wacker CM, van Rossum AC, et al. MR-IMPACT: comparison of perfusion-cardiac magnetic resonance with single-photon emission computed tomography for the detection of coronary artery disease in a multi-centre, multi-vendor, randomized trial. Eur Heart J. 2008;29:480–9.
3. Schwitter J, Wacker CM, Wilke N, et al. MR-IMPACT II: Magnetic Resonance Imaging for Myocardial Perfusion Assessment in Coronary artery disease Trial: perfusion-cardiac magnetic resonance vs. single-photon emission computed tomography for the detection of coronary artery disease: a comparative multi-centre, multivendor trial. Eur Heart J. 2013;34:775–81.
4. Shaw LJ, Vasey C, Sawada S, et al. Impact of gender on risk stratification by exercise and dobutamine stress echocardiography: long-term mortality in 4234 women and 6898 men. Eur Heart J. 2005;26:447–56.
5. Yao SS, Bangalore S, Chaudhry FA. Prognostic implications of stress echocardiography and impact on patient outcomes: an effective gatekeeper for coronary angiography and revascularization. Am Soc Echocardiogr. 2010;23:832–9.
6. Maron DJ, Hochman JS, Reynolds HR, et al. Initial invasive or conservative strategy for stable coronary disease. N Engl J Med. 2020;382:1395–407.
7. Lauer MS, Pothier CE, Magid DJ, et al. An externally validated model for predicting long-term survival after exercise treadmill testing in patients with suspected coronary artery disease and a normal electrocardiogram. Ann In-tern Med. 2007;147:821–8.

40. Correct Answer: C

Rationale

At 10-year follow-up patients in the STITCH trial with ischemic cardiomyopathy who underwent CABG plus medical therapy had improved survival compared to those who received medical therapy alone: a primary outcome event occurred in

359 patients (59%) who received CABG plus medical therapy and in 398 patients (66%) who received medical therapy (HR with CABG vs. medical therapy, 0.84; 95% CI, 0.73–0.97; $P = 0.02$, log-rank test). A total of 247 patients (40%) in the CABG group and 297 patients (49%) in the medical-therapy group died from cardiovascular causes (HR 0.79; 95% CI, 0.66–0.93; $P = 0.006$ by log-rank test). The benefits of the interventions in choices 2, 4, and 5 do not extend to reduced mortality.

Reference
1. Velazquez EJ, Lee KL, Jones RH, et al. Coronary artery bypass surgery in patients with ischemic cardiomyopathy. N Engl J Med. 2016;374:1511–20.

41. Correct Answer: D

Rationale
The 2018 AHA/ACC/Multisociety guideline advocates for CAC testing when risk is between 5% and 20% (low-intermediate and intermediate risk), when decisions about statins remain uncertain (Level IIA recommendation). CAC has proven to be incremental and independent predictors of cardiac risk, and a robust predictor in every racial/ethnic/gender and age group studied.

Reference
1. Grundy SM, Stone NJ, Bailey AL, et al. 2018 AHA/ACC/AACVPR/AAPA/ABC/ACPM/ADA/AGS/APhA/ASPC/NLA/PCNA Guideline on the management of blood cholesterol: a report of the American College of Cardiology/American Heart Association task force on clinical practice guidelines. Circulation. 2019;139(25):e1082–143.

42. Correct Answer: A

Rationale
The 2018 AHA/ACC/Multisociety guideline recommends statin for patients who have CAC score ≥100 or ≥75th percentile for age/gender/race. There is no need to do ischemic evaluation or computed tomography (CT) angiogram in asymptomatic persons.

Reference
1. Grundy SM, Stone NJ, Bailey AL, et al. 2018 AHA/ACC/AACVPR/AAPA/ABC/ACPM/ADA/AGS/APhA/ASPC/NLA/PCNA Guideline on the management of blood cholesterol: a report of the American College of Cardiology/American Heart Association task force on clinical practice guidelines. Circulation. 2019;139(25):e1082–143.

43. Correct Answer: B

Rationale

The 2018 AHA/ACC/Multisociety guideline recommends withholding statin therapy in those with CAC of zero, who do not have accelerated risk factors such as familial hyperlipidemia, diabetes, smoking, or family history. Retesting is recommended in 5 years to determine if she has developed any CAC. IMT is a Class III recommendation (not useful, may be harmful) as it is non-reproducible in most environments.

Reference

1. Grundy SM, Stone NJ, Bailey AL, et al. 2018 AHA/ACC/AACVPR/AAPA/ABC/ACPM/ADA/AGS/APhA/ASPC/NLA/PCNA guideline on the management of blood cholesterol: a report of the American College of Cardiology/American Heart Association task force on clinical practice guidelines. Circulation. 2019;139(25):e1082–143.

44. Correct Answer: A

Rationale

A head-to-head study establishes that cardiac CT is the most accurate of all imaging modalities to identify obstructive disease.

Reference

1. Neglia D, Rovai D, Caselli C, et al. EVINCI Study Investigators. Detection of significant coronary artery disease by noninvasive anatomical and functional imaging. Circ Cardiovasc Imaging. 2015;8(3):e002179.

45. Correct Answer: C

Rationale

Guidelines advocate a high-risk state when CAC is ≥100 or ≥75th Percentile for age, race/ethnicity, and gender.

Reference

1. Grundy SM, Stone NJ, Bailey AL, et al. 2018 AHA/ACC/AACVPR/AAPA/ABC/ACPM/ADA/AGS/APhA/ASPC/NLA/PCNA guideline on the management of blood cholesterol: a report of the American College of Cardiology/American Heart Association task force on clinical practice guidelines. Circulation. 2019;139(25):e1082–143.

46. Correct Answer: B

Rationale

A CAC scan affords similar doses to a mammogram (<1 mSv of radiation). In comparison, a chest X-ray is much lower (<0.1), and background radiation (at sea level) is about 3 mSv a year, and higher at elevation. A technetium nuclear scan is about 11–18 mSv and a cardiac catheterization affords 2–20 mSv.

Reference
1. Hirshfeld JW Jr, Ferrari VA, Bengel FM, et al. 2018 ACC/HRS/NASCI/SCAI/SCCT expert consensus document on optimal use of ionizing radiation in cardiovascular imaging: best practices for safety and effectiveness: a report of the American College of Cardiology task force on clinical expert consensus documents. J Am Coll Cardiol. 2018;71:e283–351.

47. Correct Answer: B

Rationale

Women with HeFH do not appear to have a higher risk of preterm delivery or of having infants with low birth weight or congenital malformations than unaffected women. Lipid lowering therapy should not be withheld in young women of childbearing age. Untreated women with HeFH are at very high risk for early onset ASCVD (atherosclerotic cardiovascular disease). Early and aggressive lipid lowering therapy can markedly attenuate this risk in both women and men alike. Although recent evidence has not confirmed the teratogenic potential of statins, until further safety data is obtained, contraception is advised for women of childbearing age taking statins. In addition, women should be advised to suspend statins if trying to conceive or if an unplanned pregnancy is discovered. Several conditions specific to women (e.g., hypertensive disorders during pregnancy, preeclampsia, gestational diabetes mellitus, delivering a preterm or low-birth-weight infant, and premature menopause [age <40 years] [6–8]) have been shown to increase ASCVD risk.

References
1. Toleikyte I, Retterstol K, Leren TP, et al. Pregnancy outcomes in familial hypercholesterolemia: a registry-based study. Circulation. 2011;124:1606–14.
2. Balla S, Ekpo EP, Wilemon KA, Knowles JW, Rodriguez F. Women living with familial hypercholesterolemia: challenges and considerations surrounding their care. Curr Atheroscler Rep. 2020;22(10):60.
3. Bateman BT, Hernandez-Diaz S, Fischer MA, Seely EW, Ecker JL, Franklin JM, Desai RJ, Allen-Coleman C, Mogun H, Avorn J, Huybrechts KF. Statins and congenital malformations: cohort study. BMJ. 2015;350:h1035.

4. Grandi SM, Vallee-Pouliot K, Reynier P, et al. Hypertensive disorders in pregnancy and the risk of subsequent cardiovascular disease. Paediatr Perinat Epidemiol. 2017;31:412–21.
5. Catov JM, Newman AB, Roberts JM, et al. Preterm delivery and later maternal cardiovascular disease risk. Epidemiology. 2007;18:733–9.
6. Muka T, Oliver-Williams C, Kunutsor S, et al. Association of age at onset of menopause and time since onset of menopause with cardiovascular outcomes, intermediate vascular traits, and all-cause mortality: a systematic review and meta-analysis. JAMA Cardiol. 2016;1:767–76.
7. Roeters van Lennep JE, Heida KY, Bots ML, et al. Cardiovascular disease risk in women with premature ovarian insufficiency: a systematic review and meta-analysis. Eur J Prev Cardiol. 2016;23:178–86.
8. Ley SH, Li Y, Tobias DK, et al. Duration of reproductive life span, age at menarche, and age at menopause are associated with risk of cardiovascular disease in women. J Am Heart Assoc. 2017;6:e006713.

48. Correct Answer: B

Rationale

A great body of research has shown the CAC score to be an effective tool to stratify risk and improve risk estimation. Over an approximate 8-year follow-up period, CAC strongly predicted risk beyond traditional risk factors in postmenopausal women in the Women's Health Initiative.

The CAC score is especially useful for patients at borderline or intermediate 10-year estimated ASCVD risk. In this group of patients, if the score is 0, statin therapy may be safely withheld unless the patient smokes or has premature cardiovascular disease. If the CAC score is 1–99, statin therapy is suggested, especially in patients older than 55. If the score is 100 or higher or patients are in the 75th percentile or higher for CAC, statin therapy is clearly indicated.

A CAC assessment-guided strategy for statin therapy appears to be cost-effective compared with initiating statin therapy in all African American individuals at intermediate risk for atherosclerotic cardiovascular disease.

References
1. Blankstein R, Gupta A, Rana JS, Nasir K. The implication of coronary artery calcium testing for cardiovascular disease prevention and diabetes. Endocrinol Metab (Seoul). 2017;32(1):47–57. https://doi.org/10.3803/EnM.2017.32.1.47. Erratum in: Endocrinol Metab (Seoul). 2017;32(4):487.
2. Poornima IG, et al. "Coronary Artery Calcification (CAC) and post-trial cardiovascular events and mortality within the Women's Health Initiative (WHI) estrogen-alone trial. J Am Heart Assoc. 2017;6(11):e006887.
3. Grundy SM, Stone NJ, Bailey AL. 2018 AHA/ACC/AACVPR/AAPA/ABC/ACPM/ADA/AGS/APhA/ASPC/NLA/PCNA guideline on the management of

blood cholesterol: a report of the American College of Cardiology/American Heart Association task force on clinical practice guidelines. Circulation. 2019;139(25):e1082–143.
4. Spahillari A, Zhu J, Ferket BS, et al. Cost-effectiveness of contemporary statin use guidelines with or without coronary artery calcium assessment in African American individuals. JAMA Cardiol. 2020;5(8):871–80.

49. Correct Answer: C

Rationale

Patients with clinical ASCVD who are judged to be very high risk include those with a history of multiple major ASCVD events or 1 major ASCVD event and multiple high-risk conditions. In these patients, additional net benefit from further LDL-C lowering when LDL-C is ≥70 mg/dL has been demonstrated by three randomized controlled trials.

The 2018 AHA/ACC /Multisociety Cholesterol Guidelines make a strong recommendation for clinicians to first add ezetimibe to maximally tolerated statin therapy as initial step in further LDL-C lowering. The stepwise addition of ezetimibe first, was based on the generic availability, tolerability, safety, and lower cost of this drug.

For those patients identified as being at very high risk with an absolute LDL-C ≥70 mg/dL on maximally tolerated statin therapy and with persistent fasting triglycerides ≥150 and <500 mg/dL, additional LDL-C lowering rather than TG-lowering therapies should be considered first.

References

1. Grundy SM, Stone NJ, Bailey AL, et al. 2018 AHA/ACC/AACVPR/AAPA/ABC/ACPM/ADA/AGS/APhA/ASPC/NLA/PCNA guideline on the management of blood cholesterol: a report of the American College of Cardiology/American Heart Association task force on clinical practice guidelines. Circulation. 2019;139(25):e1082–143.
2. Cannon CP, Blazing MA, Giugliano RP, et al. Ezetimibe added to statin therapy after acute coronary syndromes. N Engl J Med. 2015;372:2387–97.
3. Sabatine MS, Giugliano RP, Keech AC, et al. Evolocumab and clinical outcomes in patients with cardiovascular disease. N Engl J Med. 2017;376:1713–22.
4. Schwartz GG, Steg PG, Szarek M. Alirocumab after acute coronary syndrome. Reply. N Engl J Med. 2019;380(21):2077.
5. Virani SS, Morris PB, Agarwala A, et al. 2021 ACC expert consensus decision pathway on the management of ASCVD risk reduction in patients with persistent hypertriglyceridemia: a report of the American College of Cardiology Solution Set Oversight Committee. J Am Coll Cardiol. 2021;78(9):960–93.

Answers

50. Correct Answer: C

Rationale

The 2018 AHA/ACC/Multisociety Cholesterol Guidelines emphasize a clinician–patient risk discussion before initiating cholesterol treatment. Risk discussions are the cornerstone of the shared decision-making process.

Based on the concept that intensity of prevention effort should match the absolute risk of the individual patient, risk assessment is the first step in prevention of ASCVD. The guidelines recommend using a risk calculator, the Pooled Cohort Equations (PCE), to estimate the patient's risk of cardiovascular event within the next 10 years.

To further personalize risk, the current guidelines recommend evaluation of risk-enhancing factors when treatment decision is unclear. Risk enhancing factors are evidence-based characteristics, outside of traditional risk factors, which are associated with increased risk of developing ASCVD. The presence of risk-enhancing factors in patients, especially with borderline or intermediate risk, may convey higher baseline risk and more strongly favor initiation of treatment.

Lipoprotein (a) is a modified form of LDL that possesses atherogenic potential. Relative indications for its measurement are family history of premature ASCVD or personal history of ASCVD not explained by major risk factors. Lp(a) increases ASCVD risk especially at higher levels. An Lp(a) ≥50 mg/dL or ≥125 nmol/L, may be considered a risk-enhancing factor.

References

1. Grundy SM, Stone NJ, Bailey AL, et al. 2018 AHA/ACC/AACVPR/AAPA/ABC/A CPM/ ADA/AGS/APhA/ASPC/NLA/PCNA guideline on the management of blood cholesterol: a report of the American College of Cardiology/American Heart Association task force on clinical practice guidelines. Circulation. 2019;139(25):e1082–143.
2. Tsimikas S. A test in context: lipoprotein(a): diagnosis, prognosis, controversies, and emerging therapies. J Am Coll Cardiol. 2017;69(6):692–711.

51. Correct Answer: C

Rationale

The National Lipid Association has a Class I recommendation for the use of icosapent ethyl in individuals 45 years or older with clinical ASCVD. Repeating lipids is recommended 4–12 weeks after initiation or change in therapy. As there has been no change in therapy and lipids have already been checked at this visit within 4–12 weeks, repeating is not indicated. LDL goal according to the 2018 Multisociety Cholesterol guidelines for patients with clinical ASCVD and judged to be at high risk is <70 mg/dL. Intensification with PCSK9 inhibitor therapy or ezetimibe at this point is not indicated. Additionally, risk-enhancing factors, such as high-sensitivity C-reactive protein should be considered in the context of primary prevention rather than secondary prevention. CAC testing is not indicated for patients with a history of clinical ASCVD.

References
1. Orringer CE, Jacobson TA, Maki KC. National Lipid Association scientific statement on the use of icosapent ethyl in statin-treated patients with elevated triglycerides and high or very-high ASCVD risk. J Clin Lipidol. 2019;13(6):860–72.
2. Grundy SM, Stone NJ, Bailey AL, et al. 2018 AHA/ACC/AACVPR/AAPA/ABC/A CPM/ADA/AGS/APhA/ASPC/NLA/PCNA guideline on the management of blood cholesterol: a report of the American College of Cardiology/American Heart Association task force on clinical practice guidelines. Circulation. 2019;139(25):e1082–143.

52. Correct Answer: A

Rationale
Lipoprotein (a) [Lp(a)] is an independent risk factor for ASCVD. It has a strong relationship with the risk of stroke, especially in young individuals. Plasma concentrations of Lp(a) are largely determined by genetics. A family history of stroke in this patient's mother at a young age in addition to her mother's sibling with a history of myocardial infarction at an early age should raise concern for an elevated Lp(a). Per the National Lipid Association 2019 Scientific Statement, "Lp(a) testing is reasonable to refine risk assessment for ASCVD events in adults with: First-degree relatives with premature ASCVD (55 years of age in men; 65 years of age in women)."

An elevated Lp(a) is considered a risk-enhancing factor for ASCVD when levels exceed ≥ 50 mg/dL or ≥ 125 nmol/L. Other risk-enhancing factors include an apolipoprotein B100 ≥ 130 mg/dL, hsCRP ≥ 2 mg/L, and persistently elevated triglycerides ≥ 175 mg/dL.

References
1. Wilson DP, Jacobson TA, Jones PH, et al. Use of lipoprotein(a) in clinical practice: a biomarker whose time has come. A scientific statement from the National Lipid Association. J Clin Lipidol. 2019;13(3):374–92.
2. Grundy SM, Stone NJ, Bailey AL, et al. 2018 AHA/ACC/AACVPR/AAPA/ABC/ACPM/ADA/AGS/APhA/ASPC/NLA/PCNA Guideline on the management of blood cholesterol: a report of the American College of Cardiology/American Heart Association task force on clinical practice guidelines. Circulation. 2019;139(25):e1082–143.

53. Correct Answer: D

Rationale
With an elevated ASCVD risk between 7.5% and 19.9%, the patient is at intermediate 10-year risk. All individuals can benefit from shared-decision making, and for individuals in this category, this can be focused on testing to further personalize risk, such as CAC testing and assessment of risk-enhancing factors as well as what alternative options are available. For individuals who have tried and had side effects to three different statins, it is a more appropriate next step to consider an alternative class rather than challenging with a fourth statin. Ezetimibe therapy is the most appropriate non-statin therapy to choose. PCSK9 inhibitor therapy should be reserved for individuals with a clinical history of ASCVD at very high risk or those with diabetes and additional risk factor after discussion about the cost of therapy. Aspirin therapy is no longer recommended for primary prevention, and recent USPSTF guidelines discourage aspirin use in individuals ≥60 years.

References
1. US Preventive Services Task Force, Davidson KW, Barry MJ, Mangione CM, et al. Aspirin use to prevent cardiovascular disease: US preventive services task force recommendation statement. JAMA. 2022;327(16):1577–84.
2. Grundy SM, Stone NJ, Bailey AL, et al. 2018 AHA/ACC/AACVPR/AAPA/ABC/ACPM/ADA/AGS/APhA/ASPC/NLA/PCNA guideline on the management of blood cholesterol: a report of the American College of Cardiology/American Heart Association task force on clinical practice guidelines. Circulation. 2019;139(25):e1082–143.

54. Correct Answer: B

Rationale
CAC testing is recommended for individuals at intermediate risk (i.e., 7.5–19.9% 10-year risk) of ASCVD in whom the decision to initiate pharmacologic therapy is uncertain. Blaha and colleagues demonstrated that the best "negative risk marker" for lowering posttest probability of an ASCVD event was a coronary artery calcium score of 0. In individuals without a history of diabetes, family history of premature CHD, or current smoking habit, it is reasonable to delay the addition of lipid-lowering therapy.

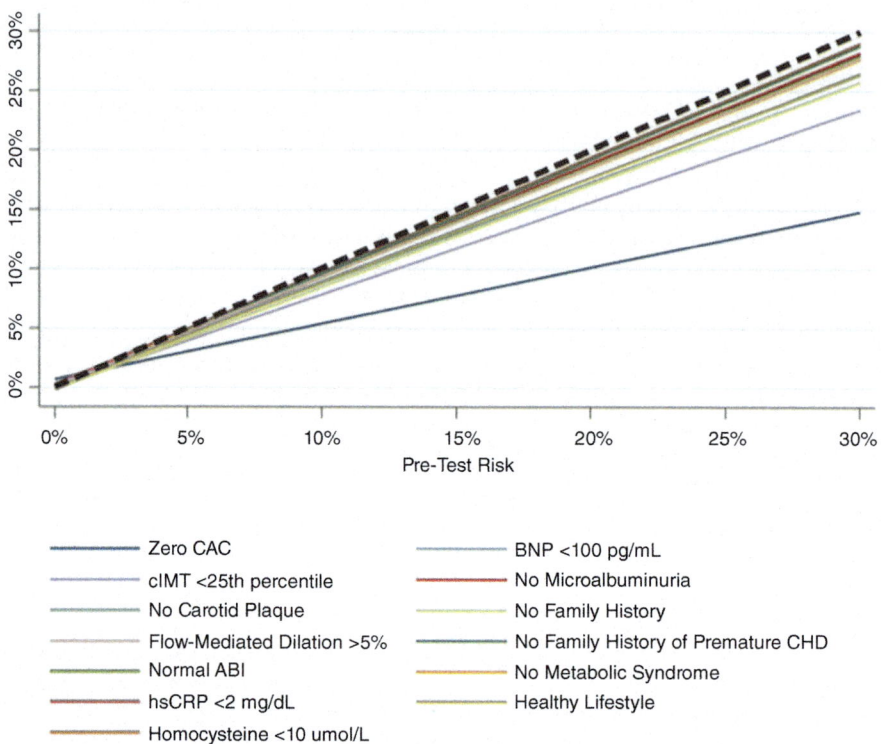

Relationship between pretest and posttest cardiovascular disease (CVD) risk after the knowledge of the negative result of each risk marker. The regression lines display the relationship between the pretest predicted 10-year ASCVD risk (*x* axis) and the posttest risk (*y* axis) after the knowledge of the negative result of each risk marker. A broken back line is displayed as reference (risk shift with no additional testing). Results were obtained by plotting the pretest and posttest risk on the basis of the diagnostic likelihood ratio of each Multi-Ethnic Study of Atherosclerosis (MESA) participant and then applying a linear fit. *ABI* ankle-brachial index, *BNP* brain natriuretic peptide, *CAC* coronary artery calcium, *CHD* coronary heart disease, *CIMT* carotid intima-media thickness, *FMD* flow-mediated dilation, *hsCRP* high-sensitivity C-reactive protein. (Figure and legend reproduced with permission from Circulation. 2016 Mar 1;133(9):849–58)

References

1. Blaha MJ, Cainzos-Achirica M, Greenland P, Role of coronary artery calcium score of zero and other negative risk markers for cardiovascular disease: the Multi-Ethnic Study of Atherosclerosis (MESA). Circulation. 2016;133(9):849–58.
2. Arnett DK, Blumenthal RS, Albert MA, et al. 2019 ACC/AHA Guideline on the primary prevention of cardiovascular disease: a report of the American College of Cardiology/American Heart Association task force on clinical practice guidelines. Circulation. 2019;140(11):e596–646.

55. Correct Answer: B

Rationale
Due to the patient's Japanese ancestry, a low or moderate-intensity statin should be initiated regardless of the ASCVD. Japanese patients may be more sensitive to statin therapy, although there is no clinical data to suggest treating high-risk Japanese patients with a high-dose statin is harmful. In regard to choice A, CAC is useful regardless of race/ethnicity but should be measured if ASCVD risk is uncertain. The patient's ASCVD risk is 20.2% (without aspirin or statin therapy), so a high-intensity statin is indicated in this patient. Choice C is not correct as the 10-year ASCVD risk score in Asian individuals may be under or overestimated depending on the population. Considering all information, choice B is the best answer for this patient.

56. Correct Answer: C

Rationale
Black have a lower odds of awareness and lower incidence of atrial fibrillation when compared with White patients. Because of the lower odds of awareness in Black, this significantly increases the risk of adverse outcomes such as strokes, as Black patients are less likely to be treated with anticoagulation therapy. Black patients are also less likely to be treated with novel oral anticoagulants and interventional therapies for atrial fibrillation when compared with White patients, making choice B incorrect. Therefore, the most appropriate answer is C.

57. Correct Answer: B

Rationale
According to the most recent data from the National Center for Health Statistics (CDC), non-Hispanic Asian have the highest uncontrolled rates of HTN (86.3%), followed by Hispanics (81.6%), Black (79.4%), and Whites (74%). Even though Whites with HTN have the lowest uncontrolled rates, they are the largest group (number in millions) compared with other groups in the United States (53.5 million overall, compared with 12 million Black, 10.6 million Hispanics, and 4.4 million Asian). These findings are likely due to the higher number of Whites in the United States. Although there are varying rates of uncontrolled HTN among the racial and ethnic groups of the United States, the rates of HTN control overall are still poor for all and require major efforts to decrease.

58. Correct Answer: A

Rationale
Initiation of pitavastatin or other high-intensity statin while following closely for adverse effects is most appropriate. High-dose (4 mg/day) compared with low-dose

(1 mg/day) pitavastatin therapy significantly reduced cardiovascular events in Japanese patients with stable CAD. Administration of maximum tolerable doses of statins, within the range of local approval, would be the preferred statin strategy in patients with established CAD regardless of baseline low-density lipoprotein cholesterol levels.

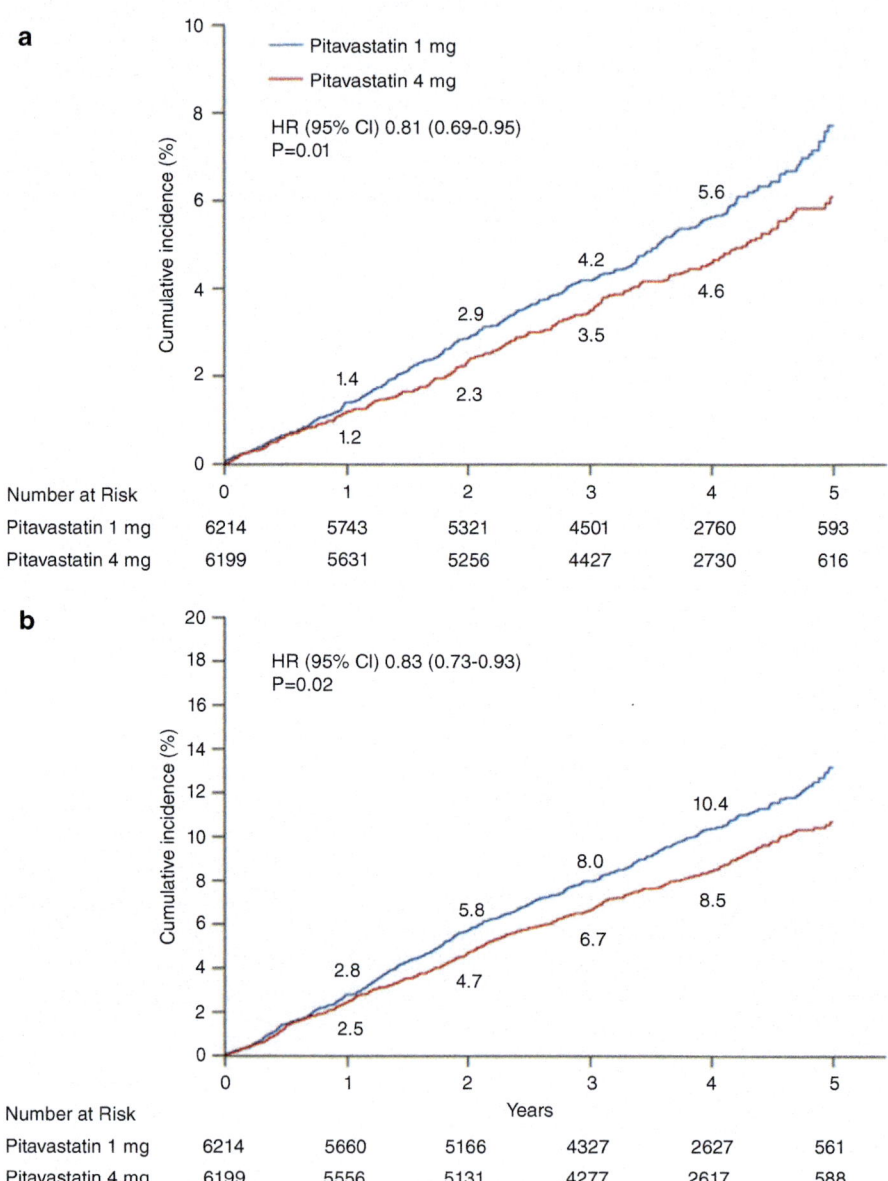

Kaplan–Meier curves for the primary end point and a secondary composite end point (primary end point plus coronary revascularization). The cumulative incidence was estimated by the Kaplan–Meier method. (**a** and **b**) Kaplan–Meier curves for the primary end point (a composite of cardiovascular death, nonfatal myocardial infarction, nonfatal ischemic stroke, or unstable angina requiring emergency hospitalization) and for a secondary composite end point (a composite of primary end point or coronary revascularization based on clinical indication), respectively. Coronary revascularization as a component of the secondary composite end point excluded target-lesion revascularization for lesions treated at the time of prior percutaneous coronary intervention. *CI* confidence interval, *HR* hazard ratio. (Figure and legend reproduced with permission from Circulation. 2018 May 8;137(19):1997–2009)

Reference
1. Taguchi I, Iimuro S, Iwata H, et al. High-dose versus low-dose pitavastatin in Japanese patients with stable coronary artery disease (REAL-CAD): a randomized superiority trial. Circulation. 2018;137(19):1997–2009.

59. Correct Answer: C

Rationale
A significant prevention target in ASCVD is the treatment of lipid disorders, as these lipid abnormalities, primarily elevated low-density lipoprotein (LDL-C), contribute to atherosclerotic plaque burden, ultimately causing CHD, cerebrovascular accident, as well as sudden cardiac death from ischemia. Although Black patients tend to have more favorable lipid profiles when compared to the national average, they suffer from higher rates of mortality due to CHD. The REGARDS study suggests Black patients are less likely to be aware of their hyperlipidemia and less likely to have adequate control than White patients. MESA, CARDIA, and other studies that have evaluated coronary calcium in diverse populations also show Black patients have less coronary calcium than similarly aged White patients.

References
1. Carnethon MR, Pu J, Howard G, et al; American Heart Association Council on Epidemiology and Prevention; Council on Cardiovascular Disease in the Young; Council on Cardiovascular and Stroke Nursing; Council on Clinical Cardiology; Council on Functional Genomics and Translational Biology; and Stroke Council. Cardiovascular health in African Americans: a scientific statement from the American Heart Association. Circulation. 2017;136(21):e393–423.
2. Arnett DK, Blumenthal RS, Albert MA, et al. 2019 ACC/AHA guideline on the primary prevention of cardiovascular disease: executive summary: a report of the American College of Cardiology/American Heart Association task force on clinical practice guidelines. J Am Coll Cardiol. 2019;74(10):1376–414.

60. Correct Answer: D

Rationale

An essential and potentially potent first step in reducing racial and ethnic disparities in ASCVDshould focus in addressing the SDH that continue to systematically and disproportionately affect minority populations in the United States. Defined as "the circumstances in which people are born, grow, live, work, and age, and the systems put in place to deal with illness" by the World Health Organization and others, SDH contribute to up to 80% of illness, encompassing adverse health behaviors, SES, and environmental factors of the individual. The American Heart Association (AHA) reports that higher prevalence of traditional ASCVD risk factors in certain racial/ethnic groups is mostly attributable to SDH.

References
1. Magnan S. Social determinants of health 101 for health care: five plus five. 2017. https://nam.edu/social-determinants-of-health-101-for-health-care-five-plus-five/.
2. Carnethon MR, Pu J, Howard G, et al. American Heart Association Council on Epidemiology and Prevention; Council on Cardiovascular Disease in the Young; Council on Cardiovascular and Stroke Nursing; Council on Clinical Cardiology; Council on Functional Genomics and Translational Biology; and Stroke Council. Cardiovascular health in African Americans: a scientific statement from the American Heart Association. Circulation. 2017;136(21):e393–423.

61. Correct Answer: A

Rationale

Hypertension is the most widely prevalent and potent risk factor in the development of ASCVD and microvascular complications. Several studies document a differential response to pharmacologic interventions in reducing high blood pressure, with thiazide-type diuretics and calcium channel blockers maybe most effective in lowering blood pressure and stroke as a first-step agent in Black patients. However, compelling indications may best determine first line medications to better address hypertension in Black patients. In this case, this patient's history of heart failure with reduced ejection fraction more than self-identified race, necessitates the use of an angiotensin-converting-enzyme inhibitors than other pharmacologic interventions.

References
1. Whelton PK, Carey RM, Aronow WS, et al. 2017 ACC/AHA/AAPA/ABC/ACPM/AGS/APhA/ASH/ASPC/NMA/PCNA guideline for the prevention, detection, evaluation, and management of high blood pressure in adults: executive summary: a report of the American College of Cardiology/American Heart Association task force on clinical practice guidelines. Circulation. 2018;138(17):e426–83.
2. Ferdinand KC. Novel interventions in addressing racial disparities in blood pressure control. Circulation. 2018;138(4):339–41.

62. Correct Answer: B

Rationale
Since heart rate (HR) shows a linear relation with oxygen uptake (VO_2) during exercise, a simple method for estimating VO_2 during physical activity, expressed as METs, in persons with and without ASCVD, including those taking β-blockers, employs the resting and exercise HRs using the HR index equation.

$$METs = (6 \times \text{Heart Rate Index}) - 5$$

where the heart rate index equals the activity HR divided by the resting HR. In this case, 120 bpm/60 bpm = 2.0 heart rate index which is multiplied by 6, yielding 12, from which we subtract 5, yielding an estimated 7 METs.

Reference
1. Wicks JR, Oldridge NB, Nielsen LK, Vickers CE. HR index—a simple method for the prediction of oxygen uptake. Med Sci Sports Exerc. 2011;43(10):2005–12.

63. Correct Answer: C

Rationale
Although 10,000 steps/day has been the traditional recommendation, ever fewer steps per day appear to confer survival benefits. The recent CARDIA study reported that participants taking ≥7000 steps/day, compared with <7000 steps/day, had a much lower risk of mortality. These findings suggest a viable alternative to a moderate-to-vigorous intensity physical activity regimen to improve survival and life expectancy.

Reference
1. Paluch AE, Gabriel KP, Fulton JE, et al. Steps per day and all-cause mortality in middle-aged adults in the coronary artery risk development in young adults study. JAMA Netw Open. 2021;4(9):e2124516.

64. Correct Answer: B

Rationale
Accordingly, a 1–2 MET increase in exercise capacity confers a reduction in mortality that compares favorably with the survival advantage provided by commonly prescribed cardioprotective medications after acute myocardial infarction. Increased cardiorespiratory fitness can decrease the risk of initial and recurrent cardiovascular events, presumably from multiple mechanisms, including anti-atherosclerotic, anti-ischemic, anti-arrhythmic, and anti-thrombotic adaptations.

References
1. Kodama S, Saito K, Tanaka S, et al. Cardiorespiratory fitness as a quantitative predictor of all-cause mortality and cardiovascular events in healthy men and women: a meta-analysis. JAMA. 2009;301(19):2024–35.
2. Boden WE, Franklin BA, Wenger NK. Physical activity and structured exercise for patients with stable ischemic heart disease. JAMA. 2013;309(2):143–4.

65. Correct Answer: D

Rationale
The favorable risk factor profiles and superb cardiac performance of long-distance runners, coupled with the finding that regular endurance exercise prevents cellular senescence in animals and humans, have led an increasing number of middle-aged and older adults to the conclusion that "more exercise is better." However, recent reports have linked extreme exercise regimens with adverse cardiovascular outcomes. This relationship has been increasingly described by a U- or reverse J-shaped dose response curve. These reports should be considered by clinicians when counseling patients regarding their exercise practices.

Reference
1. Franklin BA, Thompson PD, Al-Zaiti SS, et al. American Heart Association Physical Activity Committee of the Council on Lifestyle and Cardiometabolic Health; Council on Cardiovascular and Stroke Nursing; Council on Clinical Cardiology; and Stroke Council. Exercise-related acute cardiovascular events and potential deleterious adaptations following long-term exercise training: placing the risks into perspective-an update: a scientific statement from the American Heart Association. Circulation. 2020;141(13):e705–36.

66. Correct Answer: D

Rationale
The 2019 ACC/AHA Prevention Guidelines recommend all cardioprotective dietary patterns that are plant centered, low in saturated fat and dietary cholesterol, and emphasize fruits, vegetables, whole grains, low-fat or fat-free dairy products, lean protein sources, legumes, pulses, nuts, seeds, and liquid vegetable oils. Furthermore, they are low in red and processed meats and low in refined grains, sugar sweetened foods and beverages.

References
1. Arnett DK, Blumenthal RS, Albert MA, et al. 2019 ACC/AHA guideline on the primary prevention of cardiovascular disease: a report of the American College of Cardiology/American Heart Association task force on clinical practice guidelines. J Am Coll Cardiol. 2019. pii: S0735-1097(19)33877-X.
2. Shan Z, Li Y, Baden MY, Bhupathiraju SN, et al. Association between healthy eating patterns and risk of cardiovascular disease. JAMA Intern Med. 2020;180(8):1090–100.

67. Correct Answer: D

Rationale
The DASH dietary patterns are high in vegetables, fruits, whole grains; low-fat or non-fat dairy, seafood, skinless poultry, legumes, and nuts; moderate in alcohol (for adults); low in red and processed meats; and low in refined grains, sugar sweetened foods and beverages. In the Omni-Heart DASH trial, an additional 10% of energy intake from carbohydrate was replaced with unsaturated fat.

References
1. Dietary Guidelines Advisory Committee. 2020–2025. Scientific report of the 2020–2025 Dietary Guidelines Advisory Committee report to the secretary of agriculture and the secretary of health and human services. Washington, DC: U.S. Department of Agriculture, Agricultural Research Service.
2. Appel LJ, Sacks FM, Carey VJ, et al. Effects of protein, monounsaturated fat, and carbohydrate intake on blood pressure and serum lipids: results of the Omni Heart randomized trial. JAMA. 2005;294(19):2455–64.

68. Correct Answer: A

Rationale
This is supported by the 2019 ACC/AHA guideline on the primary prevention of cardiovascular disease.

Reference
1. Arnett DK, Blumenthal RS, Albert MA, et al. 2019 ACC/AHA guideline on the primary prevention of cardiovascular disease: a report of the American College of Cardiology/American Heart Association task force on clinical practice guidelines. J Am Coll Cardiol. 2019:S0735-1097(19)33877-X.

69. Correct Answer: D

Rationale
The National Lipid Association (NLA) recommends 5–10 g/day of viscous fiber and more if tolerated either from foods high in viscous fiber and/or psyllium or methyl cellulose supplements. NLA recommends 2–3 g of phytosterols as supplements since diet cannot contribute more than 400–800 g/day even on a vegetarian diet.

References
1. Jacobson TA, Maki KC, Orringer CE, et al. National Lipid Association recommendations for patient-centered management of dyslipidemia: part 2. J Clin Lipidol. 2015;9(6 Suppl): S1–22.e1.
2. Sikand G, Severson T. Top 10 dietary strategies for atherosclerotic cardiovascular risk reduction. Am J Prev Cardiol. 2020;4:100106. ISSN 2666–6677. https://doi.org/10.1016/j.ajpc.2020.100106.

70. Correct Answer: C

Rationale

The 2019 ACC/AHA guideline on primary prevention gives a Class III recommendation (harm) for low-dose aspirin (75–100 mg orally daily) in the primary prevention of ASCVD among adults ≥70 years of age. While low dose aspirin used to be prescribed routinely for primary prevention, this is no longer the case given data from the ASPREE trial showing no CVD (cardiovascular disease) benefit among adults ≥70 years of age on 100 mg of aspirin versus placebo, though there was an increased risk of major hemorrhage.

References
1. Arnett DK, Blumenthal RS, Albert MA, et al. 2019 ACC/AHA guideline on the primary prevention of cardiovascular disease: executive summary: a report of the American College of Cardiology/American Heart Association task force on clinical practice guidelines. J Am Coll Cardiol. 2019.
2. McNeil JJ, Wolfe R, Woods RL, et al. Effect of aspirin on cardiovascular events and bleeding in the healthy elderly. N Engl J Med. 2018;379(16):1509–18.

71. Correct Answer: B

Rationale

The 2019 ACC/AHA guideline on primary prevention states low-dose aspirin (75–100 mg orally daily) might be considered for primary prevention of ASCVD among select adults 40–70 years of age who are at higher ASCVD risk but not at increased bleeding risk. Additionally, several observational studies have demonstrated net benefit among individuals with CAC ≥100 Agatston Units, whereas randomized control trial data failed to show benefit for primary prevention aspirin among individuals with diabetes mellitus.

References
1. Arnett DK, Blumenthal RS, Albert MA, et al. 2019 ACC/AHA guideline on the primary prevention of cardiovascular disease: executive summary: a report of the American College of Cardiology/American Heart Association task force on clinical practice guidelines. J Am Coll Cardiol. 2019.
2. Ajufo E, Ayers CR, Vigen R, et al. Value of coronary artery calcium scanning in association with the net benefit of aspirin in primary prevention of atherosclerotic cardiovascular disease. JAMA Cardiol. 2021;6(2):179–87.
3. Cainzos-Achirica M, Miedema MD, McEvoy JW, et al. Coronary artery calcium for personalized allocation of aspirin in primary prevention of cardiovascular disease in 2019. Circulation. 2020;141(19):1541–53.
4. Effects of aspirin for primary prevention in persons with diabetes mellitus. N Engl J Med. 2018;379(16):1529–39.

72. Correct Answer: E

Rationale
Smoking cessation medications approved by the U.S. Food and Drug Administration and behavioral counseling are effective treatments for quitting, particularly when used in combination. E-cigarettes or electronic nicotine delivery systems (ENDS) are increasing in prevalence, particularly among young populations. Although some patients may use e-cigarettes to aid in quitting, the 2020 surgeon general's report on smoking and tobacco use notes that research is uncertain on whether e-cigarettes increase quitting rates. At present, e-cigarettes are not FDA approved to aid in smoking cessation.

References
1. Arnett DK, Blumenthal RS, Albert MA, et al. 2019 ACC/AHA guideline on the primary prevention of cardiovascular disease: executive summary: a report of the American College of Cardiology/American Heart Association task force on clinical practice guidelines. J Am Coll Cardiol. 2019.
2. U.S. Department of Health and Human Services. Smoking Cessation. A report of the Surgeon General. Atlanta, GA: U.S. Department of Health and Human Services, Centers for Disease Control and Prevention, National Center for Chronic Disease Prevention and Health Promotion, Office on Smoking and Health; 2020.

73. Correct Answer: B

Rationale
While varenicline, bupropion, and nicotine patches are all FDA (Food and Drug Administration) approved to aid in smoking cessation, bupropion is contraindicated in patients with a history of seizure disorder or binge drinking because it reduces the seizure threshold. While varenicline previously carried a black box warning for patients with a history of depression, this warning was removed by the FDA in 2016.

References
1. Anthenelli RM, Benowitz NL, West R, et al. Neuropsychiatric safety and efficacy of varenicline, bupropion, and nicotine patch in smokers with and without psychiatric disorders (EAGLES): a double-blind, randomised, placebo-controlled clinical trial. Lancet. 2016;387(10037):2507–20.
2. Barua RS, Rigotti NA, Benowitz NL, et al. 2018 ACC expert consensus decision pathway on tobacco cessation treatment. J Am Coll Cardiol. 2018;72(25):3332–65.

74. Correct Answer: B

Rationale
The estimated GFR is sustained for 3 months or more at between 45 and 59 mL/min/1.73 m^2 and the patient has a urinary albumin to creatinine ratio values of between 30 and 300 mg/g of creatinine.

Reference

1. Kidney disease improving global outcomes 2012—clinical practice Guidelines for the evaluation and management of chronic kidney disease. Kidney Int Suppl. 2013;3:1–150.

75. Correct Answer: D

Rationale

Among Medicare recipients with CKD, not on dialysis, the prevalence of CAD in 38%. The prevalence for similar patients of atrial fibrillation is 24%, congestive heart failure is 26%, and ischemic stroke is 16%. Any cardiovascular disease is present in 56% of older patients with CKD.

Reference

1. United States Renal Data System, 2018 Annual data report. www.USRDS.gov.

76. Correct Answer: C

Rationale

Inhibition of the renin-angiotensin system and the sodium-glucose co-transport in the proximal tubule of the kidneys is strongly associated with improved heat function and slowing of the progression of chronic kidney disease. The other options have far less or no benefit in patients like this.

Reference

1. Braunwald E. Gliflozins in the management of cardiovascular disease. N Engl J Med. 2022;386(21):2024–34.

77. Correct Answer: D

Rationale

Better control of blood pressure, via use of renin-angiotensin system inhibitors, would provide the best chance of delaying progression of ischemic heart disease. Statins would be of no benefit despite a lowering of LDL cholesterol. Beta-blockers in the absence of heart failure would be ineffective. Fibric acid derivatives have not shown any benefits in patients with dialysis treated with advanced CKD.

Reference

1. Baigent C, Landray MJ, Reith C, et al. SHARP Investigators. The effects of lowering LDL cholesterol with simvastatin plus ezetimibe in patients with chronic kidney disease (Study of Heart and Renal Protection): a randomised placebo-controlled trial. Lancet. 2011;377(9784):2181–92.

78. Correct Answer: C

Rationale
Moderate or severe mitral stenosis. In the 2019 AHA/ACC/HRS Focused Update of the 2014 AHA/ACC/HRS Guideline for the Management of Patients with Atrial Fibrillation, DOACs are recommended over warfarin in DOAC-eligible patients with atrial fibrillation; exceptions include those with moderate-to-severe mitral stenosis or a mechanical heart valve (Class of Recommendation I, Level of Evidence A).

Reference
1. January CT, Wann LS, Calkins H, et al. 2019 AHA/ACC/HRS focused update of the 2014 AHA/ACC/HRS guideline for the management of patients with atrial fibrillation: a report of the American College of Cardiology/American Heart Association task force on clinical practice guidelines and the Heart Rhythm Society. J Am Coll Cardiol. 2019;74(1):104–32.

79. Correct Answer: A

Rationale
CAD. In the 2020 ACC/AHA Guideline for the Management of Patients with Valvular Heart Disease, anticoagulation using a vitamin K antagonist is recommended for all patients with a mechanical prosthetic valve (Class of Recommendation I). In patients that have undergone mechanical aortic valve replacement, an INR goal of 2.5 (range of 2.0–3.0) is recommended (Class of Recommendation I), unless other risk factors are present (older-generation valve, atrial fibrillation, previous thromboembolism, hypercoagulable state, or left ventricular systolic dysfunction), in which case an INR goal of 3.0 (range of 2.5–3.5) is recommended (Class of Recommendation I).

Reference
1. Otto CM, Nishimura RA, Bonow RO, et al. 2020 ACC/AHA guideline for the management of patients with valvular heart disease: a report of the American College of Cardiology/American Heart Association Joint Committee on clinical practice guidelines. J Am Coll Cardiol. 2021;77(4):e25–197.

80. Correct Answer: C

Rationale
Six months. In the 2021 ACC/AHA/SCAI Guideline for Coronary Artery Revascularization, dual antiplatelet therapy with aspirin and a $P2Y_{12}$ inhibitor is recommended for at least 6 months after PCI with a DES for SIHD (Class of Recommendation I, Level of Evidence A). The Guideline further notes that (a) it is reasonable to consider discontinuing aspirin after 1–3 months, with continuation of a $P2Y_{12}$ inhibitor alone (Class of Recommendation IIa), and (b) it may be

reasonable to continue dual antiplatelet therapy for >6 months in those that are not at high risk of bleeding and in whom there has been no significant overt bleeding while on dual antiplatelet therapy (Class of Recommendation IIb).

Reference
1. Lawton JS, Tamis-Holland JE, Bangalore S, et al. 2021 ACC/AHA/SCAI guideline for coronary artery revascularization: a report of the American College of Cardiology/American Heart Association Joint Committee on clinical practice guidelines. J Am Coll Cardiol. 2022;79(2):e21–129.

81. Correct Answer: D

Rationale
Experienced a major bleed within the last 3 months. In the 2017 ACC Expert Consensus Decision Pathway for Periprocedural Management of Anticoagulation in Patients with Nonvalvular Atrial Fibrillation, periprocedural bridging of anticoagulation is not recommended for those on a vitamin K antagonist either (a) at low thrombotic risk or (b) at moderate thrombotic risk without prior stroke or TIA (transient ischemic attack) and/or with increased bleed risk. Patients on a vitamin K antagonist at high thrombotic risk are recommended to undergo periprocedural bridging of anticoagulation in the absence of major bleeding or intracranial hemorrhage within the prior 3 months.

Reference
1. Doherty JU, Gluckman TJ, Hucker WJ, et al. 2017 ACC expert consensus decision pathway for periprocedural management of anticoagulation in patients with nonvalvular atrial fibrillation: a report of the American College of Cardiology clinical expert consensus document task force. J Am Coll Cardiol. 2017;69(7):871–98.

82. Correct Answer: B

Rationale
Gastric. In the 2020 ACC Expert Consensus Decision Pathway on Management of Bleeding in Patients on Oral Anticoagulants, bleeding in the following locations were defined as critical site bleeds: intracranial, intraocular, spinal, pericardial, airway, intrathoracic, intraabdominal, retroperitoneal, intramuscular, and intraarticular. Gastrointestinal (intraluminal) bleeds do not constitute critical site bleeds.

Reference
1. Tomaselli GF, Mahaffey KW, Cuker A, et al. 2020 ACC expert consensus decision pathway on management of bleeding in patients on oral anticoagulants: a report of the American College of Cardiology Solution Set Oversight Committee. J Am Coll Cardiol. 2020;76(5):594–622.

83. Correct Answer: B

Rationale
False. In women, the cardio-protective effect of estrogen during premenopause years can result in an ~8–10-year lag in the onset of CAD. However, in postmenopausal women this effect is diminished and generally after the age of 55 years, the risk for CAD increases similarly in both men and women.

Reference
1. Udell JA, Lu H, Redelmeier DA. Failure of fertility therapy and subsequent adverse cardiovascular events. CMAJ. 2017;189(10):E391–7.

84. Correct Answer: E

Rationale
Fertility therapy. At this time, fertility treatment itself is not considered an independent risk or protective factor for ASCVD beyond noting the adverse pregnancy outcomes that may occur in the short term. However, there is an early signal to suggest that women who have failed fertility therapy have an increased risk for future ASCVD events. It is plausible that fertility therapy failure could be an indicator for future ASCVD risk as it poses a unique cardiometabolic stress test. This hypothesis warrants further investigation.

References
1. Udell JA, Lu H, Redelmeier DA. Failure of fertility therapy and subsequent adverse cardiovascular events. CMAJ. 2017;189(10):E391–7.
2. Grundy SM, Stone NJ, Bailey AL, et al. 2018 AHA/ACC/AACVPR/AAPA/ABC/ACPM/ADA/AGS/APhA/ASPC/NLA/PCNA guideline on the management of blood cholesterol: executive summary: a report of the American College of Cardiology/American Heart Association task force on clinical practice guidelines. J Am Coll Cardiol. 2019;73(24):3168–209.

85. Correct Answer: D

Rationale
Hormone replacement therapy. The ACC/AHA guidelines recognize premature menopause as a risk enhancer for ASCVD (arteriosclerotic cardiovascular disease) events; however, the evidence promoting hormonal replacement therapy (HRT) is controversial. In the Women's Health Initiative (WHI) study, estrogen-progestin replacement had no cardioprotective effect and signals of harm were observed with higher risk of coronary heart disease events. Nonetheless, noting the presence of premature ovarian insufficiency and the age of menopause should be part of any woman's ASCVD risk assessment.

References
1. Grundy SM, Stone NJ, Bailey AL, et al. 2018 AHA/ACC/AACVPR/AAPA/ABC/ACPM/ADA/AGS/APhA/ASPC/NLA/PCNA guideline on the management of blood cholesterol: executive summary: a report of the American College of Cardiology/American Heart Association task force on clinical practice guidelines. J Am Coll Cardiol. 2019;73(24):3168–209.
2. Rossouw JE, Anderson GL, Prentice RL, et al. Risks and benefits of estrogen plus progestin in healthy postmenopausal women: principal results from the Women's Health Initiative randomized controlled trial. JAMA. 2002;288(3): 321–33.

86. Correct Answer: B

Rationale
Among the non-pharmacologic treatments of high blood pressure is low-sodium dietary intake (<2300 mg of sodium per day). To lower dietary sodium intake, some patients may inquire about salt substitutes. Salt substitutes vary regarding their sodium chloride and potassium chloride content; their taste varies as well. Salt substitutes with no sodium may have high amounts of potassium chloride, which may exacerbate hyperkalemia in patients with renal insufficiency. Sea salt is evaporation of seawater that is minimally processed and retains trace minerals such as magnesium, potassium, calcium, and other nutrients. In most cases, sea salt does not offer substantial sodium-reduction or potential health advantages over table salt. It is often recommended that for adults with an average BP >20/10 mmHg above their BP target, that antihypertensive drug therapy be initiated with two first-line agents of different classes, either as separate agents or in a fixed-dose combination. Common examples include angiotensin-converting enzyme inhibitor/angiotensin-receptor blocker in combination with a calcium channel blocker or thiazide diuretic in the same pill. Chlorthalidone and indapamide are "thiazide-like" diuretics with longer half-lives than hydrochlorothiazide and may achieve greater BP reduction. Although some advocate chlorthalidone is preferred over hydrochlorothiazide, the data supporting such a recommendation is not always consistent. Loop diuretics (e.g., furosemide, torasemide, bumetanide, and azosemide) may be preferred in patients with heart failure and when estimated glomerular filtration rate is <30 mL/min. Due to questionable added benefit in lowering blood pressure, and increased risk of hyperkalemia, angiotensin receptor blockers should not be used in combination with direct renin inhibitors (i.e., aliskiren). Beta blockers reduce CVD in patients with reduced ejection fraction are used to treat angina pectoris and cardiac dysrhythmias and may reduce the risk of recurrent myocardial infarction after an acute myocardial infarction.

Reference
1. Bays HE, Kulkarni A, German C, et al. Ten things to know about ten cardiovascular disease risk factors—2022. Am J Prev Cardiol. 2022;10:100342.

Answers

87. Correct Answer: D

Rationale

In patients treated for obesity, semaglutide and liraglutide are examples of anti-diabetes agents with CVD outcome trial support for reduction in major adverse cardiac events (MACE) in patients with Type 2 diabetes mellitus. At higher doses, semaglutide and liraglutide are approved to treat obesity. However, at the time of this writing, no anti-obesity drug has an indicated use to reduce MACE. Semaglutide at 2.4 mg subcutaneously per week is approved for treatment of obesity. Lower doses of semaglutide and liraglutide are approved to lower glucose in patients with diabetes mellitus. Semaglutide is administered as subcutaneous injectable doses of 0.25–2.0 mg per week and oral doses of 7–14 mg per day. In patients with congestive cardiomyopathy and obesity, GLP-1 receptor agonists may be of benefit. However, most guidelines and evidence from cardiovascular outcomes studies support the use of certain sodium glucose transport 2 inhibitors, which inhibit renal tubular reabsorption, produce natriuresis, and have proven benefit in improving CVD outcomes especially in patients with congestive cardiomyopathy. Tirzepatide is a unimolecular GLP-1 and glucose-dependent insulinotropic polypeptide (GIP) agonist that reduces glucose in patients with diabetes and reduces body weight in patients with overweight or obesity. Phentermine is a sympathomimetic that is a commonly prescribed anti-obesity agent. While some data suggests phentermine may be safe in patients at low CVD risk, phentermine is contraindicated in patients with cardiovascular disease, and its long-term effects on MACE in patients at low or moderate CVD risk are unknown.

Reference
1. Bays HE, Kulkarni A, German C, Satish P, Iluyomade A, Dudum R, Thakkar A, Rifai MA, Mehta A, Thobani A, Al-Saiegh Y, Nelson AJ, Sheth S, Toth PP. Ten things to know about ten cardiovascular disease risk factors—2022. Am J Prev Cardiol. 2022;10:100342.

88. Correct Answer: B

Rationale

Coronary anatomy is often assessed by CAC, coronary computerized tomography (CCTA), cardiac resonance imaging (CMR), and cardiac catheterization. Cardiac diastolic dysfunction is often evaluated by echocardiogram and CMR (cardiac magnetic resonance). Myocardial perfusion is often assessed by single-photon emission computerized tomography (SPECT), positron emission tomography (PET), and CMR. Cardiomyocyte injury and fibrosis is often evaluated by CMR and CCTA. Microvascular dysfunction is often evaluated by PET and CMR. Hybrid imaging tests include: PET/CT and PET/MRI to assess perfusion, cardiac viability, and atherosclerosis. CT-Fractional Flow Reserve (FFR) provides anatomic (i.e., luminal and plaque) and physiologic/functional imaging data to assess obstructive CAD. Cardiac catheterization and FFR: Provides (invasive) anatomic and functional assessment of CAD. CAC added to SPECT or PET may help further identify coronary artery plaque and better stratify risk. CCTA added to CAC scoring may help improve the assessment of total plaque burden and better discriminate risk of death and/or myocardial infarction among symptomatic patients with suspected CAD.

Reference
1. Bays HE, Khera A, Blaha MJ, Budoff MJ, Toth PP. Ten things to know about ten imaging studies: a preventive cardiology perspective ("ASPC top ten imaging"). Am J Prev Cardiol. 2021;6:100176.

89. Correct Answer: A

Rationale
CCTA has over 90% sensitivity for anatomically significant CAD. CCTA has a high negative predictive value, such that if negative, the patient has low likelihood of clinically meaningful CVD risk. Exercise treadmill stress testing alone has about a 60% sensitivity and specificity for anatomically significant coronary artery disease. That is why treadmill stress testing is often performed along with an imaging study (e.g., single-photon emission computed tomography or SPECT). SPECT may have close to a 90% sensitivity, but around a 70% specificity for anatomically significant CAD. Examples of factors associated with false positive SPECT results are female sex, presence of cardiac microvascular coronary artery disease, left bundle branch block, and cardiomyopathy. Positron emission tomography (PET) and stress cardiac magnetic resonance (CMR) both have >80% sensitivity and selectivity for anatomically and functionally significant CVD. The choice of PET and CMR is largely due to location and clinician/institutional choice. Coronary calcium imaging (CAC)/score has over 90% sensitivity, but less than 50% specificity for anatomically significant CVD. That is why CAC scores are mainly used to identify high CAC risk individuals, such that more definitive diagnostic tests can then be considered.

Reference
1. Bays HE, Khera A, Blaha MJ, Budoff MJ, Toth PP. Ten things to know about ten imaging studies: a preventive cardiology perspective ("ASPC top ten imaging"). Am J Prev Cardiol. 2021;6:100176.

90. Correct Answer: D

Rationale
Distinguished nineteenth and early twentieth century physicians, such as Vasquez in France, Bollinger in Germany and Graham Steel from the UK noted that chronic heavy drinking was related to heart disease. In 1893, Graham Steel said, "Not only do I recognize alcoholism as one of the causes of heart muscle failure, but I find it a comparatively common one." In 1902 William MacKenzie used the term alcoholic heart disease.

Ideas changed dramatically when Aalsmar and Wenckebach described high output failure in polished rice eaters in Java. These people were malnourished and had vitamin B1 deficiency (thiamine, carboxylase). Subsequently, it was logically and widely assumed that heart failure in alcoholics in Western countries was due to this deficiency. However, most cases did not fit this hypothesis. They had dilated and poorly contracting hearts and did not respond to thiamine. Since the mid-twentieth century, mostly in the form of noninvasive studies of structure and function, massive circumstantial evidence supports the concept of alcoholic cardiomyopathy. Heavy drinking in susceptible persons can be a mitochondrial poison.

The data show that regression may occur with abstinence. The path to prevention is clear. Two epidemics of acute cardiomyopathy in heavy beer drinkers provide insights. The first was caused by accidental arsenic contamination of well water used to brew beer in Manchester, UK in 1900. The second was caused by deliberate introduction of small amounts of cobalt into beer to improve foaming in several sites in North America and in Europe in the 1960s. The combination of very small amounts of either cobalt or arsenic with alcohol caused severe heart failure with high mortality. Survivors continued their uncontaminated beer intake without apparent consequences. The data suggest synergistic toxicity, that is, the effects of co-factors.

References
1. Maisch B. Alcoholic cardiomyopathy: the result of dosage and individual predisposition. Herz. 2016;41(6):484–93.
2. Urbano-Márquez A, Fernández-Solà J. Effects of alcohol on skeletal and cardiac muscle. Muscle Nerve. 2004;30(6):689–707.

91. Correct Answer: D

Rationale
First presented and named in 1978 by Ettinger and colleagues, Holiday Heart Syndrome refers to supra-ventricular arrythmias occurring after large meals with much alcohol on holidays like New Year's. The supra-ventricular arrythmias comprised all types, including PAT, atrial flutter, and the most common, atrial fibrillation. These occur in people with otherwise apparently normal hearts and spontaneously regress. This close relationship supports alcohol as the major cause.

Triggers suspected for paroxysmal tachycardias include caffeine, stress, medications and alcohol. Not widely known until recently, drinking cold beverages can be a trigger. Following a case report, a number of patients reached out to the researcher via the internet. This should be sought to be elicited from patient history as an avoidable cause.

Predictors of chronic atrial fibrillation include advanced age, coronary disease, systemic hypertension, valvular disease and several non-cardiovascular diseases such as hyperthyroidism, sleep apnea, and COPD. Heavy alcohol intake is related to several of these conditions, especially systemic hypertension and cardiomyopathy. Whether light–moderate drinking of alcohol is related to risk of atrial fibrillation is unresolved.

As we write the questions for this primer and certification, we hope that we are currently near the end of the COVID 19 pandemic. The sophistication of epidemiology concepts through the media have affected patient knowledge. The discussions in the media of epidemiology methods have been extensive and have no doubt educated the general public in this area far more than what would ordinarily have been expected.

References
1. Ettinger PO, Wu CF, De La Cruz C Jr, et al. Arrhythmias and the "Holiday Heart": alcohol-associated cardiac rhythm disorders. Am Heart J. 1978;95(5):555–62.
2. Tonelo D, Providência R, Gonçalves L. Holiday heart syndrome revisited after 34 years. Arq Bras Cardiol. 2013;101(2):183–9.
3. Marcus GM, Vittinghoff E, Whitman IR, et al. Acute consumption of alcohol and discrete atrial fibrillation events. Ann Intern Med. 2021;174(11):1503–9.
4. Lugovskaya N, Vinson DR. Paroxysmal atrial fibrillation and brain freeze: a case of recurrent co-incident precipitation from a frozen beverage. Am J Case Rep. 2016;17:23–6.
5. Vinson DR. Redressing under recognition of "Cold Drink Heart": patients teaching physicians about atrial fibrillation triggered by cold drink and food. Perm J. 2020;24:19.238.

92. Correct Answer: C

Rationale
Investigators at a large integrated health system attempted to identify persons likely to be under-reporters by using all available information in a large, computerized data base. This included people with diagnoses such as acute alcoholic intoxication and alcoholic cirrhosis and were light to moderate drinkers who reported light to moderate drinking on the index exam by heavy drinking on other occasion.

Underreporting of alcohol intake can place heavy drinkers into the same category and health outcomes of light to moderate drinkers. Studies have shown that underreporting can lead to a false increase in risk and a false lower threshold.

In view of the obvious harm that uncontrolled drinking causes to many people, it is difficult to construct a model in which underreporting produces an inverse alcohol health relationship. Many alcohol researchers found it difficult to accept the possibility of health benefits. Thus, the lower risk of atherosclerotic disease was controversial from the time of the first reports in the 1970s. Prospective data from many studies were consistent and specific, though skeptics questioned the methodology on the basis of misclassifications. Contamination of an abstainer reference group by past heavy drinkers who became ill could produce a spurious inverse relationship. This explanation, sometimes called the "Sick Quitter Hypothesis," has been refuted by many studies that separated past drinkers from life-long abstainers. The inverse relationship between light drinkers and life-long abstainers persisted in virtually all of these.

Thus, the available data do not support the hypothesis that misclassification of the risk of some subjects because of alcohol related illness, under reported drinking amount, or residual confounding by smoking to result in false relationships because of modified reference groups.

Answers

References
1. Klatsky AL, Udaltsova N, Li Y, Baer D, Nicole Tran H, Friedman GD. Moderate alcohol intake and cancer: the role of underreporting. Cancer Causes Control. 2014;25(6):693–9.
2. Klatsky AL, Gunderson EP, Kipp H, Udaltsova N, Friedman GD. Higher prevalence of systemic hypertension among moderate alcohol drinkers: an exploration of the role of underreporting. J Stud Alcohol. 2006;67(3):421–8.
3. Klatsky AL. Alcohol and cardiovascular diseases: where do we stand today? J Intern Med. 2015;278(3):238–50.

93. Correct Answer: D

Rationale
According to the "Dietary Guidelines for Americans 2020–2025," US Department of Health and Human Services and US Department of Agriculture, adults of legal drinking age can choose not to drink or to drink in moderation by limiting intake to two drinks or less in a day for men and one drink or less in a day for women, when alcohol is consumed. Drinking less is better for health than drinking more.

All definitions of heavy drinking are arbitrary. NIAAA (National Institute of Alcohol Abuse and Alcoholism) defines this for men as more than 14 drinks per week. For women, this is defined as consuming more than three drinks on any day or more than seven drinks per week.

The different definitions for heavy alcohol drinking in men and women are due to more rapid absorption in the upper GI tract and the smaller body size and increased fat distribution.

Reference
1. https://www.niaaa.nih.gov/alcohol-health/overview-alcohol-consumption/moderate-binge-drinking

94. Correct Answer: A

Rationale
Elevated Lipoprotein (a) [Lp(a)] is the most common monogenic cause of ASCVD. Screening for elevated Lp(a) (lipoprotein [a]) should be considered at least once in each adult person's lifetime to identify those with very high inherited Lp(a) levels who may be at an elevated risk for ASCVD.

Reference
1. Wilson DP, Jacobson TA, Jones PH, et al. Use of lipoprotein(a) in clinical practice: a biomarker whose time has come. A scientific statement from the National Lipid Association. J Clin Lipidol. 2019;13:374–92.

95. Correct Answer: D

Rationale
The estimated global prevalence of elevated Lp(a) is approximately 20%.

Reference

1. Tsimikas S, Fazio S, Ferdinand KC, et al. NHLBI working group recommendations to reduce lipoprotein(a)-mediated risk of cardiovascular disease and aortic stenosis. J Am Coll Cardiol. 2018;71:177–92.

96. Correct Answer: B

Rationale

In a patient with the clinical phenotype of familial hypercholesterolemia (FH), a negative DNA genetic test to identify pathogenic variants of LDLR, APOB, or PCSK9 does not exclude a diagnosis of FH. It is likely that patients with phenotypic FH who have negative genetic testing for FH may have an unidentified FH mutation. Thus, many clinicians choose to utilize clinical diagnostic criteria based upon AHA, Simon Broome, and/or Dutch Lipid Clinic Network criteria over genetic testing to diagnose FH.

Reference

1. Sturm AC, Knowles JW, Gidding SS, et al. Clinical genetic testing for familial hypercholest-erolemia: JACC scientific expert panel. J Am Coll Cardiol. 2018;72:662–80.

97. Correct Answer: B

Rationale

The reduction in ASCVD risk is not only dependent upon the degree of LDL (low-density lipoprotein)-C lowering but also the timing when lipid treatment is implemented. Earlier statin initiation may reduce the lifetime exposure and burden of elevated LDL-C, with the age for onset of coronary heart disease delayed by earlier administration of statin therapy. Statin treatment should strongly be considered in patients with heterozygous familial hypercholesterolemia beginning at 8–10 years of age.

Reference

1. Nordestgaard BG, Chapman MJ, Humphries SE, et al. Familial hypercholesterolaemia is underdiagnosed and undertreated in the general population: guidance for clinicians to prevent coronary heart disease: consensus statement of the European Atherosclerosis Society. Eur Heart J. 2013;34:3478–90a.

98. Correct Answer: C

Rationale

There are data to support the use of L-arginine, beetroot, and cocoa flavonoids, among others, in the integrative approach to hypertension treatment. Red yeast rice is most commonly used for treatment of hyperlipidemia and does not have data to support its use in hypertension.

References
1. Wong AP, Kassab YW, Mohamed AL, Qader AMA. Beyond conventional therapies: complementary and alternative medicine in the management of hypertension: an evidence-based review. Pak J Pharm Sci. 2018;31:237–44
2. Therapeutic Research Center. Natural medicines [database on the Internet]. 2020. https://naturalmedicines.therapeuticresearch.com. Accessed 19 Apr 2020.

99. Correct Answer: F

Rationale
Acupuncture is described to increase endogenous opioid production and improve autonomic dysregulation. Further data is required to understand these mechanisms in more detail.

References
1. Pomeranz B. Scientific basis of acupuncture. In: Pomeranz B, Stux G, editors. Basics of acupuncture. Berlin: Springer; 1989. p. 4–55.
2. Mehta P, Polk D, Zhang X. A randomized controlled trial of acupuncture in stable ischemic heart disease patients. Int J Cardiol. 2014;176:376–4.
3. Longhurst J. Acupuncture's cardiovascular actions: a mechanistic perspective. Med Acupunct. 2013;25:101–13.

100. Correct Answer: D

Rationale
Exercise (at least 150 min of moderate intensity aerobic exercise) and the Mediterranean diet have demonstrated benefits for treatment of high cholesterol. Berberine can be used as an adjunctive therapy and also can improve regulation of blood glucose. While chelation therapy has been shown to decrease cardiovascular events, especially in those with diabetes, it is not currently approved as a modality for primary prevention in the setting of hyperlipidemia.

References
1. Banach M, Patti AM, Giglio RV, et al. on behalf of the International Lipid Expert Panel (ILEP). The role of nutraceuticals in statin intolerant patients. J Am Coll Cardiol. 2018;72:96–118.
2. Dans AL, Tan FN, Villarruz-Sulit EC. Chelation therapy for atherosclerotic cardiovascular disease (review). Cochrane Database Syst Rev. 2010;2010:1–21.
3. Arnett DK, Blumenthal RS, Albert MA, et al. 2019 ACC/AHA guideline on the primary prevention of cardiovascular disease: a report of the American College of Cardiology/American Heart Association task force on clinical practice guidelines. J Am Coll Cardiol. 2019;74:e177–232.

101. Correct Answer: B

Rationale

The DASH diet can help attain many of these goals with its focus on the consumption of low sodium (<2000 mg/day), fruits, vegetables, and low-fat dairy and was found to reduce SBP and DBP by 5.5 and 3 mmHg, respectively.

Reference

1. Appel LJ, Moore TJ, Obarzanek E, et al., for the DASH Collaborative Research Group. A clinical trial of the effects of dietary patterns on blood pressure. N Engl J Med. 1997;336:1117–24.

102. Correct Answer: B

Rationale

The ISCHEMIA trial found that in stable patients with at least moderate ischemia on a stress test that an invasive strategy was associated with more myocardial infarctions (MIs) in early follow-up due to procedural MIs, fewer MIs later on due to fewer spontaneous MIs, but no statistical overall reduction in MIs compared with conservative management. Patients who had angina had better quality of life with invasive management. The take home points from the trial are that in patients who met eligibility criteria for entry in the trial, the clear benefit from revascularization was less angina. If he has persistent angina after optimizing antianginal therapy and he is not satisfied with his quality of life, he should be advised that revascularization is likely to improve his symptoms. There is no hard rule about how long medical therapy should be tried before advancing to cath and revascularization, but all patients should be started on guideline-directed medical therapy whether or not they pursue revascularization. Although he is likely to have better symptom control with revascularization, this will not reduce his overall chances of death or MI. As in COURAGE, in ISCHEMIA there was no relationship between severity of ischemia and risk of events.

References

1. Maron DJ, Hochman JS, Reynolds HR, et al. Initial invasive or conservative strategy for stable coronary disease. N Engl J Med. 2020;382:1395–407.
2. Spertus JA, Jones PG, Maron DJ, et al. Health-status outcomes with invasive or conservative care in coronary disease. N Engl J Med. 2020;382:1408–19.
3. Reynolds HR, Shaw LJ, Min JK, et al. Outcomes in the ISCHEMIA trial based on coronary artery disease and ischemia severity. Circulation. 2021. https://doi.org/10.1161/CIRCULATIONAHA.120.049755.

103. Correct Answer: D

Rationale
The guideline for the prevention, detection, evaluation, and management of high blood pressure in adults recommends nonpharmacologic therapy for patients with stage 1 hypertension (systolic BP 130–139 mmHg or diastolic BP 80–89 mmHg) and a 10-year ASCVD risk <10%, with repeat evaluation in 3–6 months. The rationale for this approach is that the combination of lifestyle changes including weight loss, adoption of the DASH diet, a reduction in sodium and alcohol consumption, an increase in potassium intake, and an increase in physical activity can lower blood pressure to an optimal range for people with Stage 1 hypertension. Initiation of pharmacologic therapy is recommended for patients with Stage 1 hypertension who have a 10-year ASCVD risk ≥10% or for patients who have Stage 2 hypertension systolic BP ≥140 mmHg or diastolic BP ≥90 mmHg.

Reference
1. Whelton PK, Carey RM, Aronow WS, et al. 2017 ACC/AHA/AAPA/ABC/ACPM/AGS/APhA/ASH/ASPC/NMA/PCNA guideline for the prevention, detection, evaluation, and management of high blood pressure in adults: a report of the American College of Cardiology/American Heart Association task force on clinical practice guidelines. Hypertension. 2018;71:e13–115.

104. Correct Answer: D

Rationale
According to the AHA/ACC Guideline on the Management of Blood Cholesterol, in patients with severe primary hypercholesterolemia (LDL-C [low density lipoprotein cholesterol]) level ≥190 mg/dL), if the LDL-C level remains ≥100 mg/dL on high-intensity statin plus ezetimibe and the patient has multiple factors that increase subsequent risk of ASCVD (arteriosclerotic cardiovascular disease) events, a PCSK9 inhibitor may be considered. A is not correct because stress testing is not recommended for asymptomatic patients or for patients with high coronary artery calcium scores. B is not correct because neither CT nor invasive coronary angiography is recommended for asymptomatic patients or for patients with high coronary artery calcium scores. C is not correct because although bempedoic acid lowers LDL-C, it would not lower it sufficiently to achieve an LDL-C <100 mg/dL starting from an LDL-C of 152 mg/dL.

Reference
1. Grundy SM, Stone NJ, Bailey AL, et al. 2018 AHA/ACC/AACVPR/AAPA/ABC/ACPM/ADA/AGS/APhA/ASPC/NLA/PCNA guideline on the management of blood cholesterol. J Am Coll Cardiol. 2018. https://doi.org/10.1016/j.jacc.2018.11.003.

105. Correct Answer: A

Rationale
The SCOT-HEART trial found that an initial evaluation for chest pain that incorporated coronary CT angiography in addition to standard care was associated with a 41% lower rate of death from coronary artery disease or nonfatal myocardial infarction after almost 5 years of follow-up as compared with standard care alone. This observed lower rate of events has been attributed to the higher rate of initiation of preventive interventions in the group that underwent coronary CT angiography, including the initiation of statin therapy. Statin therapy is also recommended by AHA/ACC cholesterol management guidelines for patients 55 years and older at intermediate risk who have a CAC score of 1–99. B is not correct because obstructive disease has already been ruled out effectively by the CT angiogram. Similarly, C is not correct because invasive angiography is not indicated to rule out obstructive disease after having the CT angiogram results. D is not correct because preventive therapies should be initiated when nonobstructive coronary disease is documented. Reassurance alone is not adequate.

References
1. The SCOT-HEART Investigators. Coronary CT angiography and 5-year risk of myocardial infarction. N Engl J Med. 2018; 379:924–933.
2. Grundy SM, Stone NJ, Bailey AL. 2018 AHA/ACC/AACVPR/AAPA/ABC/ACPM/ADA/AGS/APhA/ASPC/NLA/PCNA guideline on the management of blood cholesterol. J Am Coll Cardiol. 2018. https://doi.org/10.1016/j.jacc.2018.11.003.

106. Correct Answer: C

Rationale
The ACC/AHA Primary Prevention Guidelines recommend at least 150 min/week of moderate-intensity physical activity (PA) or 75 min/week of vigorous activity or combination (where 1 min of vigorous activity equals 2 min of moderate intensity) [1]. The Department of Health and Human Services recommends 150–300 min/week of moderate-intensity or 75–150 min vigorous-intensity activity [2]. Thus, answer A is wrong. In a pooled analysis of two large prospective cohort studies, the lowest risk of mortality was actually seen among participants who reported two to four times the recommended minimum of leisure time activity (meaning 300–599 min/week of moderate-intensity and 150–299 min/week of vigorous-intensity) without further incremental benefit beyond that point [3]. Importantly though even higher levels of activity beyond this was not associated with increased harm. However, meta-analyses have shown that even some activity, even less than recommended, is beneficial compared to being sedentary [3, 4], so B is wrong. This is why the ACC/AHA guidelines additional state that for adults unable to meet the

minimum recommended amount that engaging in some moderate- or vigorous-intensity PA, even if less than recommended, can be beneficial to reduce ASCVD [1]. Sedentary behavior confers risk even among those who are active (although attenuated) [5] so D is wrong. Counseling is effective in increasing physical activity behavior in randomized controlled trials, with a number needed to treat (with counseling) of only 12 to achieve 1 additional sedentary individual to meet PA recommendations [6]. Therefore, E is wrong. C is the correct answer—fitness is associated with survival even in older adults. In fact, in older adults, fitness was prognostic of mortality risk regardless of CVD risk factor burden, whereas traditional risk factors were not [7].

References
1. Arnett DK, Blumenthal RS, Albert MA, et al. 2019 ACC/AHA guideline on the primary prevention of cardiovascular disease: executive summary: a report of the American College of Cardiology/American Heart Association task force on clinical practice guidelines. Circulation. 2019;140:e563–95.
2. Piercy KL, Troiano RP, Ballard RM, et al. The physical activity guidelines for Americans. JAMA. 2018;320:2020–8.
3. Lee DH, Rezende LFM, Joh HK, et al. Long-term leisure-time physical activity intensity and all-cause and cause-specific mortality: a prospective cohort of US adults. Circulation. 2022.
4. Sattelmair J, Pertman J, Ding EL, et al.. Dose response between physical activity and risk of coronary heart disease: a meta-analysis. Circulation. 2011;124:789–95.
5. Biswas A, Oh PI, Faulkner GE, et al. Sedentary time and its association with risk for disease incidence, mortality, and hospitalization in adults: a systematic review and meta-analysis. Ann Intern Med. 2015;162:123–32.
6. Orrow G, Kinmonth AL, Sanderson S, Sutton S. Effectiveness of physical activity promotion based in primary care: systematic review and meta-analysis of randomised controlled trials. BMJ. 2012;344:e1389.
7. Whelton SP, McAuley PA, Dardari Z, et al. Fitness and mortality among persons 70 years and older across the spectrum of cardiovascular disease risk factor burden: the FIT project. Mayo Clinic Proc. 2021;96:2376–85.

107. Correct Answer: A

Rationale
The Dept of Health and Human services recommended muscle strengthening activities in addition to PA. Answer B is wrong because moderate-intensity activity achieves cardiovascular benefit, PA does not have to be vigorous to have benefit. In the aforementioned pooled cohort analysis, among individuals achieving ≥300 min/week of moderate-intensity PA, additional vigorous-intensity PA did not appear to be associated with lower mortality beyond the moderate-intensity. In sum the findings suggest that any combination of moderate-intensity or vigorous-intensity, providing sufficient volume, can provide nearly the same maximum mortality reduction. Answer C is wrong, as moderate intensity is defined as 3–5.9 METs with vigorous

being ≥6 METs. Healthy adults do not need medical screening before starting exercise, only those with cardiovascular symptoms, so answer D is wrong. Answer E is wrong, because even trading sedentary behavior for light activity is associated with lower mortality risk—all steps count.

References
1. Piercy KL, Troiano RP, Ballard RM, et al. The physical activity guidelines for Americans. JAMA. 2018;320:2020–8.
2. Lee DH, Rezende LFM, Joh HK, et al. Long-term leisure-time physical activity intensity and all-cause and cause-specific mortality: a prospective cohort of US adults. Circulation. 2022.
3. Beddhu S, Wei G, Marcus RL, et al. Light-intensity physical activities and mortality in the United States general population and CKD subpopulation. Clin J Am Soc Nephrol. 2015;10:1145–53.

108. Correct Answer: B

Rationale
Using the Pooled Cohort Risk Equations, this patient has an estimated 10-year ASCVD risk of 5.1% which places her at "borderline" risk. Therefore, answer A is incorrect. However, she is at high lifetime risk of 39%. Furthermore, she has several risk-enhancing factors, including South Asian ethnicity, premature menopause, a pregnancy associated condition associated with increased ASCVD risk (gestational diabetes), and family history of premature coronary artery disease. Although PCOS was not specifically mentioned in the 2019 ACC/AHA Primary Prevention Guideline as a risk enhancer, this is also associated with increased CVD risk in women. In the setting of borderline risk with risk enhancing factors, statin therapy for prevention can be considered (Class IIb recommendation). If there is still uncertainty about risk and the net benefit of statin therapy, a CAC score is reasonable to guideline clinician-patient risk decisions (Class IIa recommendation). Therefore, B is the correct answer. With a 10-year risk score of 5.1% the patient is not considered "high-risk"; furthermore, stress testing is not indicated in asymptomatic individuals. Therefore, answer C is incorrect. Aspirin therapy is not routinely recommended for primary prevention. If patients are at higher ASCVD risk with a low risk of bleeding, aspirin therapy may be considered with a Class IIb recommendation. Therefore, answer D is incorrect. A CAC score ≥100 might be considered as a threshold at enough elevated risk to have a favorable net benefit level for aspirin therapy in primary prevention if bleeding risk is otherwise low. However, in this question, the CAC score has not yet been provided.

References
1. Arnett DK, Blumenthal RS, Albert MA, et al. 2019 ACC/AHA guideline on the primary prevention of cardiovascular disease: executive summary: a report of the American College of Cardiology/American Heart Association task force on clinical practice guidelines. Circulation. 2019;140:e563–95.

2. Guan C, Zahid S, Minhas AS, et al. Polycystic ovary syndrome: a "risk-enhancing" factor for cardiovascular disease. Fertil Steril. 2022;117:924–35.
3. Cainzos-Achirica M, Miedema MD, McEvoy JW, et al. Coronary artery calcium for personalized allocation of aspirin in primary prevention of cardiovascular disease in 2019: the MESA Study (Multi-Ethnic Study of Atherosclerosis). Circulation. 2020;141:1541–53.
4. Orringer CE, Blaha MJ, Blankstein R, et al. The National Lipid Association scientific statement on coronary artery calcium scoring to guide preventive strategies for ASCVD risk reduction. J Clin Lipidol. 2021;15:33–60.

109. Correct Answer: F

Rationale
Women may experience unique reproductive risk factors throughout their lifespan, that men do not experience, that may be "risk-enhancing" factors that elevate their CVD risk. This includes menarche when early <12 or late >17 compared to normal menarche at age 12–13. Therefore, answer F is wrong because this is normal age of menarche. Additionally, polycystic ovary syndrome, infertility, spontaneous pregnancy loss, multi-parity, adverse pregnancy outcomes (like preeclampsia and gestational diabetes), lack of breastfeeding, and early menopause (before age 45) have all been associated with elevated CV [cardiovascular] risks, for the rest of the answers are correct.

References
1. Guan C, Zahid S, Minhas AS, et al. Polycystic ovary syndrome: a "risk-enhancing" factor for cardiovascular disease. Fertil Steril. 2022;117:924–35.
2. Elder P, Sharma G, Gulati M, Michos ED. Identification of female-specific risk enhancers throughout the lifespan of women to improve cardiovascular disease prevention. Am J Prev Cardiol. 2020;2:100028.
3. O'Kelly AC, Michos ED, Shufelt CL, et al. Pregnancy and reproductive risk factors for cardiovascular disease in women. Circ Res. 2022;130:652–72.
4. Okoth K, Chandan JS, Marshall T, et al. Association between the reproductive health of young women and cardiovascular disease in later life: umbrella review. BMJ. 2020;371:m3502.
5. Charalampopoulos D, McLoughlin A, Elks CE and Ong KK. Age at menarche and risks of all-cause and cardiovascular death: a systematic review and meta-analysis. Am J Epidemiol. 2014;180:29–40.
6. Yang L, Li L, Millwood IY, Peters SAE, et al. and China Kadoorie Biobank Study Collaborative Group. Age at menarche and risk of major cardiovascular diseases: evidence of birth cohort effects from a prospective study of 300,000 Chinese women. Int J Cardiol. 2017;227:497–502.
7. Zhang X, Liu L, Song F, et al. Ages at menarche and menopause, and mortality among postmenopausal women. Maturitas. 2019;130:50–6.
8. Canoy D, Beral V, Balkwill A, et al. and Million Women Study. Age at menarche and risks of coronary heart and other vascular diseases in a large UK cohort. Circulation. 2015;131:237–44.

9. Peters SA, Woodward M. Women's reproductive factors and incident cardiovascular disease in the UK Biobank. Heart (British Cardiac Society). 2018;104:1069–75.
10. Lau ES, Wang D, Roberts M, et al. Infertility and risk of heart failure in the Women's Health Initiative. J Am Coll Cardiol. 2022;79:1594–603.
11. Wang YX, Minguez-Alarcon L, Gaskins AJ, et al. Pregnancy loss and risk of cardiovascular disease: the Nurses' Health Study II. Eur Heart J. 2022;43:190–9.
12. Catov JM, Newman AB, Sutton-Tyrrell K, et al. Parity and cardiovascular disease risk among older women: how do pregnancy complications mediate the association? Ann Epidemiol. 2008;18:873–9.
13. Ness RB, Harris T, Cobb J, et al. Number of pregnancies and the subsequent risk of cardiovascular disease. N Engl J Med. 1993;328:1528–33.
14. Parikh NI, Cnattingius S, Dickman PW, et al. Parity and risk of later-life maternal cardiovascular disease. Am Heart J. 2010;159:215–21.e6.
15. Li W, Ruan W, Lu Z, Wang D. Parity and risk of maternal cardiovascular disease: a dose-response meta-analysis of cohort studies. Eur J Prev Cardiol. 2019;26:592–602.
16. Hauspurg A, Ying W, Hubel CA, et al. Adverse pregnancy outcomes and future maternal cardiovascular disease. Clin Cardiol. 2018;41:239–46.
17. Parikh NI, Gonzalez JM, Anderson CAM, et al., American Heart Association Council on E, Prevention, Council on Arteriosclerosis T, Vascular B, Council on C, Stroke N and the Stroke C. Adverse pregnancy outcomes and cardiovascular disease risk: unique opportunities for cardiovascular disease prevention in women: a scientific statement from the American Heart Association. Circulation. 2021;143:e902–16.
18. Tschiderer L, Seekircher L, Kunutsor SK, et al. Breastfeeding is associated with a reduced maternal cardiovascular risk: systematic review and meta-analysis involving data from 8 studies and 1 192 700 parous women. J Am Heart Assoc. 2022;11:e022746.
19. Wellons M, Ouyang P, Schreiner PJ, et al. Early menopause predicts future coronary heart disease and stroke: the Multi-Ethnic Study of Atherosclerosis. Menopause. 2012;19:1081–7.

110. Correct Answer: C

Rationale

Answer A is wrong. Although women are less likely to have obstructive CAD than men, studies have shown that even when accounting this, women are under-enrolled in trials relative to their disease burden in the population (i.e., lower participant to prevalence ratio).

Answer B is wrong. Black individuals represented only 4% of participants in cardiometabolic clinical trials, which is much lower than their US population census percentage of population (13%).

Answer C is correct. There is a correlation, albeit modest, between gender and racial/ethnic characteristics of study investigators and greater enrollment of diverse participants into clinical trials. Diversifying investigators and clinical trial staff may assist with connecting to the language, customs, and beliefs of study populations and increase recruitment of participants from diverse backgrounds.

Answer D is incorrect. In an analysis of NIH-sponsored CV clinical trials with published trial protocols, the majority of these trials did not specify a Black enrollment target, did not meet their targets, and largely did not report specific plans to enroll Black adults in their studies.

References
1. Michos ED, Reddy TK, Gulati M, et al. Improving the enrollment of women and racially/ethnically diverse populations in cardiovascular clinical trials: an ASPC practice statement. Am J Prev Cardiol. 2021;8:100250.
2. Khan SU, Khan MZ, Raghu Subramanian C, et al. Participation of women and older participants in randomized clinical trials of lipid-lowering therapies: a systematic review. JAMA Netw Open. 2020;3:e205202.
3. Khan MS, Shahid I, Siddiqi TJ, et al. Ten-year trends in enrollment of women and minorities in pivotal trials supporting recent US Food and Drug Administration approval of novel cardiometabolic drugs. J Am Heart Assoc. 2020;9:e015594.
4. Khan SU, Michos ED. Women in stroke trials—a tale of perpetual inequity in cardiovascular research. JAMA Neurol. 2021;78:654–6.
5. Khan SU, Raghu Subramanian C, et al. Association of women authors with women enrollment in clinical trials of atrial fibrillation. J Am Heart Assoc. 2022:e024233.
6. Reza N, Tahhan AS, Mahmud N, et al. Representation of women authors in international heart failure guidelines and contemporary clinical trials. Circ Heart Fail. 2020;13:e006605.
7. Whitelaw S, Thabane L, Mamas MA, et al. Characteristics of heart failure trials associated with under-representation of women as lead authors. J Am Coll Cardiol. 2020;76:1919–30.
8. Kelsey MD, Patrick-Lake B, Abdulai R, et al. Inclusion and diversity in clinical trials: actionable steps to drive lasting change. Contemp Clin Trials. 2022;116:106740.
9. Prasanna A, Miller HN, Wu Y, et al. Recruitment of Black adults into cardiovascular disease trials. J Am Heart Assoc. 2021;10:e021108.

111. Correct Answer: C

Rationale
Meta-analysis of statin therapy has shown that women benefit similar to men in MACE reduction, even in primary prevention. Therefore, answer A is incorrect. Eligible patients should be treated with statin therapy regardless of sex. Unfortunately, women are less likely be prescribed statins and are more likely to report statin associated muscle symptoms.

Women with FH [familial hypercholesterolemia] lose their female protection against CVD [cardiovascular disease] with the same age of onset of CVD as men. Early treatment is imperative in both men and women. Answer B is incorrect.

Answer C is correct. Indeed, better controlled studies have demonstrated no clear relationship of congenital anomalies with statin use in pregnancy. Statins are probably not teratogenic. Accordingly, the FDA [Food and Drug Administration] has recently lifted its highest risk warning about the use of statins in pregnancy. However, until more information is available, statins should generally be avoided in pregnancy due to insufficient data, but statins may be considered in the highest-risk women such as those with recent acute coronary syndrome (ACS), as part of shared decision making. Additionally, whether statins can reduce preeclampsia risk in pregnancy is an area of active study (NCT03944512).

Answer D is wrong. Ezetimibe confers similar LDL-C reduction in women as in men (about 16 mg/dL lowering), with similar (if not even greater) relative risk reduction in MACE than men among patients with ACS. In the IMPROVE trial of ezetimibe in ACS on a background of statin therapy, there was no significant interaction by sex (p-interaction 0.26). When the total number of primary events was considered, there was a trend for even greater MACE reduction in women [RR 0.81 (0.71–0.94) than men [RR 0.94 (0.87–1.02)], p-interaction by sex = 0.08.

Answer E is wrong. In the FOURIER trial, evolocumab reduced CV events to a similar degree in women; no interaction by sex. For the primary outcome, the HR for evolocumab compared to placebo was 0.81 (0.69–0.95) in women and 0.86 (0.80–0.94) in men, p-interaction for sex = 0.48.

References

1. Kostis WJ, Cheng JQ, Dobrzynski JM, et al. Meta-analysis of statin effects in women versus men. J Am Coll Cardiol. 2012;59:572–82.
2. Nanna MG, Wang TY, Xiang Q, Goldberg AC, Robinson JG, Roger VL, Virani SS, Wilson PWF, Louie MJ, Koren A, et al. Sex differences in the use of statins in community practice. Circ Cardiovasc Qual Outcomes. 2019;12:e005562.
3. Karalis DG, Wild RA, Maki KC, et al. Gender differences in side effects and attitudes regarding statin use in the Understanding Statin Use in America and Gaps in Patient Education (USAGE) study. J Clin Lipidol. 2016;10:833–41.
4. Ahmad Z, Li X, Wosik J, et al. Premature coronary heart disease and autosomal dominant hypercholesterolemia: increased risk in women with LDLR mutations. J Clin Lipidol. 2016;10:101–8.e1–3.
5. Krogh HW, Mundal L, Holven KB, Retterstol K. Patients with familial hypercholesterolaemia are characterized by presence of cardiovascular disease at the time of death. Eur Heart J. 2016;37:1398–405.
6. Karalis DG, Hill AN, Clifton S, Wild RA. The risks of statin use in pregnancy: a systematic review. J Clin Lipidol. 2016;10:1081–90.
7. Vahedian-Azimi A, Makvandi S, et al. Fetal toxicity associated with statins: a systematic review and meta-analysis. Atherosclerosis. 2021;327:59–67.
8. U.S. Food and Drug Administration. Statins: drug safety communication—FDA requests removal of strongest warning against using cholesterol-lowering statins during pregnancy.

Answers

112. Correct Answer: B

Rationale
Based on the 2019 National Lipid Association Scientific Statement, the use of icosapent ethyl is recommended for the lowering of ASCVD risk in patients aged ≥45 years with clinical ASCVD or aged ≥50 years with diabetes that require medication plus ≥1 additional risk factor and with fasting triglycerides 135–499 mg/dL while on high-intensity or maximally tolerated statin therapy. It does not recommend adding ezetimibe or a PCSK9 inhibitor in this situation nor changing his statin to a PCSK9 inhibitor or a different high-intensity statin.

Reference
1. Orringer CE, Jacobson TA, Maki KC. National Lipid Association scientific statement on the use of icosapent ethyl in statin-treated patients with elevated triglycerides and high or very-high ASCVD risk. J Clin Lipidol. 2019;13(6):860–72.

113. Correct Answer: A

Rationale
The use of dual antiplatelet therapy (aspirin and clopidogrel) may be considered for 21 days if initiated within 24 h after a minor stroke or high-risk TIA according to results of the CHANCE (Clopidogrel in High-Risk Patients with Acute Nondisabling Cerebrovascular Events) and POINT (Platelet-Oriented Inhibition in New TIA and Minor Ischemic Stroke) trials. The rate of recurrent stroke and major ischemic events was lower in the first 90 days when this regimen was used compared to aspirin monotherapy.

References
1. Wang Y, Wang Y, Zhao X, et al. CHANCE Investigators. Clopidogrel with aspirin in acute minor stroke or transient ischemic attack. N Engl J Med. 2013;369(1):11–9.
2. Johnston SC, Easton JD, Farrant M, et al; Clinical Research Collaboration, Neurological Emergencies Treatment Trials Network, and the POINT Investigators. Clopidogrel and aspirin in acute ischemic stroke and high-risk TIA. N Engl J Med. 2018;379(3):215–25.

114. Correct Answer: D

Rationale
In 2017, the AHA/ACC hypertension guideline defined hypertension as BP consistently ≥130/80 mmHg. The 2021 AHA/ASA secondary stroke guidelines support a goal BP <130/80 mmHg in neurologically stable patients in the outpatient setting.

The effect of intensive antihypertensive therapy for secondary prevention of stroke has been evaluated, as a primary outcome, in the SPS3 trial (Secondary Prevention of Small Subcortical Strokes) and RESPECT trial (Recurrent Stroke Prevention Clinical Outcome) and, as a secondary outcome, in the PAST-BP trial (Prevention After Stroke-Blood Pressure) and PODCAST (Prevention of Decline in Cognition After Stroke Trial). A meta-analysis of these 4 trials supports a benefit of treating patients with prior stroke or TIA to achieve a goal BP of <130/80 mmHg by showing a significant reduction in recurrent stroke risk with an intensive versus standard target (RR, 0.78 [95% CI, 0.64–0.96]). In addition, for those with a history of lacunar stroke such as in this patient, a systolic blood pressure lowering target of <130 mmHg is reasonable.

References
1. Whelton PK, Carey RM, Aronow WS, et al. 2017 ACC/AHA/AAPA/ABC/ACPM/AGS/APhA/ASH/ASPC/NMA/PCNA guideline for the prevention, detection, evaluation, and management of high blood pressure in adults: executive summary: a report of the American College of Cardiology/American Heart Association task force on clinical practice guidelines. Circulation. 2018;138(17):e426–83.
2. Kleindorfer DO, Towfighi A, Chaturvedi S, et al. 2021 guideline for the prevention of stroke in patients with stroke and transient ischemic attack: a guideline from the American Heart Association/American Stroke Association. Stroke. 2021;52(7):e364–467.
3. Gorelick PB, Whelton PK, Sorond F, Carey RM. Blood pressure management in stroke. Hypertension. 2020;76(6):1688–95.

115. Correct Answer: C

Rationale
Low-salt and Mediterranean diets are recommended for stroke risk reduction. In patients with stroke and TIA, it is reasonable to counsel individuals to follow a Mediterranean-type diet, typically with emphasis on monounsaturated fat, plant-based foods, and fish consumption, with either high extra virgin olive oil or nut supplementation, in preference to a low-fat diet, to reduce risk of recurrent stroke. It is also reasonable to recommend that individuals reduce their sodium intake by at least 1 g/day sodium (2.5 g/day salt) to reduce the risk of CVD events (including stroke). Decreasing rather than eliminating salt from the diet is recommended. While high potassium consumption is associated with lower stroke rates, there are currently no evidence supporting potassium-based interventions for stroke reduction. Even though adopting a diet low in saturated fat is beneficial, the consumption of certain monounsaturated fats such as found in nuts and fish are part of the Mediterranean diet and are recommended. There is no indication for significant caloric restriction intake in this case because his BMI is within normal.

References
1. Kleindorfer DO, Towfighi A, Chaturvedi S, et al. 2021 guideline for the prevention of stroke in patients with stroke and transient ischemic attack: a guideline from the American Heart Association/American Stroke Association. Stroke. 2021;52(7):e364–467.
2. Rees K, Takeda A, Martin N, et al. Mediterranean-style diet for the primary and secondary prevention of cardiovascular disease. Cochrane Database Syst Rev. 2019;3(3):CD009825.
3. He FJ, Tan M, Ma Y, MacGregor GA. Salt reduction to prevent hypertension and cardiovascular disease: JACC state-of-the-art review. J Am Coll Cardiol. 2020;75(6):632–47.
4. Vinceti M, Filippini T, Crippa A, et al. Meta-analysis of potassium intake and the risk of stroke. J Am Heart Assoc. 2016;5(10):e004210.

116. Correct Answer: D

Rationale
The 2019 AHA/ACC/Multisociety guideline on primary prevention of cardiovascular disease only recommends considering aspirin in "select adults 40–70 years of age who are at higher ASCVD (atherosclerotic cardiovascular disease) risk but not an increased bleeding risk." Persons over 70 and persons at increased bleeding risk should not be recommended aspirin for primary prevention.

Reference
1. Arnett DK, Blumenthal RS, Albert MA et al. 2019 ACC/AHA guideline on the primary prevention of cardiovascular disease: a report of the American College of Cardiology/American Heart Association task force on clinical practice guidelines. Circulation. 2019;140(11):e596–646.

117. Correct Answer: A

Rationale
Persons with myocardial infarction should be treated with dual antiplatelet therapy (P2Y$_{12}$ inhibitor + aspirin 75–100 mg daily) for at least 12 months, including those treated with medical therapy, bare metal or drug eluting stent, or coronary artery bypass surgery.

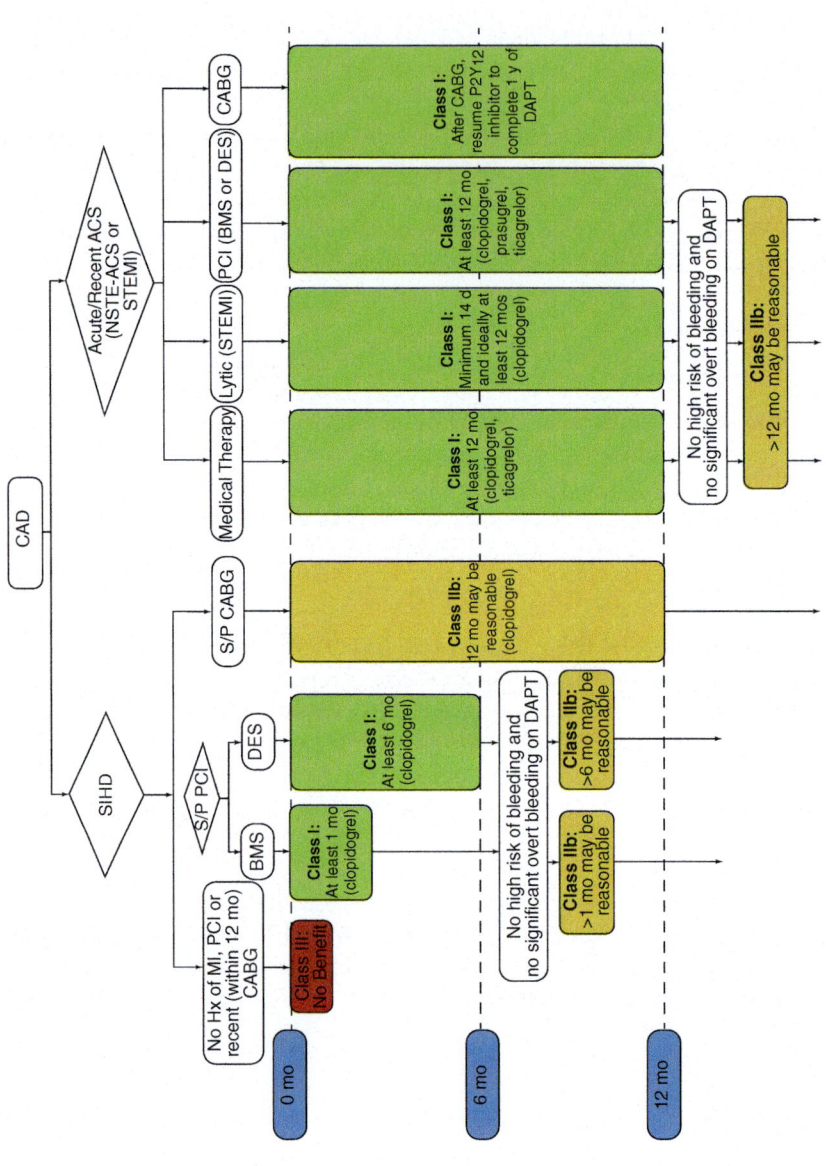

Master treatment algorithm for duration of P2Y$_{12}$ inhibitor therapy in patients with CAD treated with dual antiplatelet therapy. (Reproduced with permission from J Am Coll Cardiol. 2016 Sep, 68 (10) 1082–1115)

Reference
1. Levine GN Bates ER, Bittl JA, et al. 2016 ACC/AHA guideline focused update on duration of dual antiplatelet therapy in patients with coronary artery disease: a report of the American College of Cardiology/American Heart Association task force on clinical practice guidelines. J Am Coll Cardiol. 2016;68(10):1082–115.

118. Correct Answer: B

Rationale
In persons treated medically or with coronary stent implantation after acute coronary syndrome, ticagrelor may be preferred to clopidogrel. In those treated with stent implantation, prasugrel may be preferred over clopidogrel in those not at high bleeding risk and who do not have prior stroke or TIA [transient ischemic attack]. Prasugrel should not be given to persons with prior stroke or TIA due to increased risk of intracranial hemorrhage in persons with prior stroke or TIA in the TRITON-TIMI 38 trial. In persons requiring "triple therapy" (aspirin, P2Y12 inhibitor, and anticoagulant), clopidogrel is the $P2Y_{12}$ inhibitor of choice.

References
1. Montalescot G, Wiviott SD, Braunwald E, et al. Prasugrel compared with clopidogrel in patients undergoing percutaneous coronary intervention for ST-elevation myocardial infarction (TRITON-TIMI 38): double-blind, randomised controlled trial. Lancet. 2009;373:723.
2. Levine GN, et al. 2016 ACC/AHA guideline focused update on duration of dual antiplatelet therapy in patients with coronary artery disease: a report of the American College of Cardiology/American Heart Association task force on clinical practice guidelines. J Am Coll Cardiol. 2016;68(10):1082–115.

119. Correct Answer: B

Rationale
Bleeding risk should be evaluated to help guide choice and duration of both antiplatelet and antithrombotic therapy. Risk factors for bleeding include: history of prior bleeding, use of oral anticoagulation, older age, female sex, lower body weight, chronic kidney disease, diabetes, anemia, chronic steroid use, and chronic NSAID therapy.

Reference
1. Levine GN, Bates ER, Bittl JA, et al. 2016 ACC/AHA guideline focused update on duration of dual antiplatelet therapy in patients with coronary artery disease: a report of the American College of Cardiology/American Heart Association task force on clinical practice guidelines. J Am Coll Cardiol. 2016;68(10):1082–115.

120. Correct Answer: B

Rationale

Patients with chronic inflammatory diseases have an increased risk of major adverse cardiovascular events and cardiovascular mortality. The 2019 AHA/ACC/Multisociety guidelines state ASCVD risk is likely underestimated in these patients leading to potential undertreatment with pharmacological therapy. Further testing to document subclinical coronary disease (e.g., CAC scoring) in those considered at borderline or intermediate risk is appropriate to guide pharmacologic initiation. Given these patients have a higher prevalence of obesity and diabetes, counseling on diet and exercise is also important but should not be the sole intervention in this patient. This patient may benefit from statin therapy (A) but testing for subclinical atherosclerosis will help guide pharmacologic intervention and dosing.

Reference
1. Arnett DK, Blumenthal RS, Albert MA, et al. 2019 ACC/AHA guideline on the primary prevention of cardiovascular disease: executive summary: a report of the American College of Cardiology/American Heart Association task force on clinical practice guidelines. J Am Coll Cardiol. 2019;74(10):1376–414.

121. Correct Answer: D

Rationale

The CANTOS trial is a double blind RCT published in 2017 that enrolled over 10,000 patients with stable CAD under optimal cardiovascular treatment and hs-CRP levels >2 mg/L. Participants were randomized to receive either placebo or canakinumab, an anti-IL-1β antibody. Participants achieving levels of hs-CRP <2 mg/L after initiation of Canakinumab had a significant reduction in cardiovascular mortality. Importantly, Canakinumab did not affect circulating levels of circulating cholesterol. ESR (erythrocyte sedimentation rate) was not evaluated during this study.

Reference
1. Ridker PM, Everett BM, Thuren T, et al. CANTOS Trial Group. Antiinflammatory therapy with canakinumab for atherosclerotic disease. N Engl J Med. 2017;377(12):1119–31.

122. Correct Answer: C

Rationale

Inflammasomes are protein complexes that are responsible for the activation of inflammatory response. The NLRP3 inflammasome is well studied and highly prevalent in human coronary plaques. Its inhibition has been shown to blunt atherosclerosis in murine models and its activation has been shown to be proatherogenic. Canakinumab and colchicine both inhibit the NLRP3 inflammasome through different pathways. IL-1β reduction is a mechanism of canakinumab, and microtubule assembly disruption is a mechanism of Colchicine. Reduction of absolute immune cell counts is not a function of either therapy.

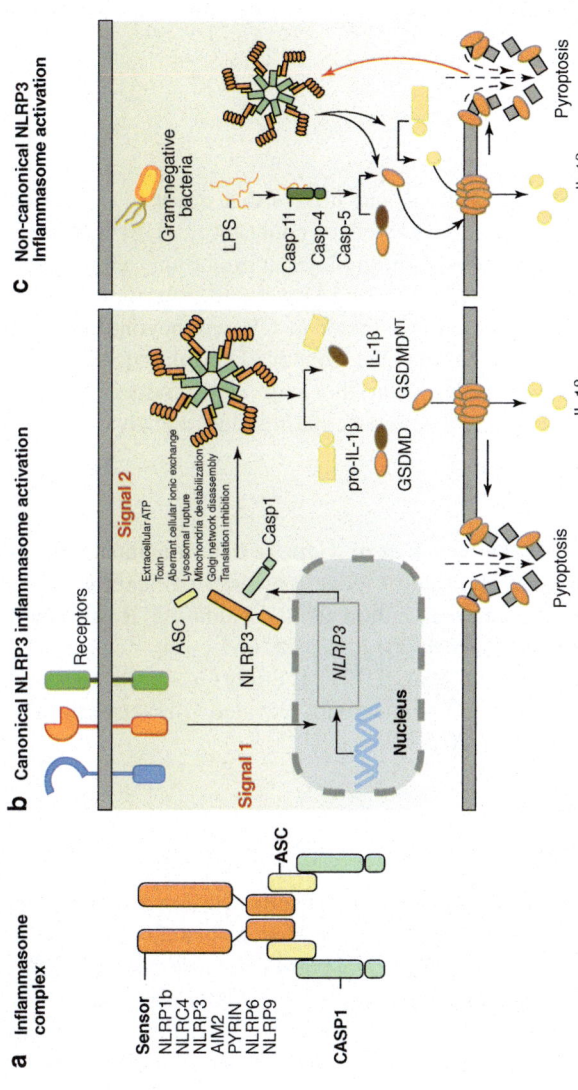

NLRP3 inflammasome assembly. (**a**) Inflammasome complex. Inflammasomes are composed of cytosolic sensors, which trigger caspase-1 activation. The identified cytosolic sensors are the NLR family pyrin domain-containing 1b (NLRP1b), NLR family CARD domain-containing protein 4 (NLRC4), and NLR family pyrin domain-containing 3 (NLRP3), absent in melanoma-2 (AIM2) receptor and pyrin receptor (PYRIN), NLR family pyrin domain-containing 6 (NLRP6) and NLR family pyrin domain-containing 9 (NLRP9). First, the sensors recruit the adaptor apoptosis-associated speck-like protein containing a CARD (ASC) via domain–domain (PYRIN-PYRIN) interaction. Then, ASC recruits and interacts with the caspase-1 CARD domain by domain–domain interaction, resulting in the assembly of a functionally mature inflammasome. (**b**) Canonical NLRP3 inflammasome activation. The canonical NLRP3 inflammasome requires two parallel and complementary steps: (1) priming (signal 1) after sensing invaders or sterile insult, which induces the transcription of NLRP3 inflammasome components (NLRP3, pro-IL1β, …) and (2) activation, which results in the assembly of the NLRP3 inflammasome, Gasdermin D (GSDMD)-dependent pore formation, pyroptosis, and IL-1β release. (**c**) Noncanonical NLRP3 inflammasome activation. The non-canonical NLRP3 inflammasome is engaged in response to Gram-negative bacteria by the binding of LPS on the protease caspase-11 (mouse) or caspase-4/-5 (human). Activated caspase-11 or caspase-4/-5 cleaves GSDMD and induces pore formation, potassium efflux, culminating in NLRP3 inflammasome activation. (Figure and legend reproduced with permission from Paget et al. *Cells* **2022**, *11*(7), 1188; https://doi.org/10.3390/cells11071188)

References
1. Guo H, Callaway JB, Ting JP. Inflammasomes: mechanism of action, role in disease, and therapeutics. Nat Med. 2015;21(7):677–87.
2. Pandey A, Shen C, Feng S, Man SM. Cell biology of inflammasome activation. Trends Cell Biol. 2021;31(11):924–39.
3. Paget C, Doz-Deblauwe E, Winter N, Briard B. Specific NLRP3 inflammasome assembling and regulation in neutrophils: relevance in inflammatory and infectious diseases. Cells. 2022;11(7):1188.

123. Correct Answer: B

Rationale
More than half of the myocardial infarctions and strokes that occur in the United States occur in patients with average or low levels of cholesterol. JUPITER was a primary prevention study that found inflammation plays an important role in potentiating MACE in those with low LDL-C. A, C, and D were all important findings that supported inflammation as a residual risk factor in CV risk beyond dyslipidemia. Indeed, a follow-up study found that the genetic determinants of statin-induced hs-CRP reduction are different from those of statin-induced LDL-C reduction [1] suggesting different pathways impact statin induced changes in lipid and inflammatory markers.

References
1. Chasman DI, Giulianini F, MacFadyen J, et al. Genetic determinants of statin-induced low-density lipoprotein cholesterol reduction: the Justification for the Use of Statins in Prevention: an Intervention Trial Evaluating Rosuvastatin (JUPITER) trial. Circ Cardiovasc Genet. 2012;5(2):257–64.
2. Ridker PM, Danielson E, Fonseca FA, et al. JUPITER Study Group. Rosuvastatin to prevent vascular events in men and women with elevated C-reactive protein. N Engl J Med. 2008;359(21):2195–207.

124. Correct Answer: D

Rationale
IL-6 is a cytokine pivotal to the immune system and is activated downstream of the NLRP3 inflammasome. In CANTOS, the degree of clinical benefit was directly related to the degree IL-6 was reduced by individual participants, suggesting inhibition of IL-6 may be atheroprotective. Indeed, those who achieved greater than median reduction in IL-6 after canakinumab induction had a 36% decrease in MACE.

Reference
1. Ridker PM, Everett BM, Thuren T, et al. CANTOS Trial Group. Antiinflammatory therapy with canakinumab for atherosclerotic disease. N Engl J Med. 2017;377(12):1119–31.

Answers   155

125. Correct Answer: A

Rationale

Psoriasis is a chronic inflammatory condition associated with increased risk of premature major adverse cardiovascular events (MACE) and cardiovascular mortality. Several studies have found patients with moderate-severe psoriasis have similar risk of MACE as those with known diabetes. The 2018 AHA/ACC/multisociety guidelines suggest chronic inflammatory diseases as risk-enhancing factors. Recent studies including and [2] found treatment with biologic therapy reduced noncalcified coronary plaque and lipid-rich necrotic core over 1 year. Both coronary markers are strongly associated with increased risk of MACE. The same cardioprotective benefit has not been found in those on topical/phototherapy treatments alone, suggesting early initiation of biologic therapy may benefit patients with severe psoriasis.

References
1. Elnabawi YA, Dey AK, Goyal A, et al. Coronary artery plaque characteristics and treatment with biologic therapy in severe psoriasis: results from a prospective observational study. Cardiovasc Res. 2019;115(4):721–8.
2. Choi H, Uceda DE, Dey AK, et al. Treatment of psoriasis with biologic therapy is associated with improvement of coronary artery plaque lipid-rich necrotic core: results from a prospective, observational study. Circ Cardiovasc Imaging. 2020;13(9):e011199.

126. Correct Answer: A

Rationale

The KDIGO guideline recommends initiating a sodium glucose transport protein inhibitor (SGLT2i) for patients with Type 2 diabetes and CKD across all albuminuria levels and eGFR stages ($\geq$30 mL/min per 1.73 m^2), but especially among those with uACR >200 mg/g. This can be safely done by exchanging the dipeptidyl peptidase-4 inhibitor (DPP-4) for the SGLT-2i without exposing the patient to (unlikely) hypoglycemia.

Reference
1. Zoungas S, de Boer IH. SGLT2 inhibitors in diabetic kidney disease. Clin J Am Soc Nephrol. 2021;16(4):631–3.

127. Correct Answer: C

Rationale

Kidney Disease Improving Global Outcomes (KDIGO) recommends patients >50 years old with >stage II CKD (but not ESKD) be treated with a statin ± ezetimibe. KDIGO recommends using formulations and doses of statins that were studied in clinical trials enrolling CKD populations (i.e., atorvastatin 20 mg (4D Trial) or rosuvastatin 10 mg (AURORA)). As per the SHARP trial, the addition of ezetimibe to a statin (simvastatin in the case of the trial) reduced LDL-C by 32% and was associated with a 17% reduction in the MACE composite.

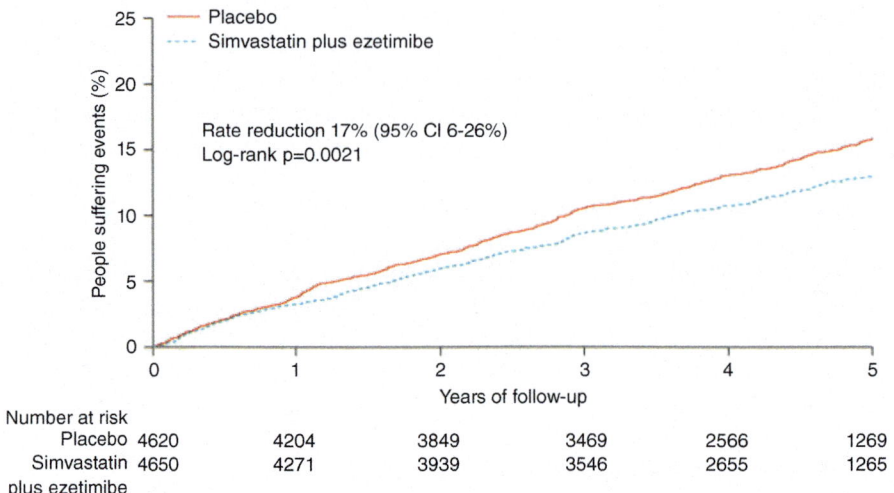

Life-table plot of effects of allocation to simvastatin plus ezetimibe versus placebo on major atherosclerotic events in the SHARP trial. (Reproduced with permission from Lancet 2011; 25;377(9784):2181–92)

References
1. Kidney Disease: Improving Global Outcomes (KDIGO) Lipid Work Group. KDIGO clinical practice guideline for lipid management in chronic kidney disease. Kidney Int. 2013;3:259–305.
2. Baigent C, Landray MJ, Reith C, et al. The SHARP Investigators. The effects of lowering LDL cholesterol with simvastatin plus ezetimibe in patients with chronic kidney disease (Study of Heart and Renal Protection): a randomised placebo-controlled trial. Lancet. 2011;377(9784):2181–92.

128. Correct Answer: C

Rationale

KDIGO guidelines recommend treating all adult kidney transplant patients with a statin, regardless of age. This data comes from the ALERT trial which randomized patients to fluvastatin or placebo and showed a 38% reduction in cardiac death despite missing its primary MACE endpoint.

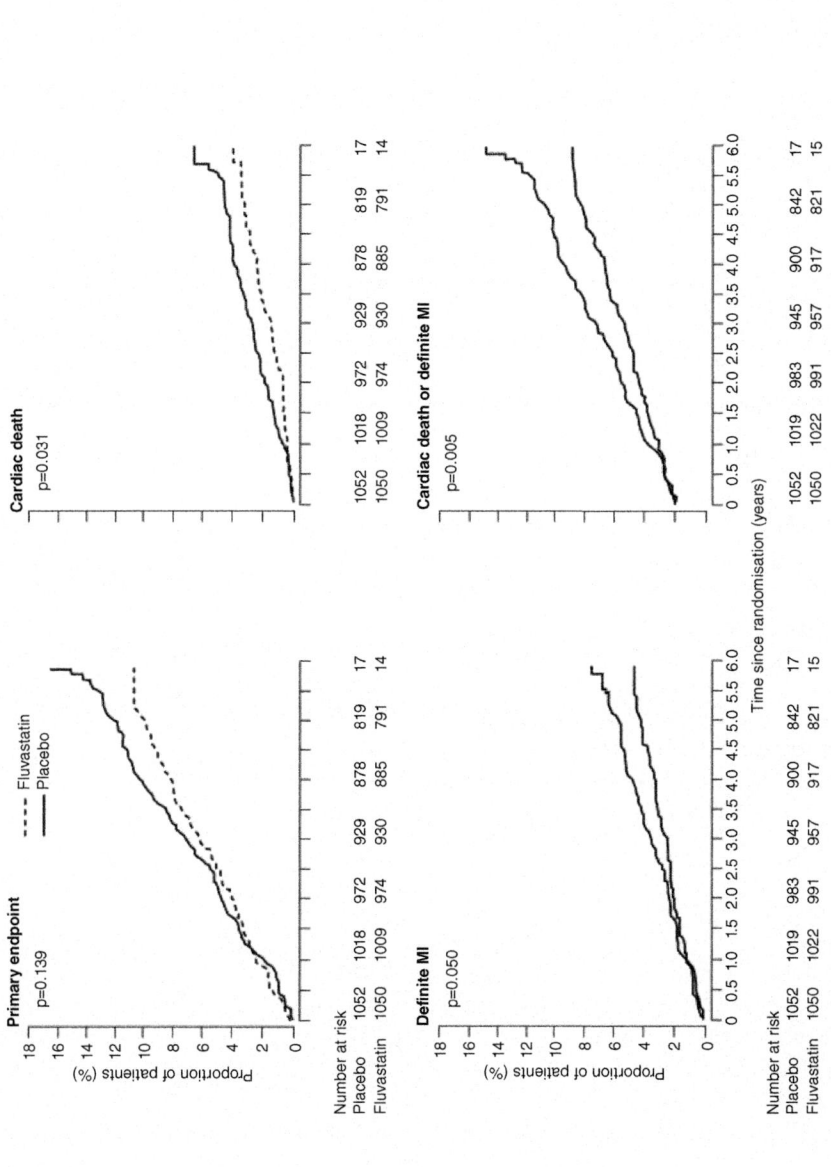

Cumulative rates for primary composite endpoints. Analyses by intention-to-treat and stratified by country and coronary heart disease status at baseline. (Reproduced with permission from Holdaas et al. Lancet. 2003 Jun 14;361(9374):2024–31)

References
1. Kidney Disease: Improving Global Outcomes (KDIGO) Lipid Work Group. KDIGO clinical practice guideline for lipid management in chronic kidney disease. Kidney Int. 2013;3:259–305.
2. Holdaas H, Fellström B, Jardine AG, et al. Assessment of LEscol in Renal Transplantation (ALERT) Study Investigators. Effect of fluvastatin on cardiac outcomes in renal transplant recipients: a multicentre, randomised, placebo-controlled trial. Lancet. 2003;361(9374):2024–31.

129. Correct Answer: C

Rationale
Over ¼ of patients commencing an SGLT-2i will experience an acute dip in eGFR after the first 4 weeks. Outcome data reveal that patients who experience a dip of <20% in their eGFR after commencement of SGLT-2i are not at increased risk of AKI. The drop in eGFR relates to restoration of tubuloglomerular feedback and is protective long-term and SGLT-2i do not cause electrolyte disturbance as can occur with ACE/ARB commencement. Patients who experience a dip do not have no long-term sequelae and do not require further monitoring and should have their SGLT-2i continued. Routine checks of eGFR are not required in patients commencing SGLT-2i unless there is heightened concerned for AKI.

References
1. Kraus BJ, Weir MR, Bakris GL, et al. Characterization and implications of the initial estimated glomerular filtration rate 'dip' upon sodium-glucose cotransporter-2 inhibition with empagliflozin in the EMPA-REG OUTCOME trial. Kidney Int. 2021;99:750–62.
2. Heerspink HJL, Cherney DZI. Clinical implications of an acute dip in eGFR after SGLT2 inhibitor initiation. Clin J Am Soc Nephrol. 2021;16(8):1278–80.

130. Correct Answer: E

Rationale
The amount of daily walking and/or exercise should be at least three times per week, not at least once per week. Each of the other choices are appropriate recommended approaches to support optimal blood pressure control. Optimal blood pressure control necessitates an appropriate sensitivity to, and an understanding of, demographic, socio-cultural and other factors. For patients with elevated blood pressure, initiation of non-pharmacologic therapy should be instituted to include smoking cessation in tobacco users, daily walking and/or exercise three times per week, and a vegetable-rich diet.

Answers

Reference

1. Virani SS, Alonso A, Benjamin EJ, et al. American Heart Association Council on Epidemiology and Prevention Statistics Committee and Stroke Statistics Subcommittee. Heart disease and stroke statistics-2020 update: a report from the American Heart Association. Circulation. 2020;141(9):e139–596. https://doi.org/10.1161/CIR.0000000000000757.

131. Correct Answer: C

Rationale

The most recent recommendations for the management of high blood pressure by the American College of Cardiology/American Heart Association include classifying a blood pressure level of 130–139/80–89 mmHg as Stage 1 hypertension and a blood pressure level ≥140/90 mmHg as Stage 2 hypertension.

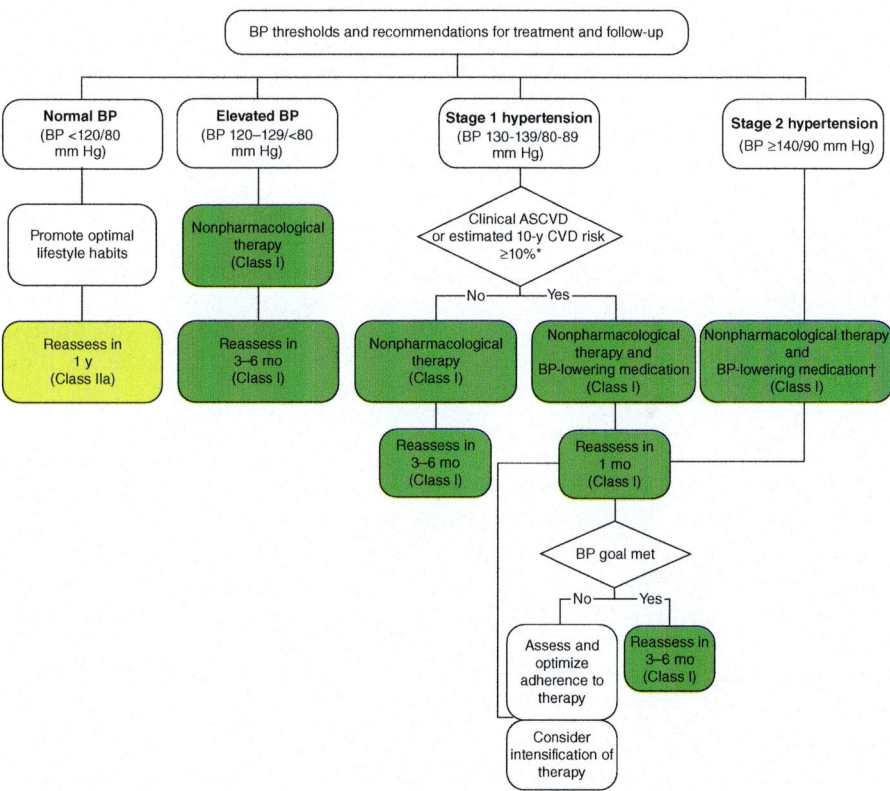

Blood pressure (BP) thresholds and recommendations for treatment and follow-up. Colors correspond to Class of Recommendation. *Using the ACC/AHA Pooled Cohort Equations. Note that patients with DM or CKD are automatically placed in the high-risk category. For initiation of RAS inhibitor or diuretic therapy, assess blood tests for electrolytes and renal function 2–4 weeks after initiating therapy. †Consider initiation of pharmacological therapy for Stage 2 hypertension with two antihypertensive agents of different classes. Patients with Stage 2 hypertension and BP ≥160/100 mmHg should be promptly treated, carefully monitored, and subject to upward medication dose adjustment as necessary to control BP. Reassessment includes BP measurement, detection of orthostatic hypotension in selected patients (e.g., older or with postural symptoms), identification of white coat hypertension or a white coat effect, documentation of adherence, monitoring of the response to therapy, reinforcement of the importance of adherence, reinforcement of the importance of treatment, and assistance with treatment to achieve BP target. *ACC* American College of Cardiology, *AHA* American Heart Association, *ASCVD* atherosclerotic cardiovascular disease, *BP* blood pressure, *CKD* chronic kidney disease, *DM* diabetes mellitus, *RAS* renin-angiotensin system. (Figure and legend reproduced with permission from Whelton et al. J Am Coll Cardiol. 2018 May 15;71(19):e127–e248)

Reference
1. Whelton PK, Carey RM, Aronow WS, et al. 2017 ACC/AHA/AAPA/ABC/ACPM/AGS/APhA/ASH/ASPC/NMA/PCNA guideline for the prevention, detection, evaluation, and management of high blood pressure in adults: a report of the American College of Cardiology/American Heart Association task force on clinical practice guidelines. Hypertension. 2018;71(6):e13–115.

132. Correct Answer: C

Rationale
For persons with blood pressure of ≥130/80 mmHg being treated with lifestyle management, it is recommended to initiate concurrent pharmacologic therapy if the estimated 10-year atherosclerotic cardiovascular disease risk is ≥10%.

Reference
1. Whelton PK, Carey RM, Aronow WS, et al. 2017 ACC/AHA/AAPA/ABC/ACPM/AGS/APhA/ASH/ASPC/NMA/PCNA guideline for the prevention, detection, evaluation, and management of high blood pressure in adults: a report of the American College of Cardiology/American Heart Association task force on clinical practice guidelines. Hypertension. 2018;71(6):e13–115.

133. Correct Answer: B

Rationale
For improving blood pressure control, one should both reduce dietary sodium intake and increase dietary potassium intake. All of the answers are correct except for reducing dietary sodium intake and reducing dietary potassium intake. Both are incorrect. The appropriate action is to reduce dietary sodium intake and increase, not reduce, dietary potassium intake.

Reference:
1. Virani SS, Alonso A, Benjamin EJ, et al. American Heart Association Council on Epidemiology and Prevention Statistics Committee and Stroke Statistics Subcommittee. Heart disease and stroke statistics-2020 update: a report from the American Heart Association. Circulation. 2020;141(9):e139–596.

134. Correct Answer: D

Rationale

As seen in the MESA (Multi-Ethnic Study of Atherosclerosis) cohort follow-up, a comprehensive approach to adopting "Life's Simple 7" reduced incident heart failure by 60% compared to subjects who did not.

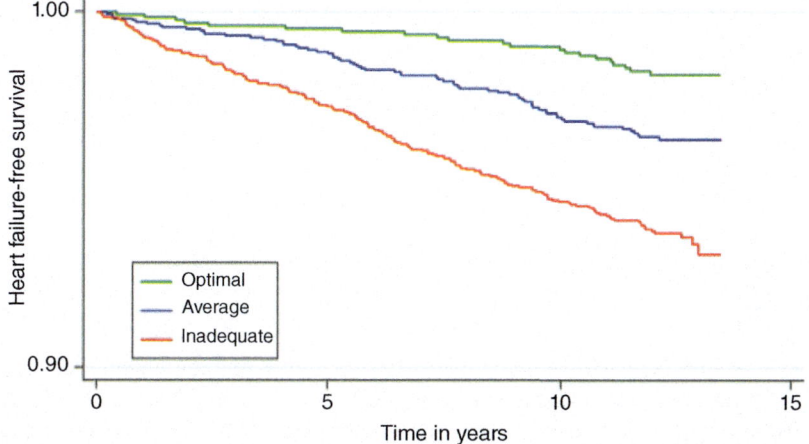

Kaplan–Meier analysis of time to incident heart failure by categories of the Life's Simple 7 Score. The Life's Simple 7 score ranged from 0 to 14 and was classified into inadequate (0–8), average (9–10), and optimal (11–14) based on points assigned to each category of the Life's Simple 7 metrics. (Figure and legend reproduced with permission from J Am Heart Assoc. 2017 Jun 27;6(6):e005180)

Reference
1. Ogunmoroti O, Oni E, Michos ED, et al. Life's simple 7 and incident heart failure: the Multi-Ethnic Study of Atherosclerosis. J Am Heart Assoc. 2017;6(6):e005180.

135. Correct Answer: D

Rationale

Recent studies have demonstrated very impressive reductions in new heart failure events in patients with Type 2 diabetes mellitus treated with any of several SGLT-2 inhibitors. These findings have since been extended to patients without diabetes, a remarkable management breakthrough that has begun to revolutionize the management and prevention of heart failure. GLP-1 agonists (a) have been shown to decrease cardiovascular disease events in patients with diabetes, but specifically not heart failure. Neither sulfonylureas (b) nor metformin (c) have been demonstrated to prevent heart failure in randomized control clinical trials.

References
1. Zinman B, Wanner C, Lachin JM, et al. Empagliflozin, cardiovascular outcomes, and mortality in type 2 diabetes. N Engl J Med. 2015;373:2117–28.
2. Neal B, Perkovic V, Mahaffey KW, et al. Canagliflozin and cardiovascular and renal events in type 2 diabetes. N Engl J Med. 2017;377:644–57.
3. Wiviott SD, Raz I, Bonaca MP, et al. Dapagliflozin and cardiovascular outcomes in type 2 diabetes. N Engl J Med. 2019;380:347–57.

136. Correct Answer: A

Rationale

In a Swedish Cohort follow-up, the DASH diet reduced incident heart failure by 20–40%. While the Mediterranean Diet (b) is a highly recommended diet for general prevention of cardiovascular events, heart failure has not been clearly documented as one of them. Neither choice (c) nor choice (d) is a recommended diet for the prevention of cardiovascular disease.

Answers

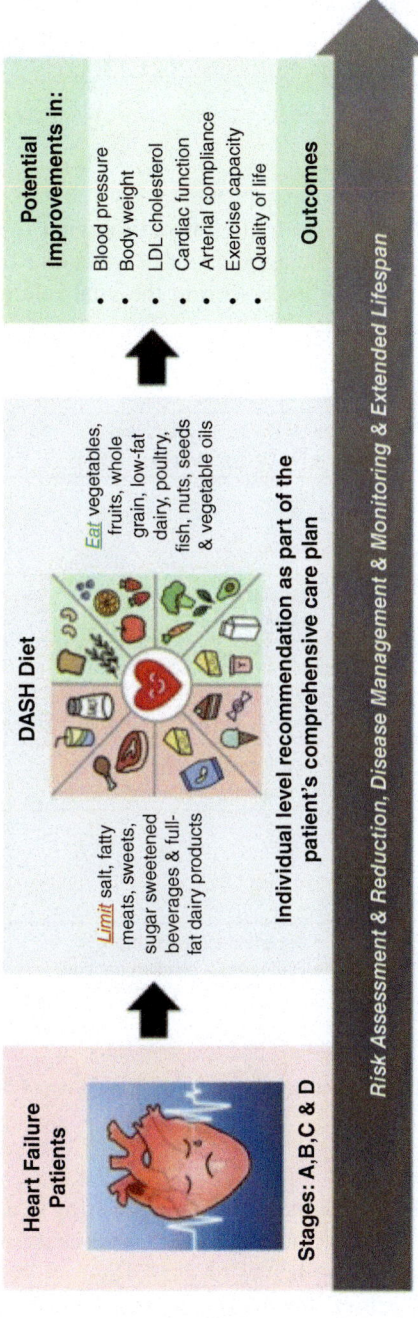

The potential role of the DASH diet in heart failure management. Assessment of patients with heart failure (HF) stages (A–D) is followed by comprehensive clinical care management, which includes an individual-level DASH diet recommendation. Once successfully adopted and adhered to, the DASH diet can improve patients' physical and functional capacities through reductions in blood pressure, body weight, and LDL cholesterol concentration and improvements in cardiac function, arterial compliance, exercise capacity, and quality of life. The positive effects of the DASH diet implemented as part of a comprehensive care plan for risk reduction and disease management and monitoring can contribute to improved health outcomes. (Figure and legend reproduced with permission from Nutrients. 2021 Dec 10;13(12):4424)

References
1. Levitan EB, Wolk A, Mittleman MA. Consistency with the DASH diet and incidence of heart failure. Arch Intern Med. 2009;169:851–7.
2. Wickman BE, Enkhmaa B, Ridberg R, et al. Dietary management of heart failure: DASH diet and precision nutrition perspectives. Nutrients. 2021;13(12):4424.

137. Correct Answer: C

Rationale

A meta-analysis of 18 randomized controlled clinical trials showed the vital role played by hypertension control in significantly reducing incident heart failure by 42%. That result is an important piece of evidence underscoring the vital role of hypertension control in the prevention of heart failure.

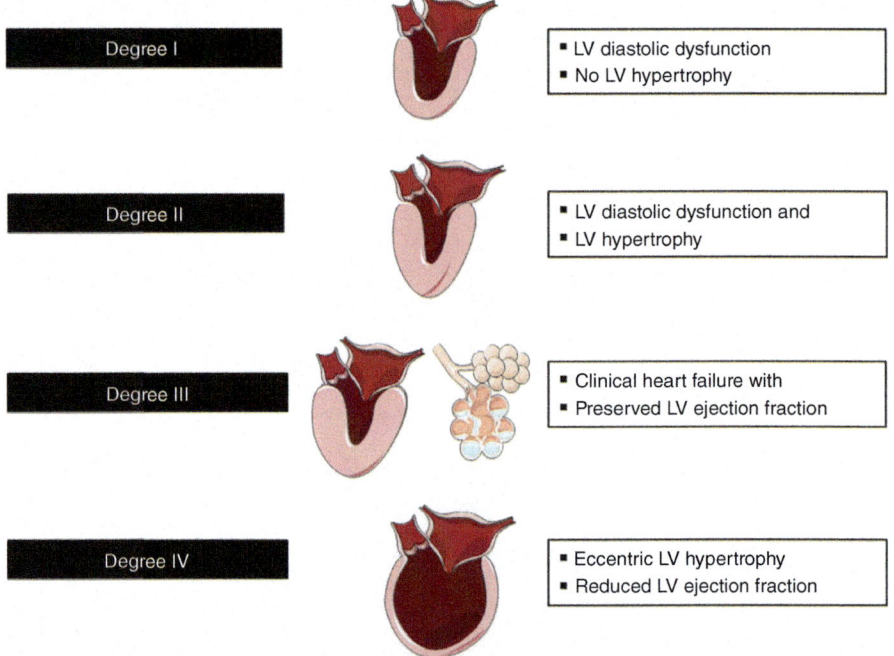

Hypertension staging and risk of heart failure. (Reproduced with permission from J Am Coll Cardiol HF. 2017 Aug, 5 (8) 543–55)

References
1. Thomopoulos C, Parati G, Zanchetti A. Effects of blood pressure-lowering treatment. 6. Prevention of heart failure and new-onset heart failure—meta-analyses of randomized trials. J Hypertens. 2016;34:373–84.
2. Messerli FH, Rimoldi SF, Bangalore S. The transition from hypertension to heart failure: contemporary update. JACC Heart Fail. 2017;5(8):543–51.

138. Correct Answer: B

Rationale

The Women's Health Study was a 10-year trial of aspirin versus placebo and found no CVD event reduction benefit in general. However, women carrying the *LPA* intron 25 genotype (rs10455872) had a significantly greater CVD event rate when randomized to placebo but a significant reduction in CVD events when randomized to aspirin.

Reference

1. Chasman DI, Shiffman D, Zee RY, et al. Polymorphism in the apolipoprotein(a) gene, plasma lipoprotein(a), cardiovascular disease, and low-dose aspirin therapy. Atherosclerosis. 2009;203(2):371–6.

139. Correct Answer: C

Rationale

The 9p21 polymorphism was discovered through analysis of multiple Genome Wide Association studies. The genetic region contains an anti-sense non-coding RNA (ANRIL) involved in the inflammatory process.

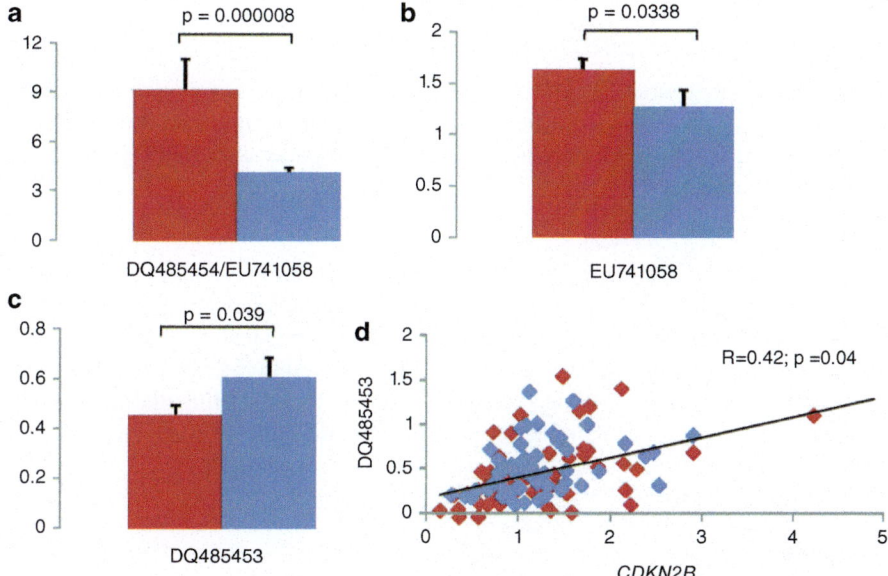

Differential expression profiles of the short and the long transcript variants of *ANRIL* in control subjects homozygous for the risk versus reference alleles. (**a**) through (**c**), Relative copy numbers of the short and the long variants of *ANRIL* as detected by quantitative RT-PCR. Column heights indicate the mean of relative transcript abundance detected in probability values were obtained using a one-tailed homoscedastic *t* test. (**d**) Scatter plot depicts a linear association between relative expression levels of *CDKN2B* and DQ485453 variant of *ANRIL*. Subjects homozygous for the risk alleles are in red and homozygous for the reference allele are in blue. (Figure and legend reproduced with permission from Arterioscler Thromb Vasc Biol. 2009;29(10):1671–7)

Reference
1. Jarinova O, Stewart AF, Roberts R, et al. Functional analysis of the chromosome 9p21.3 coronary artery disease risk locus. Arterioscler Thromb Vasc Biol. 2009;29(10):1671–7.

140. Correct Answer: A

Rationale
The cardiovascular risk of African American patients is, on average, very high. However, triglycerides tend to be lower and HDL-C higher than for other ethnic and racial groups.

Reference
1. Carnethon MR, Pu J, Howard G, et al. American Heart Association Council on Epidemiology and Prevention; Council on Cardiovascular Disease in the Young; Council on Cardiovascular and Stroke Nursing; Council on Clinical Cardiology; Council on Functional Genomics and Translational Biology; and Stroke Council. Cardiovascular health in African Americans: a scientific statement from the American Heart Association. Circulation. 2017;136(21):e393–423.

141. Correct Answer: C

Rationale
There have been several studies that have looked at the impact of Waist-Hip ratio versus BMI. Although not a universally agreed upon distinction, the waist hip ratio captures information that would help in identifying patients at risk for metabolic syndrome and diabetes.

References
1. Moosaie F, Fatemi Abhari SM, et al. Waist-to-height ratio is a more accurate tool for predicting hypertension than waist-to-hip circumference and BMI in patients with type 2 diabetes: a prospective study. Front Public Health. 2021;9:726288.
2. Sayeed MA, Mahtab H, Latif ZA, et al. Waist-to-height ratio is a better obesity index than body mass index and waist-to-hip ratio for predicting diabetes, hypertension and lipidemia. Bangladesh Med Res Counc Bull. 2003;29(1):1–10.

142. Correct Answer: C

Rationale
There was a clear relation between exercise level and waist hip ratio and risk of AF. Among participants in cross country skiing, there is a 30% increased risk of AF that was increased in those with fastest race times and also those who entered more races. Skiers with atrial fibrillation had a higher incidence of stroke than did skiers and non-skiers without atrial fibrillation (men: HR, 2.28; 95% CI, 1.93–2.70; women: HR, 3.51; 95% CI, 2.17–5.68; skiers with atrial fibrillation vs. skiers without atrial fibrillation). After the diagnosis of atrial fibrillation, skiers with atrial fibrillation had a lower incidence of stroke (HR, 0.73; 95% CI, 0.50–0.91) and lower mortality compared with non-skiers with atrial fibrillation (HR, 0.57; 95% CI, 0.49–0.65).

Answers

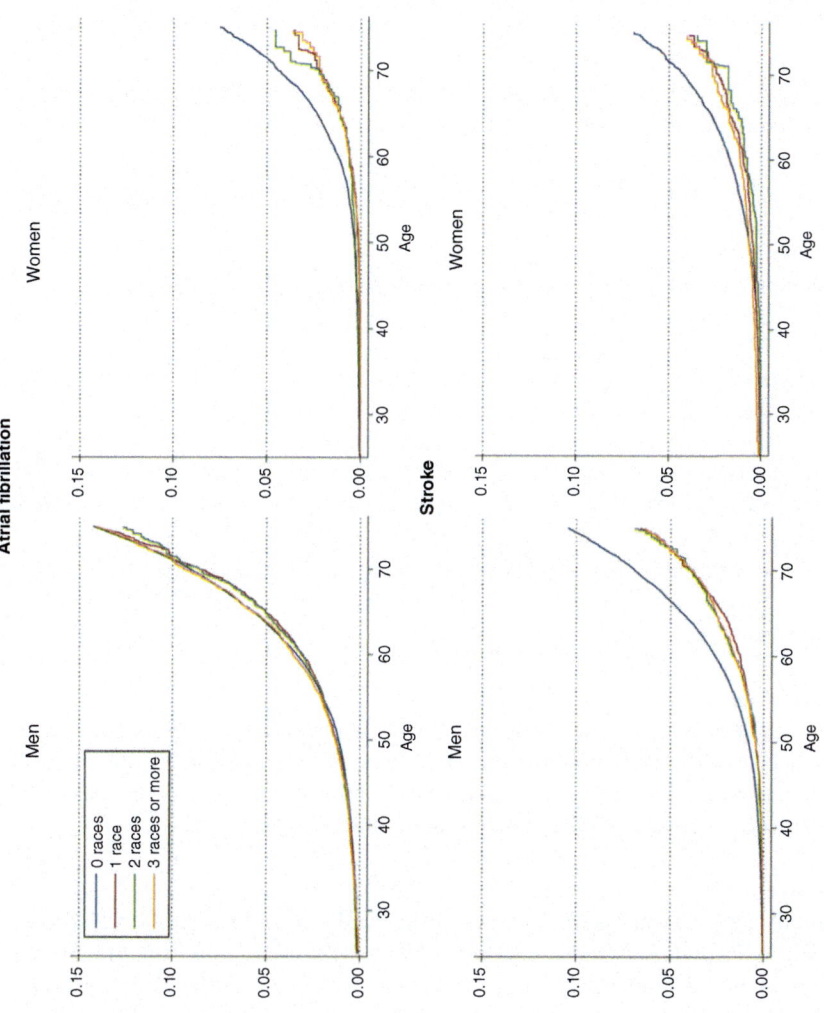

Sex-specific Kaplan–Meier failure estimates of atrial fibrillation and stroke by number of completed races in Vasaloppet (1989–2011). (Reproduced with permission from Svedberg et al. Circulation. 2019;140:910–920)

References
1. Chung MK, Eckhardt LL, Chen LY, et al. American Heart Association Electrocardiography and Arrhythmias Committee and Exercise, Cardiac Rehabilitation, and Secondary Prevention Committee of the Council on Clinical Cardiology; Council on Arteriosclerosis, Thrombosis and Vascular Biology; Council on Cardiovascular and Stroke Nursing; and Council on Lifestyle and Cardiometabolic Health. Lifestyle and risk factor modification for reduction of atrial fibrillation: a scientific statement from the American Heart Association. Circulation. 2020;141(16):e750–72.
2. Svedberg N, Sundström J, James S, et al. Long-term incidence of atrial fibrillation and stroke among cross-country skiers. Circulation. 2019;140(11):910–20.

143. Correct Answer: B

Rationale
In both the Emerging Risk Factors Collaboration and the REGARDS study, at similar Lp(a) levels there was a greater risk of CAD versus stroke.

References
1. Emerging Risk Factors Collaboration, Erqou S, Kaptoge S, Perry PL, et al. Lipoprotein(a) concentration and the risk of coronary heart disease, stroke, and nonvascular mortality. JAMA. 2009;302(4):412–23.
2. Colantonio LD, Bittner V, Safford MM, et al. Lipoprotein(a) and the risk for coronary heart disease and ischemic stroke events among Black and White adults with cardiovascular disease. J Am Heart Assoc. 2022;11(11):e025397.

144. Correct Answer: C

Rationale
The pooled cohort risk calculator is only for use in primary prevention. It has factors for diabetes as well as other ethnic groups. Although the precision of estimated risks in matching actual risks varies by population and risk group, it is not contraindicated for use in those with diabetes or other ethnic groups.

Reference
1. Grundy SM, Stone NJ, Bailey AL, et al. 2018 AHA/ACC/AACVPR/AAPA/ABC/ACPM/ADA/AGS/APhA/ASPC/NLA/PCNA guideline on the management of blood cholesterol: a report of the American College of Cardiology/American Heart Association task force on clinical practice guidelines. Circulation. 2019;139(25):e1082–143.

145. Correct Answer: B

Rationale
In persons at borderline (5–<7.5%) or intermediate (7.5–<20%) risk the clinician should next consider the presence of risk enhancing factors which aid in formulating the treatment decision.

Reference
1. Grundy SM, Stone NJ, Bailey AL, et al. 2018 AHA/ACC/AACVPR/AAPA/ABC/ACPM/ADA/AGS/APhA/ASPC/NLA/PCNA guideline on the management of blood cholesterol: a report of the American College of Cardiology/American Heart Association task force on clinical practice guidelines. Circulation. 2019;139(25):e1082–143.

146. Correct Answer: C

Rationale
When coronary calcium scores are considered to further refine the treatment decision, the 2018 guidelines notes that a calcium score of 0 may be used to withhold or delay statin therapy except in those with diabetes, premature family history of ASCVD, or who are heavy cigarette smokers; the lifetime risk of ASCVD is presumably high in these groups of patients.

Reference
1. Grundy SM, Stone NJ, Bailey AL, et al. 2018 AHA/ACC/AACVPR/AAPA/ABC/ACPM/ADA/AGS/APhA/ASPC/NLA/PCNA guideline on the management of blood cholesterol: a report of the American College of Cardiology/American Heart Association task force on clinical practice guidelines. Circulation. 2019;139(25):e1082–143.

147. Correct Answer: C

Rationale
Coronary calcium has been shown to improve the c-statistic, improving risk discrimination, beyond standard risk factors, by a much greater extent than carotid ultrasound or ankle brachial index. The 2018 guidelines only note coronary calcium for consideration of risk stratification beyond global risk assessment and risk enhancing factors. An ankle brachial index of <0.9 is diagnostic of peripheral arterial disease and is considered a risk enhancing factor in the guidelines.

References
1. Yeboah J, McClelland RL, Polonsky TS, et al. Comparison of novel risk markers for improvement in cardiovascular risk assessment in intermediate-risk individuals. JAMA. 2012;308(8):788–95.
2. Grundy SM, Stone NJ, Bailey AL, et al. 2018 AHA/ACC/AACVPR/AAPA/ABC/ACPM/ADA/AGS/APhA/ASPC/NLA/PCNA guideline on the management of blood cholesterol: a report of the American College of Cardiology/American Heart Association task force on clinical practice guidelines. Circulation. 2019;139(25):e1082–143.

148. Correct Answer: A

Rationale
A large cohort study in the United Kingdom showed peripheral arterial disease (16%) and heart failure (15%) to be the most common first manifestation of cardiovascular disease, followed by stable angina, nonfatal myocardial infarction, and stroke.

Answers

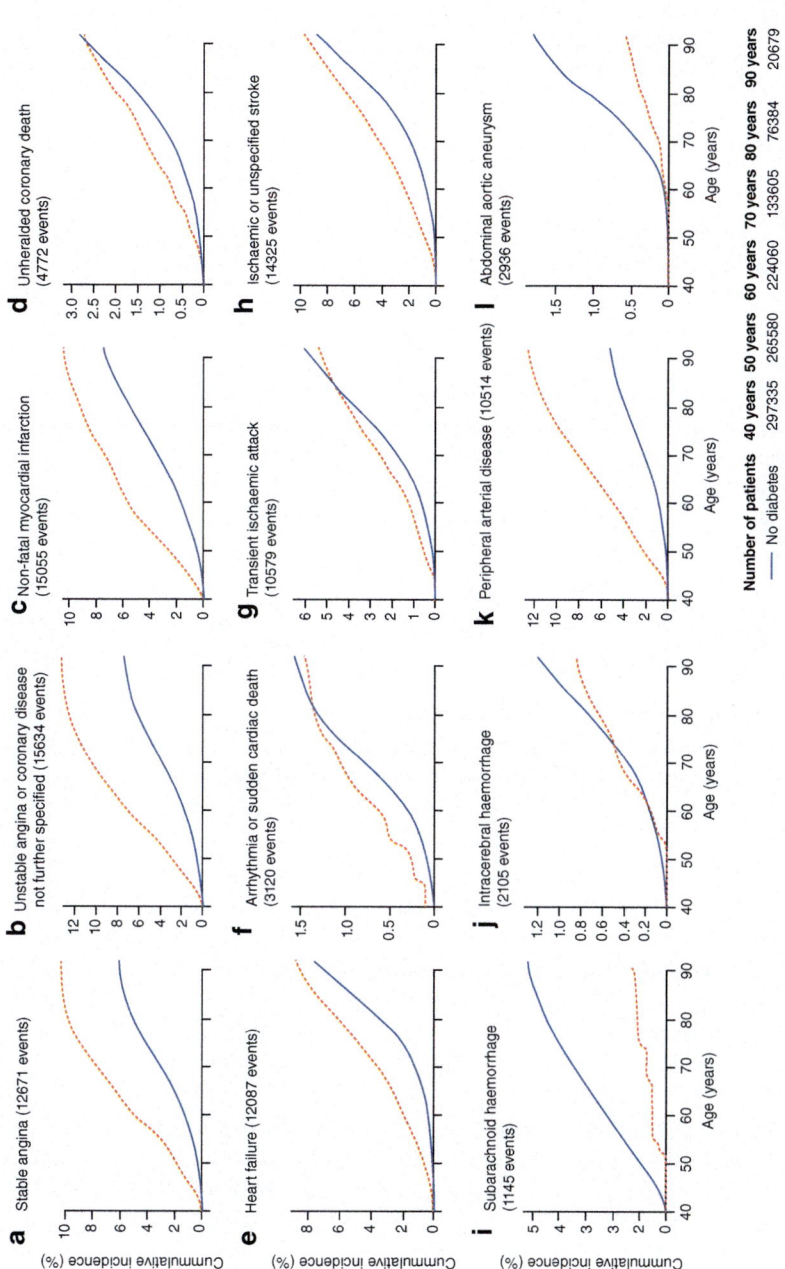

Cumulative incidence curves for the incidence of first presentation of 12 cardiovascular diseases in patients aged ≥40 years, by diabetes status. (Figure and legend reproduced with permission from Shah et al. Lancet Diabetes Endocrinol. 2015 Feb;3(2):105–13)

Reference
1. Shah AD, Langenberg C, Rapsomaniki E, Denaxas S, Pujades-Rodriguez M, Gale CP, Deanfield J, Smeeth L, Timmis A, Hemingway H. Type 2 diabetes and incidence of cardiovascular diseases: a cohort study in 1·9 million people. Lancet Diabetes Endocrinol. 2015;3(2):105–13.

149. Correct Answer: C

Rationale
Recent US data show only 10–20% of US adults to be at target for LDL-C (if considering <100 mg/dL or <70 mg/dL if with CVD, blood pressure (<130/80 mmHg), and HbA1c (<7.0%).

References
1. Fan W, Song Y, Inzucchi SE, et al. Composite cardiovascular risk factor target achievement and its predictors in US adults with diabetes: the Diabetes Collaborative Registry. Diabetes Obes Metab. 2019;21(5):1121–7.
2. Andary R, Fan W, Wong ND. Control of cardiovascular risk factors among US adults with type 2 diabetes with and without cardiovascular disease. Am J Cardiol. 2019;124(4):522–7.

150. Correct Answer: C

Rationale
A recent pooling of more than 2000 subjects with diabetes showed a 62% lower cardiovascular disease and 62% lower coronary heart disease rates when these three measures were at target compared to when none were at target.

Reference
1. Wong ND, Zhao Y, Patel R, et al. Cardiovascular risk factor targets and cardiovascular disease event risk in diabetes: a pooling project of the atherosclerosis risk in communities study, Multi-Ethnic Study of Atherosclerosis, and Jackson Heart Study. Diabetes Care. 2016;39(5):668–76.

151. Correct Answer: D

Rationale
Both B and C are appropriate. Patient has DM and multiple risk factors so should be on a high intensity statin. Also, elevated triglycerides (not likely to be controlled by a high intensity statin), is a candidate for icosapent ethyl based on REDUCE-IT. A PCSK9 inhibitor is not recommended by guidelines for persons with diabetes without a history of ASCVD (atherosclerotic cardiovascular disease) and who have not been tried on a high intensity statin.

References
1. Grundy SM, Stone NJ, Bailey AL, et al. 2018 AHA/ACC/AACVPR/AAPA/ ABC/ACPM/ADA/AGS/APhA/ASPC/NLA/PCNA guideline on the management of blood cholesterol: a report of the American College of Cardiology/ American Heart Association task force on clinical practice guidelines. Circulation. 2019;139(25):e1082–143.
2. American Diabetes Association Professional Practice Committee. Cardiovascular disease and risk management: standards of medical care in diabetes-2022. Diabetes Care. 2022;45(Suppl 1):S144–74.

152. Correct Answer: E

Rationale
Several population-specific risk assessment tools exist. These include the Framingham Risk Score, AHA/American College of Cardiology pooled cohort equation, Prospective Cardiovascular Munster Score, Systemic Coronary Risk Evaluation, and FINRISK (Finland Cardiovascular Risk Study) risk calculator. All of these underestimate the cardiovascular risk of South Asian persons. The UK QRISK2 risk assessment tool included patients of south Asian descent and was found to estimate this patient's cardiovascular risk more accurately.

Reference
1. Volgman AS, Palaniappan LS, Aggarwal NT, et al. American Heart Association Council on Epidemiology and Prevention; Cardiovascular Disease and Stroke in Women and Special Populations Committee of the Council on Clinical Cardiology; Council on Cardiovascular and Stroke Nursing; Council on Quality of Care and Outcomes Research; and Stroke Council. Atherosclerotic cardiovascular disease in South Asian in the United States: epidemiology, risk factors, and treatments: a scientific statement from the American Heart Association. Circulation. 2018;138(1):e1–34.

153. Correct Answer: A

Rationale
South Asian (including Asian Indian) persons make up 20% of the world population and constitute an important and growing portion of the US population. Small cohort studies have shown that this ethnic group is not only at an elevated risk for cardiovascular disease but also has a higher proportional mortality when compared with other ethnicities. South Asian tend to have a higher prevalence of obesity, dyslipidemia, and diabetes mellitus. Therefore, awareness and early screening are especially important in this group to prevent cardiovascular events.

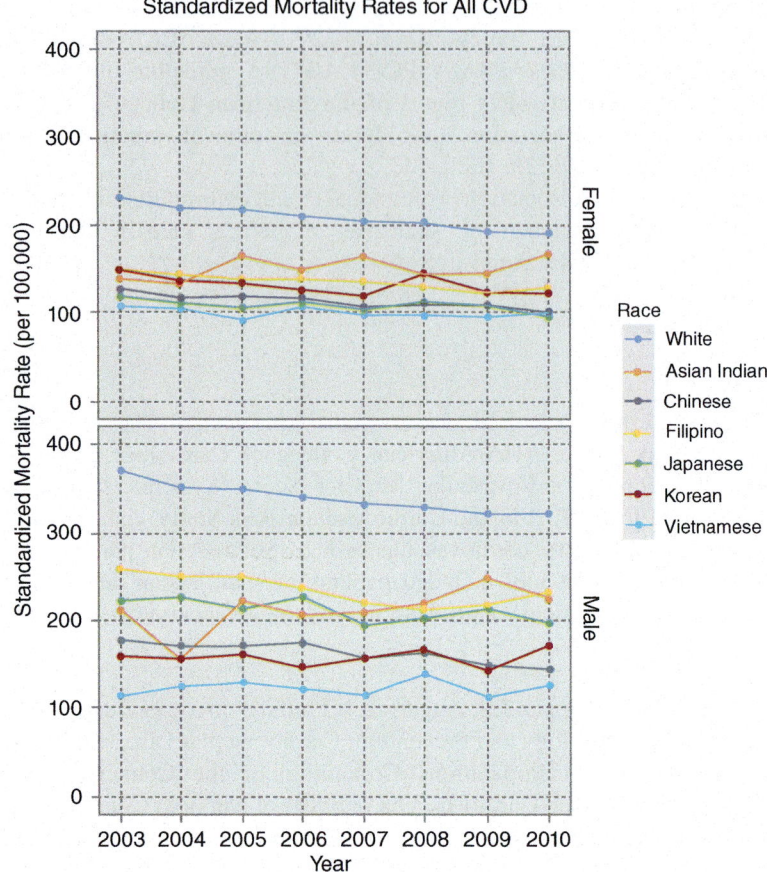

Standardized Mortality Rates for All CVD (cardiovascular disease) by Asian-American subgroups by year (2003–2010). Age-adjusted mortality rates from all CVD yearly from 2003 to 2010 for Asian-American subgroups compared with non-Hispanic Whites. (Figure and legend reproduced from Jose et al. J Am Coll Cardiol. 2014 Dec 16;64(23):2486–94)

Reference

1. Jose PO, Frank AT, Kapphahn KI, et al. Cardiovascular disease mortality in Asian Americans. J Am Coll Cardiol. 2014;64(23):2486–94.

154. Correct answer: E

Rationale

13.7% of all adults in the United States were active smokers in 2018. People with mixed race heritage, non-Hispanic American Indians and Alaskan natives make up the largest cohorts of all smokers (19.1% and 22.6%, respectively). Hispanic and Asian patients only account for 9.8% and 7.1% of all smokers. Men are more commonly smokers than women.

Smoking can affect virtually any organ system including the lung, brain, and cardiovascular system. More than 16 million Americans suffer from comorbidities that are directly attributed to smoking. Smoking leads to more than 480,000 deaths per year in the United States, resulting in a predicted life expectancy that is 10 years shorter than nonsmokers. It is the leading cause of preventable death in the United States.

References
1. https://www.cdc.gov/tobacco/data_statistics/fact_sheets/fast_facts/index.htm.
2. Creamer MR, Wang TW, Babb S, et al. Tobacco product use and cessation indicators among adults—United States, 2018. MMWR Morb Mortal Wkly Rep. 2019;68(45):1013–9.

155. Correct Answer: D

Rationale

Ketogenic is generally defined as a very low carbohydrate diet (<20–50 g glucose/day) that favors foods that are high in protein and fat. It avoids processed foods with a high glycemic index. A very low carbohydrate diet can help lower blood pressure, postprandial blood glucose and triglyceride levels. Ketogenic diets can promote short term weight loss. The long-term efficacy of a ketogenic diet for weight loss has not been determined in trials yet. Increased intake of saturated fats can lead to an increase of LDL-C levels. This can be attenuated by replacing saturated fats with monosaturated fatty acids.

Reference
1. Bays HE, Agarwala A, German C, et al. Ten things to know about ten cardiovascular disease risk factors—2022. Am J Prev Cardiol. 2022;10:100342. https://doi.org/10.1016/j.ajpc.2022.100342.

156. Correct Answer: D

Rationale

A randomized control trial enrolling 262 persons with Type 2 diabetes showed that the combination of aerobic and resistance training (−0.34%) reduced A1c levels more than aerobic (−0.16%) or resistance (−0.24%) training alone compared to a non-exercise control group. Stretching was not included as part of the trial protocol.

Reference
1. Church TS, Blair SN, Cocreham S, et al. Effects of aerobic and resistance training on hemoglobin A_{1c} levels in patients with type 2 diabetes: a randomized controlled trial. JAMA. 2010;304(20):2253–62.

157. Correct Answer: C

Rationale
The metabolic syndrome is a group of conditions that in combination have been shown to increase cardiovascular risk. It is defined by the following five criteria, three of which must be positive to meet the criteria: increased waist circumference, elevated triglycerides >150 mg/dL, elevated blood pressure, elevated glucose, and low HDL-C (high-density lipoprotein-cholesterol) <40 mg/dL in men; <50 mg/dL in women. Per the 2018 ACC/AHA guidelines, metabolic syndrome is a risk-enhancing factor and the pooled cohort equations may underestimate risk in this population. Statin therapy is recommended in non-diabetic adults with intermediate risk 7.5–19.9% who have a risk enhancing factor. The following are also ASCVD risk enhancing factors: hs-CRP (high sensitivity C-reactive protein) >2 mg/L, South Asian ancestry, and premature family history (father >55 years old, mother >65 years old).

Reference
1. Grundy SM, Stone NJ, Bailey AL, et al. 2018 AHA/ACC/AACVPR/AAPA/ABC/ACPM/ADA/AGS/APhA/ASPC/NLA/PCNA guideline on the management of blood cholesterol: a report of the American College of Cardiology/American Heart Association task force on clinical practice guidelines. Circulation. 2019;139(25):e1082–143.

158. Correct Answer: A

Rationale
There is evidence that statins increase risk of developing diabetes in individuals with risk factors for developing diabetes, components of the metabolic syndrome, and higher-intensity statin use. The mechanism for this relationship is unclear and a direct causal relationship of statins causing diabetes is considered unlikely. Per the 2018 ACC/AHA Cholesterol Guidelines, in patients with new onset diabetes on statin-therapy, it is a Class I B-R recommendation to continue statin therapy because of the net benefit to continuing the statin versus the risk gained by the new-onset diabetes. Lifestyle modifications are also encouraged as part of this recommendation.

Answers

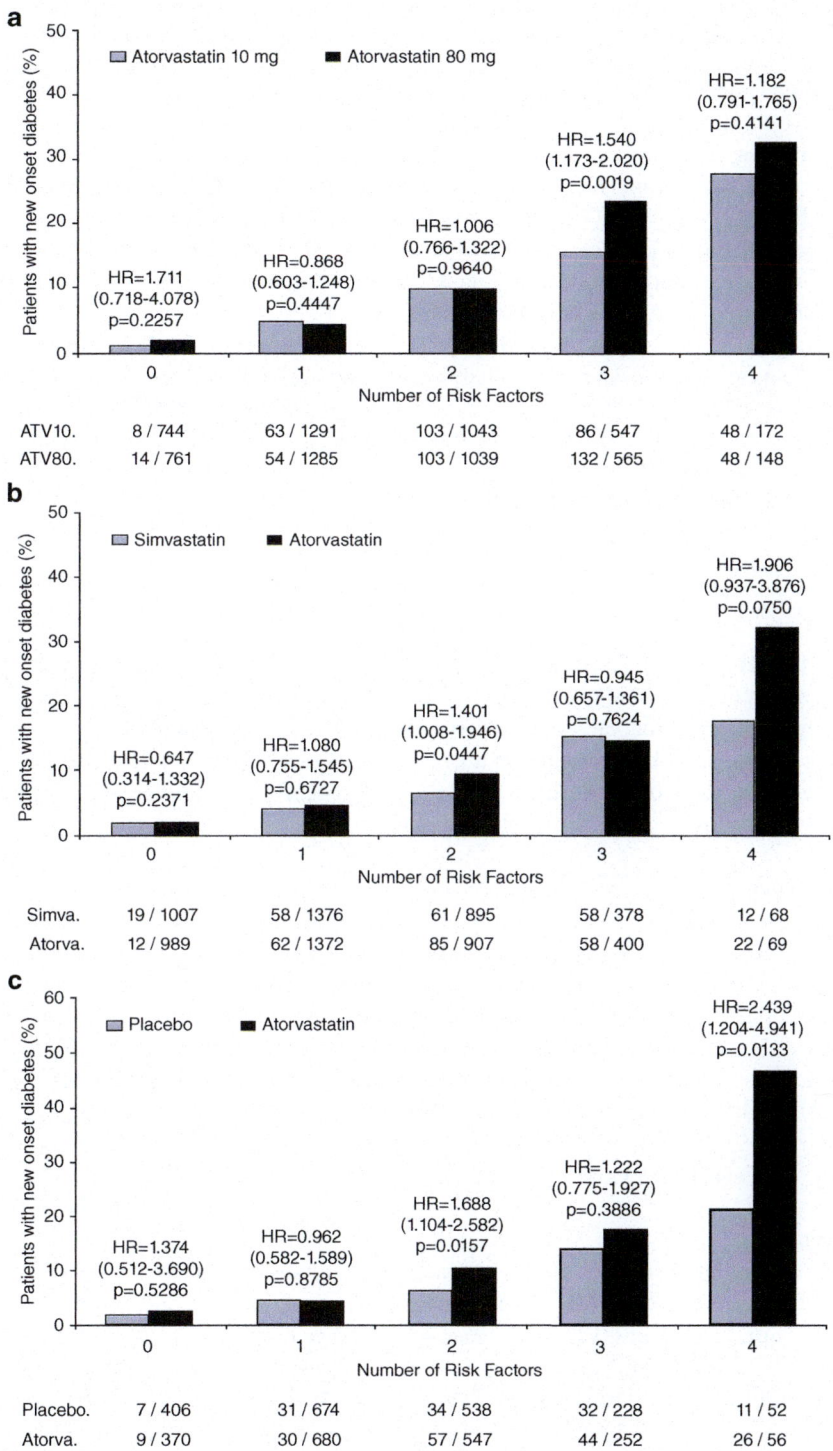

Incident diabetes in (**a**) the TNT trial, (**b**) the IDEAL trial, and (**c**) the SPARCL trial according to number of metabolic syndrome risk factors and treatment group. *Atorva* atorvastatin, *ATV10* atorvastatin 10 mg, *ATV 80* atorvastatin 80 mg, *Simva* simvastatin. (Figure and legend reproduced with permission from J Am Coll Cardiol. 2011 Apr, 57 (14) 1535–154)

References
1. Grundy SM, Stone NJ, Bailey AL, et al. 2018 AHA/ACC/AACVPR/AAPA/ABC/ACPM/ADA/AGS/APhA/ASPC/NLA/PCNA guideline on the management of blood cholesterol: a report of the American College of Cardiology/American Heart Association task force on clinical practice guidelines. Circulation. 2019;139(25):e1082–143.
2. Waters DD, Ho JE, Boekholdt SM, DeMicco DA, et al. Cardiovascular event reduction versus new-onset diabetes during atorvastatin therapy: effect of baseline risk factors for diabetes. J Am Coll Cardiol. 2013;61(2):148–52.
3. Preiss D, Seshasai SR, Welsh P, et al. Risk of incident diabetes with intensive-dose compared with moderate-dose statin therapy: a meta-analysis. JAMA. 2011;305(24):2556–64.

159. Correct Answer: C

Rationale
The DASH (Dietary Approaches to Stop Hypertension), Mediterranean diet, and vegan/vegetarian diets have all been shown to improve weight loss and glycemic control in Type 2 diabetes patients. It is a Class Ia recommendation to develop a tailored nutrition plan focusing on a heart-healthy diet in adults with Type 2 diabetes. Low-fat diets have not been shown to consistently reduce weight or improve glycemic control in Type 2 diabetic patients.

References
1. Huo R, Du T, Xu Y, et al. Effects of Mediterranean-style diet on glycemic control, weight loss and cardiovascular risk factors among type 2 diabetes individuals: a meta-analysis. Eur J Clin Nutr. 2015;69:1200–8.
2. Azadbakht L, Fard NRP, Karimi M, et al. Effects of the Dietary Approaches to Stop Hypertension (DASH) eating plan on cardiovascular risks among type 2 diabetic patients: a randomized crossover clinical trial. Diabetes Care. 2011;34:55–7.

160. Correct Answer: A

Rationale
This document comprises the most recent recommendations of the USPSTF for aspirin use to prevent CVD. The task force does not recommend aspirin use for primary prevention of CVD in all those aged ≥60 years; it does recommend against aspirin use for primary prevention of CVD in those aged ≥60 years with no evidence or history of vascular disease. It also allows for aspirin for those with increased risk for CVD (≥10% 10-year risk). The document notes that the adverse effects of aspirin, including bleeding, increase with age and may outweigh its benefits in

persons 40–59 years old. Low-dose aspirin of 81 mg is favored, but dosage from 81 to 500 mg/day have been used for primary prevention.

Reference
1. US Preventive Services Task Force. Aspirin use to prevent cardiovascular disease. JAMA. 2022;327:1577–84.

161. Correct Answer: A

Rationale
A. It is fundamental and well established that the mechanism of aspirin's antiplatelet therapy is irreversible inhibition of platelet cyclooxygenase-1 (COX-1). The remaining choices are all true. Aspirin does improve patency of saphenous vein bypass grafts. Aspirin does reduce risk of vascular events in high-risk patients with stable angina, atrial fibrillation, and peripheral artery disease. Prasugrel is contraindicated in patients with prior history of stroke or TIA because of increased bleeding risk in this group of patients. Also, in patients with an MI 1–3 years earlier, initiation of ticagrelor long term lowers subsequent CV death, MI (myocardial infarction), and stroke.

References
1. Eikelboom JW, Hirsh J, Spencer FA, Baglin TP, Weitz JI. Antiplatelet drugs: antithrombotic therapy and prevention of thrombosis, 9th ed: American College of Chest Physicians Evidence-Based Clinical Practice Guidelines. Chest. 2012;141(2 Suppl):e89S–119S.
2. Gavaghan TP, Gebski V, Baron DW. Immediate postoperative aspirin improves vein graft patency early and late after coronary artery bypass graft surgery. A placebo-controlled, randomized study. Circulation. 1991;83(5):1526–33.
3. Antithrombotic Trialists' Collaboration. Collaborative meta-analysis of randomised trials of antiplatelet therapy for prevention of death, myocardial infarction, and stroke in high-risk patients. BMJ. 2002;324(7329):71–86.
4. Wiviott SD, Braunwald E, McCabe CH, et al. TRITON-TIMI 38 Investigators. Prasugrel versus clopidogrel in patients with acute coronary syndromes. N Engl J Med. 2007;357(20):2001–15.
5. Bonaca MP, Bhatt DL, Cohen M, et al. PEGASUS-TIMI 54 Steering Committee and Investigators. Long-term use of ticagrelor in patients with prior myocardial infarction. N Engl J Med. 2015;372(19):1791–800.

162. Correct Answer: A

Rationale
Aspirin resistance remains a complex phenomenon with multiple potential causes classified as true resistance and pseudo-resistance. Those listed in choice "A" are examples of pseudo-resistance. Statement "B" is false regarding the mechanism of action of the thienopyridines, which is irreversible blockade of platelet receptor

P2Y$_{12}$. "C" is false; the combined therapeutic effects of aspirin and clopidogrel exceed the individual therapeutic effects of each drug. The risk of bleeding is higher (not lower) with prasugrel than clopidogrel. Statement "E" is false; ticagrelor is more potent than clopidogrel in reducing vascular events in ACS.

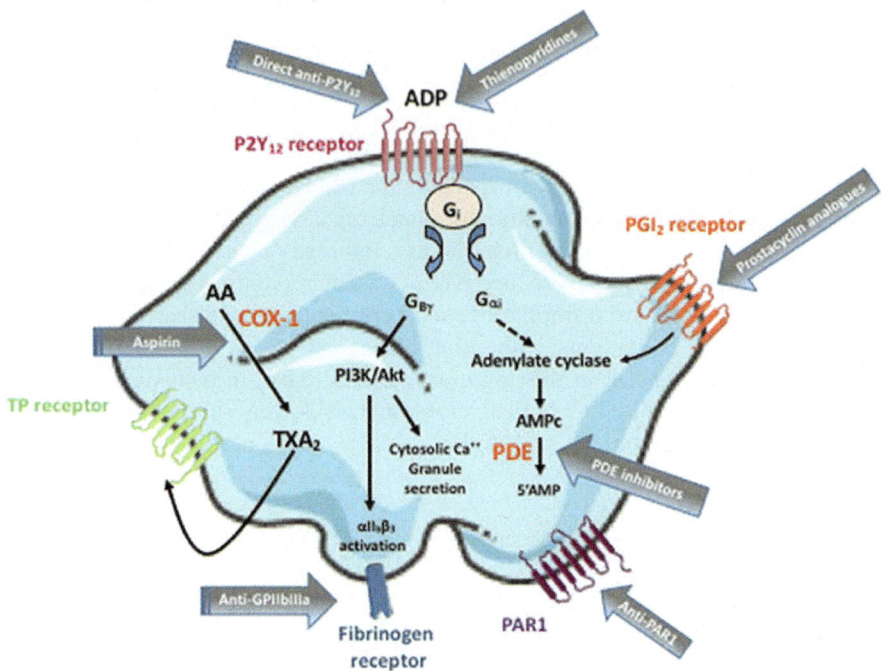

Targets of the commercialized antiplatelet agents. Arachidonic acid (AA) is produced by membrane phospholipids upon the action of phospholipase A$_2$. It is metabolized in cyclic endoperoxides by the cycloxygenase-1 (COX-1) enzyme, then in thromboxane A$_2$ (TXA$_2$) by the thromboxane synthase. TXA$_2$ activates the Thromboxane Prostanoid (TP) receptor in return. ADP, by activating P2Y$_{12}$ receptor, induces an inhibition of adenylate cyclase which downregulates cAMP (a powerful platelet inhibitor) synthesis. It also stimulates the phosphoinositide 3-kinase (PI3K) via G$_{\beta\gamma}$ protein complex resulting in Akt stimulation, which activates a number of downstream substrate proteins thereby increasing the cytosolic Ca^{2+} levels and inducing granule secretion. Inversely, prostacyclin (PGI2) binds to its receptor on platelet surface and increases cAMP intraplatelet level. cAMP is metabolized by phosphodiesterases (PDE) in 5′AMP. Blocking ADP binding site with a P2Y$_{12}$ receptor antagonist (including thienopyridines and direct anti-P2Y$_{12}$), stimulating PGI$_2$ receptor or inhibiting PDE maintains cAMP intraplatelet concentration at a high level thus keeping platelets in a resting state. Following coagulation activation, thrombin is generated and cleaves its receptor on platelet surface, that is, the protease-activated receptor 1 (PAR1), resulting in its activation. TP, P2Y$_{12}$, or PAR1 activation leads to a conformational change of the glycoprotein (GP)IIbIIIa (also called the integrin αII$_b$β$_3$) on platelet surface which links fibrinogen resulting in platelet aggregation. This figure does not aim to represent platelet physiology with the different signaling pathways. It rather illustrates in a very simple manner the targets of the currently available antiplatelet drugs. (Figure and legend reproduced from *Front. Cardiovasc. Med.* 9:805525. https://doi.org/10.3389/fcvm.2022.805525)

References
1. Grosser T, Fries S, Lawson JA, et al. Drug resistance and pseudoresistance: an unintended consequence of enteric coating aspirin. Circulation. 2013;127(3):377–85.
2. Hollopeter G, Jantzen HM, Vincent D, et al. Identification of the platelet ADP receptor targeted by antithrombotic drugs. Nature. 2001;409(6817):202–7.
3. Clopidogrel Trial Investigators. Effects of clopidogrel in addition to aspirin in patients with acute coronary syndromes without ST-segment elevation. NEJM. 2001;345:494–502.
4. Amsterdam EA, Wenger NK, Brindis RG, et al. ACC/AHA Task Force Members. 2014 AHA/ACC guideline for the management of patients with non-ST-elevation acute coronary syndromes: a report of the American College of Cardiology/American Heart Association task force on practice guidelines. Circulation. 2014;130(25):e344–426.
5. Sabatine MS, Mega JL. Pharmacogenomics of antiplatelet drugs. Hematol Am Soc Hematol Educ Program. 2014;2014(1):343–7.
6. Jourdi G, Godier A, Lordkipanidzé M, et al. Antiplatelet therapy for atherothrombotic disease in 2022-from population to patient-centered approaches. Front Cardiovasc Med. 2022;9:805525. https://doi.org/10.3389/fcvm.2022.805525.

163. Correct Answer: B

Rationale

"A" is incorrect; ticagrelor has more potent effects than clopidogrel in reducing vascular events in patients with ACS. "B" is correct. "C" is false; the dosing schedule of ticagrelor is twice daily. "D" is incorrect; ticagrelor exerts its antiplatelet effect by *reversible* inhibition of the platelet $P2Y_{12}$ receptor. "E" is incorrect; prasugrel causes especially high bleeding rates in patients ≥75 years old and those with low body weight.

References
1. Wiviott SD, Braunwald E, McCabe CH, et al. Prasugrel is more effective than clopidogrel in reducing vascular events in patients with non-STE ACS. NEJM. 2007;357:2001–15.
2. Feldman M, Cryer B. Aspirin absorption rates and platelet inhibition times with 325-mg buffered aspirin tablets (chewed or swallowed intact) and with buffered aspirin solution. Am J Cardiol. 1999;84(4):404–9.
3. Amsterdam EA, Wenger NK, Brindis RG, et al. Non-ST-elevation acute coronary syndromes: a report of the American College of Cardiology/American Heart Association task force on practice guidelines. Circulation. 2014;130:e344–426.

4. Storey RF, Husted S, Harrington RA, et al. Inhibition of platelet aggregation by AZD6140, a reversible oral P2Y12 receptor antagonist, compared with clopidogrel in patients with acute coronary syndromes. J Am Coll Cardiol. 2007;50(19):1852–6.
5. Wallentin L, Becker RC, Budaj A, et al. Ticagrelor versus clopidogrel in patients with acute coronary syndromes. N Engl J Med. 2009;361(11):1045–57.

164. Correct Answer: C

Rationale

The 2018 American College of Cardiology/American Heart Association guideline on the management of blood cholesterol states that it is reasonable to perform a CAC score for certain at-risk patients, particularly those with a 10-year ASCVD risk between ≥7.5% and <20%, to aid in the decision-making to use statin therapy, especially when needed beyond the consideration of risk enhancing factors.

Reference

1. Grundy SM, Stone NJ, Guideline Writing Committee for the 2018 Cholesterol Guidelines. 2018 Cholesterol clinical practice guidelines: synopsis of the 2018 American Heart Association/American College of Cardiology/Multisociety Cholesterol Guideline. Ann Intern Med. 2019;170(11):779–83.

165. Correct Answer: B

Rationale

Per the 2018 guidelines, if the coronary calcium score is zero, it is reasonable to withhold statin therapy and reassess in 5–10 years, as long as higher risk conditions are absent (diabetes mellitus, family history of premature CHD [coronary heart disease], cigarette smoking).

Reference

1. Grundy SM, Stone NJ, Bailey AL, et al. 2018 AHA/ACC/AACVPR/AAPA/ABC/ACPM/ADA/AGS/APhA/ASPC/NLA/PCNA guideline on the management of blood cholesterol: a report of the American College of Cardiology/American Heart Association task force on clinical practice guidelines. Circulation. 2019;139(25):e1082–143.

166. Correct Answer: C

Rationale

The MESA risk score is an estimate of 10-year CHD risk obtained using traditional risk factors and the coronary calcium score. None of the other options listed incorporate coronary calcium scoring.

Answers

MESA 10-Year CHD Risk with Coronary Artery Calcification

The Multi-Ethnic Study of Atherosclerosis

Back to CAC Tools

Gender	Male ● Female ○
Age (45-85 years)	70 Years
Coronary Artery Calcification	0 Agatston
Race/Ethnicity	Choose One: Caucasian ○ Chinese ○ African American ○ Hispanic ●
Diabetes	Yes ○ No ●
Currently Smoke	Yes ○ No ●
Family History of Heart Attack	Yes ○ No ● History in parents, siblings, or children
Total Cholesterol	190 mg/dL
HDL Cholesterol	50 mg/dL
Systolic Blood Pressure	130 mmHg
Lipid Lowering Medication	Yes ○ No ●
Hypertension Medication	Yes ○ No ●

Calculate 10-year CHD risk

The estimated 10-year risk of a CHD event for a person with this risk factor profile including coronary calcium is 3.1%. The estimated 10-year risk of a CHD event for a person with this risk factor profile if we did not factor in their coronary calcium score would be 9.3%.

Figure reproduced with permission from McClelland et al. J Am Coll Cardiol. 2015 Oct 13;66(15):1643–53

References
1. Blaha MJ, Whelton SP, Al Rifai M, et al. Comparing risk scores in the prediction of coronary and cardiovascular deaths: coronary artery calcium consortium. JACC Cardiovasc Imaging. 2021;14(2):411–21.
2. McClelland RL, Jorgensen NW, Budoff M, et al. 10-Year coronary heart disease risk prediction using coronary artery calcium and traditional risk factors: derivation in the MESA (Multi-Ethnic Study of Atherosclerosis) with validation in the HNR (Heinz Nixdorf Recall) Study and the DHS (Dallas Heart Study). J Am Coll Cardiol. 2015;66(15):1643–53.

167. Correct Answer: B

Rationale
Coronary plaques with positive remodeling have a higher lipid content and macrophage count which is thought to make the plaque more vulnerable to rupture. Coronary plaques which demonstrate negative remodeling may result in a higher degree of stenosis but tend to be more stable than those which demonstrate positive remodeling. Additionally, spotty calcifications within non-calcified plaque are a high-risk finding by coronary CTA.

References
1. Akers EJ, Nicholls SJ, Di Bartolo BA. Plaque calcification: do lipoproteins have a role? Arterioscler Thromb Vasc Biol. 2019; 39(10):1902–10.
2. Onea HL, Spinu M, Homorodean C, et al. Distinctive morphological patterns of complicated coronary plaques in acute coronary syndromes: insights from an optical coherence tomography study. Diagnostics (Basel). 2022;12(11):2837.

168-1. Correct Answer: B

Rationale
MRI-PDFF, or MRI Proton Density Fat Fraction, provides an excellent assessment of liver fat but does not give fibrosis information. MRE or magnetic resonance elastography, is the best imaging measure of liver fibrosis. At this time, however, a limited number of MRE facilities are available and the test is very costly. Thus, the preferred imaging technique to assess for advanced fibrosis is VCTE, or vibration-controlled transient elastography, known commercially as the FibroScan.

FIB-4 is an index estimate of liver fibrosis using the four variables: age, platelet count, and the aminotransferases AST and ALT. The reason patients with diabetes mellitus should be assessed for advanced fibrosis with FIB-4 even in the absence of elevated transaminases is that they have an extremely high prevalence of NASH with fibrosis, perhaps 40%. Also, T2D is now considered to be a major risk enhancer for progression of NAFLD to NASH and cirrhosis. Otherwise, all patients with the NASH phenotype of insulin resistance, pre-diabetes, obesity, hypertension, and dyslipidemia should be considered for evaluation in the presence of persistently elevated aminotransferases, that is, >6 months.

168-2. Correct Answer: E

Rationale

Vitamin E has limited evidence to support its use for NASH, but it is in patients without T2D, not those with T2D. Pioglitazone and GLP1-RA, though not FDA indicated for the treatment of NASH, have demonstrated efficacy in some studies. As GLP1-RA also convey CV benefit in patients with T2D, they represent the preferred therapeutic. Regarding the other choices, it is important to remember that NASH is a consequence of multiple metabolic derangements, all of which carry risk for CVD. Thus, each risk factor for NASH, and CVD, must be treated aggressively and according to standard of care. Weight loss is particularly beneficial as data have demonstrated that greater weight loss is associated with a greater chance of reducing not just liver fat, but fibrosis as well. A minimum 5% weight loss is essential, but a >10% weight loss is preferred.

168-3. Correct Answer: C

Rationale

C is correct. These options represent the values that define intermediate risk for progression to cirrhosis. For FIB-4, low risk is defined as <1.3; intermediate risk 1.3–2.67, and high risk >2.67. For liver stiffness measurement (LSM) based on FibroScan, low risk is defined as <8 kPa; intermediate risk 8–12 kPa; and high risk >12 kPa. Risk is enhanced if any of these additional features is also present: T2D or pre-DM, age >50, BMI >40 kg/m^2, multiple metabolic risk factors, and genetic markers such as PNLPA3. Such individuals should be referred to gastroenterology or hepatology for further evaluation, including a possible liver biopsy.

References
1. Cusi K, Isaacs S, Barb D, et al. American Association of Clinical Endocrinology clinical practice guideline for the diagnosis and management of nonalcoholic fatty liver disease in primary care and endocrinology clinical settings co-sponsored by the American Association for the Study of Liver Diseases (AASLD). Endocr Pract. 2022;28:528–62.
2. Duell PB, Welty FK, Miller M, et al. American Heart Association Council on Arteriosclerosis, Thrombosis and Vascular Biology; Council on Hypertension; Council on the Kidney in Cardiovascular Disease; Council on Lifestyle and Cardiometabolic Health; and Council on Peripheral Vascular Disease. Nonalcoholic fatty liver disease and cardiovascular risk: a scientific statement from the American Heart Association. Arterioscler Thromb Vasc Biol. 2022;42(6):e168–85.

169. Correct Answer: B

Rationale

Among the non-pharmacologic treatments of high blood pressure is low-sodium dietary intake (<2300 mg of sodium per day). To lower dietary sodium intake, some patients may inquire about salt substitutes. Salt substitutes vary regarding their sodium chloride and potassium chloride content; their taste varies as well. Salt substitutes with no sodium may have high amounts of potassium chloride, which may exacerbate hyperkalemia in patients with renal insufficiency. Sea salt is evaporation of seawater that is minimally processed and retains trace minerals such as magnesium, potassium, calcium, and other nutrients. In most cases, sea salt does not offer substantial sodium-reduction or potential health advantages over table salt. It is often recommended that for adults with an average BP >20/10 mmHg above their BP target, that antihypertensive drug therapy be initiated with two first-line agents of different classes, either as separate agents or in a fixed-dose combination. Common examples include angiotensin-converting enzyme inhibitor/angiotensin-receptor blocker in combination with a calcium channel blocker or thiazide diuretic in the same pill. Chlorthalidone and indapamide are "thiazide-like" diuretics with longer half-lives than hydrochlorothiazide and may achieve greater BP reduction. While some advocate chlorthalidone is preferred over hydrochlorothiazide, the data supporting such a recommendation is not always consistent. Loop diuretics (e.g., furosemide, torasemide, bumetanide, and azosemide) may be preferred in patients with heart failure and when estimated glomerular filtration rate is <30 mL/min. Due to questionable added benefit in lowering blood pressure, and increased risk of hyperkalemia, angiotensin receptor blockers should not be used in combination with direct renin inhibitors (i.e., aliskiren). Beta blockers reduce CVD in patients with reduced ejection fraction, are used to treat angina pectoris and cardiac dysrhythmias, and may reduce the risk of recurrent myocardial infarction after an acute myocardial infarction.

Reference

1. Bays HE, Kulkarni A, German C, et al. Ten things to know about ten cardiovascular disease risk factors—2022. Am J Prev Cardiol. 2022;10:100342.

170. Correct Answer: D

Rationale

In patients treated for obesity, semaglutide and liraglutide are examples of anti-diabetes agents with cardiovascular disease (CVD) outcome trial support for reduction in major adverse cardiac events (MACE) in patients with Type 2 diabetes mellitus. At higher doses, semaglutide and liraglutide are approved to treat obesity. However, at the time of this writing, no anti-obesity drug has an indicated use to reduce MACE. Semaglutide at 2.4 mg subcutaneously per week is approved for treatment of obesity. Lower doses of semaglutide and liraglutide are approved to lower glucose in patients with diabetes mellitus. Semaglutide is administered as subcutaneous injectable doses of 0.25–2.0 mg per week and oral doses of 7–14 mg per day. In patients with congestive cardiomyopathy and obesity, GLP-1 receptor agonists may be of benefit. However, most guidelines and evidence from cardiovascular outcomes studies support the use of certain sodium glucose transport 2 inhibitors, which inhibit renal tubular reabsorption, produce natriuresis, and have proven benefit in improving CVD outcomes especially in patients with congestive cardiomyopathy. Tirzepatide is a unimolecular GLP-1 and glucose-dependent insulinotropic polypeptide (GIP) agonist that reduces glucose in patients with diabetes and reduces body weight in patients with overweight or obesity. Phentermine is a sympathomimetic that is a commonly prescribed anti-obesity agent. While some data suggests phentermine may be safe in patients at low cardiovascular disease risk, phentermine is contraindicated in patients with cardiovascular disease, and its long-term effects on MACE in patients at low or moderate CVD risk are unknown.

Reference
1. Bays HE, Kulkarni A, German C, et al. Ten things to know about ten cardiovascular disease risk factors—2022. Am J Prev Cardiol. 2022;10:100342.

171. Correct Answer: B

Rationale
Coronary anatomy is often assessed by CAC, coronary computerized tomography (CCTA), cardiac resonance imaging (CMR), and cardiac catheterization. Cardiac diastolic dysfunction is often evaluated by echocardiogram and CMR. Myocardial perfusion is often assessed by single-photon emission computerized tomography (SPECT), positron emission tomography (PET), and CMR. Cardiomyocyte injury and fibrosis is often evaluated by CMR and CCTA. Microvascular dysfunction is often evaluated by PET and CMR. Hybrid imaging tests include: PET/CT and PET/MRI to assess perfusion, cardiac viability, and atherosclerosis. CT-Fractional Flow Reserve (FFR) provides anatomic (i.e., luminal and plaque) and physiologic/functional imaging data to assess obstructive CAD. Cardiac catheterization and FFR: Provides (invasive) anatomic and functional assessment of CAD. CAC added to SPECT or PET may help further identify coronary artery plaque and better stratify risk. CCTA added to CAC scoring may help improve the assessment of total plaque burden and better discriminate risk of death and/or myocardial infarction among symptomatic patients with suspected coronary artery disease.

Reference
1. Bays HE, Khera A, Blaha MJ, et al. Ten things to know about ten imaging studies: a preventive cardiology perspective ("ASPC top ten imaging"). Am J Prev Cardiol. 2021;6:100176.

172. Correct Answer: A

Rationale

Coronary computed tomography angiography (CCTA) has over 90% sensitivity for anatomically significant coronary artery disease. CCTA has a high negative predictive value, such that if negative, the patient has low likelihood of clinically meaningful CVD risk. Exercise treadmill stress testing alone has about a 60% sensitivity and specificity for anatomically significant coronary artery disease. That is why treadmill stress testing is often performed along with an imaging study (e.g., Single-photon emission computed tomography or SPECT). SPECT may have close to a 90% sensitivity, but around a 70% specificity for anatomically significant coronary artery disease. Examples of factors associated with false positive SPECT results are female sex, presence of cardiac microvascular coronary artery disease, left bundle branch block, and cardiomyopathy. Positron emission tomography (PET) and stress cardiac magnetic resonance (CMR) both have >80% sensitivity and selectivity for anatomically and functionally significant CVD. The choice of PET and CMR is largely due to location and clinician/institutional choice. Coronary calcium imaging (CAC)/score has over 90% sensitivity, but less than 50% specificity for anatomically significant cardiovascular disease CVD. That is why CAC scores are mainly used to identify high coronary artery disease risk individuals, such that more definitive diagnostic tests can then be considered.

Reference
1. Bays HE, Khera A, Blaha MJ, et al. Ten things to know about ten imaging studies: a preventive cardiology perspective ("ASPC top ten imaging"). Am J Prev Cardiol. 2021;6:100176.

173. Correct Answer: B

Rationale

The 2022 American College of Cardiology Expert Consensus Decision Pathway (ACC ECDP) recommends that intensity of statin therapy be based on the calculation of 10-year ASCVD risk among patients with Type 2 diabetes mellitus. This is in contrast to the 2018 ACC/AHA Multisociety guidelines that recommends a moderate intensity statin without calculating the 10-year ASCVD risk if the LDL-C is ≥70 mg/dL (unless there are multiple risk factors present). According to the 2022 ACC ECDP, if the calculated 10-year ASCVD risk is ≥7.5% or if patient has diabetes-specific risk enhancers, a high intensity statin is recommended.

References
1. Lloyd-Jones DM, Morris PB, Ballantyne CM, et al. 2022 ACC expert consensus decision pathway on the role of nonstatin therapies for LDL-cholesterol lowering in the management of atherosclerotic cardiovascular disease risk: a report of the American College of Cardiology Solution Set Oversight Committee. J Am Coll Cardiol. 2022;80(14):1366–418.
2. Grundy SM, Stone NJ, Bailey AL, et al. 2018 AHA/ACC/AACVPR/AAPA/ABC/ACPM/ADA/AGS/APhA/ASPC/NLA/PCNA guideline on the management of blood cholesterol: a report of the American College of Cardiology/American Heart Association task force on clinical practice guidelines. Circulation. 2019;139(25):e1082–143.

174. Correct Answer: B

Rationale
The 2022 ACC ECDP defines 'very high risk' ASCVD as two major ASCVD events (including ACS within the prior 12 months, prior MI, prior ischemic stroke, or PAD defined by claudication with ABI <0.85 or prior peripheral revascularization or amputation) or one major ASCVD event and multiple high-risk conditions. For patients with very high-risk ASCVD or ASCVD with FH, the threshold for the addition of either ezetimibe or PCSK9 inhibitor is ≥55 mg/dL. Additional non-statin therapies should be considered if the patient remains above the threshold. Rosuvastatin 40 mg is more effective in reducing LDL-C than atorvastatin 80 mg.

175. Correct Answer: A

Rationale
The 2022 ACC ECDP emphasizes the importance of subclinical atherosclerosis in guiding clinical management. Among patients with a CAC score of ≥1000 AU, the addition of ezetimibe is reasonable. If there is <50% reduction in LDL-C or the LDL-C remains ≥70 mg/dL despite the addition of a high-intensity statin and ezetimibe, the addition of a PCSK9 inhibitor can be considered. In the given patient, however, despite a 0 calcium score, she has a positive family history of premature CHD which is one of the exceptions for delaying the use of a statin. Thus, statin therapy would be recommended.

References
1. Lloyd-Jones DM, Morris PB, Ballantyne CM, et al. 2022 ACC expert consensus decision pathway on the role of nonstatin therapies for LDL-cholesterol lowering in the management of atherosclerotic cardiovascular disease risk: a report of the American College of Cardiology Solution Set Oversight Committee. J Am Coll Cardiol. 2022;80(14):1366–418.
2. Grundy SM, Stone NJ, Bailey AL, et al. 2018 AHA/ACC/AACVPR/AAPA/ABC/ACPM/ADA/AGS/APhA/ASPC/NLA/PCNA guideline on the management of blood cholesterol: a report of the American College of Cardiology/American Heart Association task force on clinical practice guidelines. Circulation. 2019;139(25):e1082–143.

176. Correct Answer: C

Rationale

Of the above options, only an Lp(a) of 100 mg/dL is a risk-enhancing factor. Family history of premature ASCVD is defined by premature ASCVD in a first degree relative for a male, age <55 years old, or female, age <65 years old. An HDL-C level <40 mg/dL in men (or <50 mg/dL in women) is considered risk enhancing as part of a diagnosis of metabolic syndrome which requires three of the following: increased waist circumference (by ethnically appropriate cutpoints), elevated triglycerides [≥150 mg/dL, nonfasting], elevated blood pressure, elevated glucose, and low HDL-C. Lp(a) is considered risk enhancing at levels ≥50 mg/dL. Updated 10-year risk can be estimated based Lp(a) level using the following formula: Updated 10-year risk estimate = Predicted 10-year risk estimate $\times [1.11^{(Lp(a) \text{ level in nmol/L}/50)}]$. A triglyceride level ≥175 mg (non-fasting) is considered risk enhancing when elevated on three separate occasions.

References
1. Arnett DK, Blumenthal RS, Albert MA, et al. 2019 ACC/AHA guideline on the primary prevention of cardiovascular disease: a report of the American College of Cardiology/American Heart Association Task Force on Clinical Practice Guidelines [published correction appears in Circulation. 2019;140(11):e649–50] [published correction appears in Circulation. 2020;141(4):e60] [published correction appears in Circulation. 2020;141(16):e774]. Circulation. 2019;140(11):e596–646.
2. Reyes-Soffer G, Ginsberg HN, Berglund L, et al. Lipoprotein(a): a genetically determined, causal, and prevalent risk factor for atherosclerotic cardiovascular disease: a scientific statement From the American Heart Association. Arterioscler Thromb Vasc Biol. 2022;42(1):e48–60.

177. Correct answer: A

Rationale

Early lipid screening at the age of 2 years is recommended in children with a strong family history of early onset ASCVD (male, age <55 years; female, age <65 years) in a parent, grandparent, aunt, uncle or sibling, a parent with a total cholesterol ≥240 mg/dL, or if the child has cardiac risk factors such as diabetes mellitus or obesity.

Reference
1. McGowan MP, Hosseini Dehkordi SH, et al. Diagnosis and treatment of heterozygous familial hypercholesterolemia. J Am Heart Assoc. 2019;8(24):e013225.

Answers

178. Correct Answer: C

Rationale

Data from the MESA cohort suggests that the radiation exposure with a single computed tomography scan for coronary artery calcium scoring is approximately 1 mSv. The average radiation exposure from background radiation sources in the United States is approximately 3 mSv per year per person.

References
1. Messenger B, Li D, Nasir K, et al. Coronary calcium scans and radiation exposure in the multi-ethnic study of atherosclerosis. Int J Cardiovasc Imaging. 2016;32(3):525–9. https://doi.org/10.1007/s10554-015-0799-3.
2. Akram S, Chowdhury YS. Radiation exposure of medical imaging. In: StatPearls. Treasure Island (FL): StatPearls Publishing; 2021.

179. Correct Answer: B

Rationale

Initiation of a very-low fat diet (<30 g per day) is the best next step to attempt to reduce persistent severe hypertriglyceridemia despite maximal dose statin therapy in this patient. Addition of a fibrate is also a reasonable step. However, fenofibrate would be preferred over gemfibrozil due to the higher risk of severe myopathy with combined gemfibrozil and statin use. Amlodipine is not associated with hypertriglyceridemia but anti-hypertensive medications such as beta-blockers and thiazide diuretics are associated with increases in triglyceride levels. Increases in carbohydrates, especially refined carbohydrates, in the diet may exacerbate hypertriglyceridemia.

Reference
1. Grundy SM, Stone NJ, Bailey AL, et al. 2018 AHA/ACC/AACVPR/AAPA/ABC/ACPM/ADA/AGS/APhA/ASPC/NLA/PCNA guideline on the management of blood cholesterol: executive summary: a report of the American College of Cardiology/American Heart Association task force on clinical practice guidelines [published correction appears in J Am Coll Cardiol. 2019;73(24):3234–7]. J Am Coll Cardiol. 2019;73(24):3168–209. https://doi.org/10.1016/j.jacc.2018.11.002.

180. Correct Answer: C

Rationale

Although there remain no current universally accepted criteria for familial hyperlipidemia, the Dutch Criteria and Simone Broom Criteria have been shown to have similar predictive power in identifying familial hypercholesteremia and incorporate genetic testing towards a diagnosis. National Lipid Association expert opinion guidelines states patients ≥20 years of with an LDL ≥190 mg/dL or ≥220 mg/dL should be screened for family hypercholesteremia. The Dutch Criteria uses a scored system using family history, personal history, clinical exam, genetic testing of LDL-R mutation, and LDL-C value to scale the likelihood of familial hypercholesteremia, although genetic testing alone will not suffice in a definitive diagnosis. The Simone Broom Criteria alternative is diagnosed based on any one of the criteria to make a definite or possible diagnosis. The patient falls under "possible" familial hypercholesteremia based on both the Dutch and Simone Broom Criteria. Genetic testing should be considered as may further stratify the patient into a definitive diagnosis.

References
1. McGowan MP, Hosseini Dehkordi SH, et al. Diagnosis and treatment of heterozygous familial hypercholesterolemia. J Am Heart Assoc. 2019;8(24):e013225.
2. Goldberg AC, Hopkins PN, Toth PP, et al. Familial hypercholesterolemia: screening, diagnosis, and management of pediatric and adult patients: clinical guidance from the National Lipid Association Expert Panel on Familial Hypercholesterolemia. J Clin Lipidol. 2011;5:S1–8.
3. World Health Organization. Familial hypercholesterolaemia (FH): report of a second WHO consultation. 1998. whqlibdoc.who.int/hq/1999/WHOHGN_FH_CONS 99.2.pdf. Accessed 5 Nov 2022.
4. Scientific Steering Committee on behalf of the Simon Broome Register Group. Risk of fatal coronary heart disease in familial hypercholesterolaemia. BMJ. 1991;303:893–6.

181. Correct Answer: B

Rationale
In 2019, the REDUCE-IT trial was a multicenter, double-blind, placebo-randomized control trial which compared placebo on optimal statin therapy to icosapent ethyl on optimal therapy in patient with established cardiovascular disease or diabetes mellitus on patients who had a TG of 135−499 mg/dL and LDL-C of 41−100 mg/dL. On primary endpoint of gardio, there was an absolute risk reduction of 4.8% and number need to treat of 21 with reducing cardiovascular death, nonfatal myocardial infarction, nonfatal stroke, coronary revascularization, or unstable angina with icosapent ethyl compared to placebo. Furthermore, patients with prior myocardial infarction have further benefits which icosapent ethyl applied to a maximally tolerated statin. There remains concern regarding the cost-effectiveness of icosapent ethyl at this time.

References
1. Bhatt DL, Steg PG, Miller M, et al. Cardiovascular risk reduction with icosapent ethyl for hypertriglyceridemia. N Engl J Med. 2019;380(1):11−22.
2. Gaba P, Bhatt DL, Steg PG, et al. Prevention of cardiovascular events and mortality with icosapent ethyl in patients with prior myocardial infarction. J Am Coll Cardiol. 2022;79(17):1660−71.

182. Correct Answer: B

Rationale
The American Heart Association in 2021 published a Scientific Statement regarding how to clinically implement Lp(a) Levels regarding risk assessment. They recommended that if Lp(a) levels are measured, they can be used to modify patients at borderline or intermediate 10-year risk under the Pooled Cohort Equation. Adjustment of the 10-year predictive risk can be performed by multiplying the 10-year risk by $1.11^{(Lp(a)\ level\ in\ nmol/50)}$.

References
1. Reyes-Soffer G, Ginsberg HN, Berglund L, et al. Lipoprotein(a): a genetically determined, causal, and prevalent risk factor for atherosclerotic cardiovascular disease: a scientific statement from the American Heart Association. Arterioscler Thromb Vasc Biol. 2022;42(1):e48–60.
2. Patel AP, Wang M, Pirruccello JP, Ellinor PT, Ng K, Kathiresan S, Khera AV. Lp(a) (lipoprotein[a]) concentrations and incident atherosclerotic cardiovascular disease: new insights from a large national biobank. Arterioscler Thromb Vasc Biol. 2021;41:465–74.

183. Correct Answer: D

Rationale
Coronary flow reserve (CFR)/myocardial flow reserve (MFR) when applied to a patient's PET myocardial perfusion scan can predominantly reclassify patients at intermediate risk for MACE to low or high risk based on the original results from the PET myocardial perfusion scan. A CFR of <1.5 has been associated with a six-fold increase in MACE independent of other factors compared to individuals with a normal CFR ≥2.0. The patient described here has a low-risk perfusion scan with an elevated risk MACE based on CFR. Thus, the patient is now at an intermediate risk of annual MACE. Although the risk has been elevated, 2014 guidelines do not base CFR as a factor that modifies a patient's perioperative risk and should not be actively used to assess patients risk prior to surgery.

References
1. Ziadi MC. Myocardial flow reserve (MFR) with positron emission tomography (PET)/computed tomography (CT): clinical impact in diagnosis and prognosis. Cardiovasc Diagn Ther. 2017;7(2):206–18.
2. Murthy VL, Naya M, Foster CR, et al. Improved cardiac risk assessment with noninvasive measures of coronary flow reserve. Circulation. 2011;124(20):2215–24.
3. Fleisher LA, Fleischmann KE, Auerbach AD, et al. ACC/AHA guideline on perioperative cardiovascular evaluation and management of patients undergoing

noncardiac surgery: executive summary: a report of the American College of Cardiology/American Heart Association task force on practice guidelines. Circulation. 2014;130(24):2215–45.

184. Correct Answer: B

Rationale
The lifetime prevalence of major depression disorder in the United States is 20.6%.

Reference
1. Hasin DS, Sarvet AL, Meyers JL, et al. Epidemiology of adult DSM-5 major depressive disorder and its specifiers in the United States. JAMA Psychiatry. 2018;75:336–46.

185. Correct Answer: C

Rationale
Short, brief, well-validated 2-item screening tools such as the Patient Health Questionnaire-2 for depression and the Generalized Anxiety Disorder Questionnaire-2 can be administered by nurses or medical assistants and a positive screen for these conditions can open up a discussion about additional symptoms and referral for additional assessment and management of psychiatric conditions if indicated.

Reference
1. Levine GN, Cohen BE, Commodore-Mensah Y, et al. Psychological health, well-being, and the mind-heart-body connection. A scientific statement from the American Heart Association. Circulation. 2021;e763–3783.

186. Correct Answer: D

Rationale
The Enhancing Recovery in Coronary Heart Disease (ENRICHD) study was a multicenter randomized clinical trial of 2481 post-MI patients that examined the benefit of cognitive behavioral therapy for depression on reducing cardiovascular outcomes but did not show significant improvements in cardiac events or mortality. The Recurrent Coronary Prevention Project was an intervention trial on type A behavior and did show a benefit in reducing cardiovascular outcomes. The Montreal Heart Attack Readjustment Trial intervened on anxiety and did not show benefits in cardiovascular outcomes.

References
1. Berkman LF, Blumenthal J, Burg M, et al. Enhancing Recovery in Coronary Heart Disease Patients Investigators (ENRICHD). Effects of treating depression and low perceived social support on clinical events after myocardial infarction: the Enhancing Recovery in Coronary Heart Disease Patients (ENRICHD) Randomized Trial. JAMA. 2003;289:3106–16.
2. Friedman M, Thoresen CE, Gill JJ, et al. Alteration of type A behavior and its effect on cardiac recurrences in post myocardial infarction patients: summary results of the recurrent coronary prevention project. Am Heart J. 1986;112(4):653–65.
3. Frasure-Smith N, Lespérance F, et al. Long-term survival differences among low-anxious, high-anxious, and repressive copers enrolled in the Montreal heart attack readjustment trial. Psychosom Med. 2002;64(4):571–9.

187. Correct Answer: D

Rationale
All of the above are true. Multiple studies have shown optimism is associated with healthier behaviors and a lower risk of CVD and all-cause mortality; a recent meta-analysis of over 200,000 individuals across 15 observation studies showed higher levels of optimism were associated with a 35% decreased risk of incident CVD even and a 14% decreased risk of all-cause mortality. A high sense of purpose in life has also been associated with improved cardiovascular health, longevity, and reduced CVD risk, including a meta-analysis of 10 studies involving >130,000 participants showing a high purpose in life was associated with a 17% decreased risk of both CVD events and all-cause mortality. Happiness, as a form of positive emotional state, has also been shown to be associated with lower risks of incident CHD in one prospective cohort study, as well as lower mortality risks among individuals with diabetes in the NHANES (National Health and Nutritional Examination Study) follow-up.

Reference
1. Levine GN, Cohen BE, Commodore-Mensah Y, et al. Psychological health, well-being, and the mind-heart-body connection. A scientific statement from the American Heart Association. Circulation. 2021;e763–3783.

188. Correct Answer: B

Rationale
There are two forms of androgen deficiency, primary and secondary. This patient presents with symptoms of androgen deficiency due to secondary (pituitary–hypothalamic) hypogonadism with low testosterone levels, normal LH and FSH. Obesity

is associated with lower serum testosterone levels. Low testosterone is also associated with increased risk of diabetes. Primary (testicular) hypogonadism, on the contrary, commonly presents with elevated LH and FSH and is seen in patients with genetic abnormalities, Klinefelter syndrome, testicular trauma, infection, chemotherapy/radiation, or autoimmune etiology.

The latest Endocrine Society Clinical Practice Guideline recommends testosterone therapy for men with symptomatic testosterone deficiency to improve secondary sex characteristics and correct symptoms of hypogonadism after discussing the potential benefits and risks of therapy and instituting appropriate monitoring for the patient. Hemoglobin/hematocrit and PSA levels should be monitored when administering testosterone therapy. Appropriately prescribed testosterone therapy provides benefits, especially in primary hypogonadism.

Testosterone supplementation has been shown to increase muscle mass, strength, and exercise capacity. The Testosterone in Older Men with Mobility Limitations (TOM) trial, a placebo-controlled, randomized trial, investigated the effects of testosterone on lower extremity strength and physical function in men aged 65 and older with low testosterone levels. Testosterone treatment improved their fitness, but the study was stopped early due to significantly higher rate of adverse cardiovascular events in the testosterone group. Although conflicting results exist, several other studies suggest that testosterone replacement increases the risk of cardiovascular events, leading to the FDA warning statement about potential cardiovascular risk of testosterone replacement therapy. Their cardiovascular safety remains largely unclear at this time. Informed decision, discussion about the risks/benefits is advised when considering testosterone replacement therapy.

Testosterone modulates vascular tone, increases erythropoiesis, and affects platelet aggregability. However, there are conflicting results on the effect of testosterone therapy on progression of atherosclerosis, inflammation, and insulin sensitivity. The metabolic effects of testosterone are complex and further studies are needed to elucidate cardiovascular safety of testosterone replacement therapy.

Although in a randomized, double blind, placebo-controlled trial "Testosterone Treatment to Prevent or Revert Type 2 Diabetes (T4DM)," treatment with testosterone reduced the risk of Type 2 Diabetes in men with impaired glucose tolerance or newly diagnosed Type 2 Diabetes, the Endocrine Society Clinical Practice Guideline recommends against testosterone therapy as a means of improving glycemic control in diabetic patients with low testosterone.

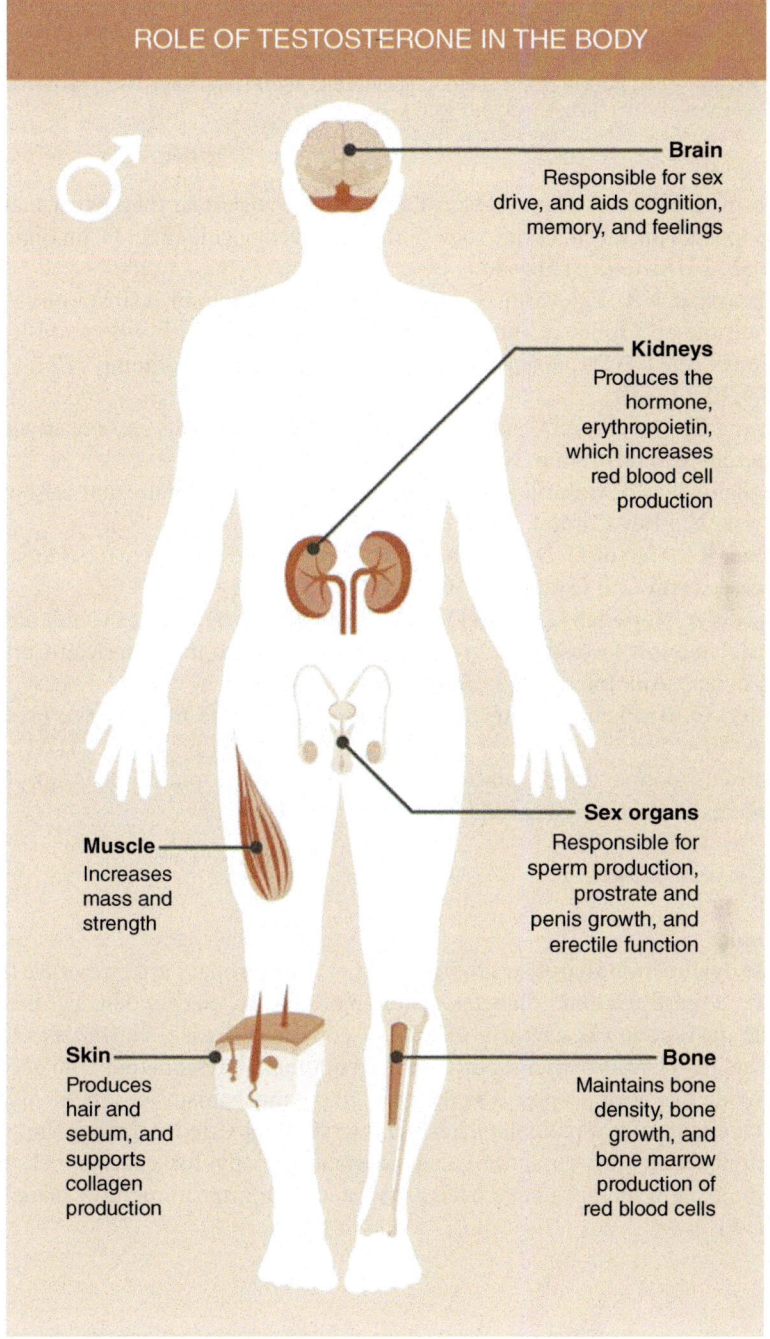

Testosterone has multiple effects on the body. Testosterone affects the brain with stimulation of libido and aggression; muscle strength and mass; bone growth and density; sex organ growth, along with spermatogenesis and erectile function; kidney production of erythropoietin; and skin effects, including hair growth. *T* testosterone. (Figure and legend reproduced with permission from J Am Coll Cardiol. 2016 Feb, 67 (5) 545–557)

References
1. Bhasin S, Brito JP, Cunningham GR, et al. Testosterone therapy in men with hypogonadism: an endocrine society clinical practice guideline. J Clin Endocrinol Metab. 2018;103(5):1715–44.
2. LeBrasseur NK, Lajevardi N, Miciek R, et al. Effects of testosterone therapy on muscle performance and physical function in older men with mobility limitations (the TOM Trial): design and methods. Contemp Clin Trials. 2009;30:133–40.
3. Basaria S, Coviello AD, Travison TG, et al. Adverse events associated with testosterone administration. NEJM. 2010;363:109–22.
4. Gagliano-Jucá T, Basaria S. Testosterone replacement therapy and cardiovascular risk. Nat Rev Cardiol. 2019;16(9):555–74.
5. Kloner RA, Carson C, Dobs A, Kopecky S, et al. Testosterone and cardiovascular disease. J Am Coll Cardiol. 2016;67(5):545–57.
6. Qaseem A, Horwitch CA, Vijan S, et al. Testosterone treatment in adult men with age-related low testosterone: a clinical guideline from the American College of Physicians. Ann Intern Med. 2020;172(2):126–33.
7. Wittert G, Bracken K, Robledo KP, et al. Testosterone treatment to prevent or revert type 2 diabetes in men enrolled in a lifestyle programme (T4DM): a randomised, double-blind, placebo-controlled, 2-year, phase 3b trial. Lancet Diabetes Endocrinol. 2021;9(1):32–45.

189. Correct Answer: C

Rationale
Erectile dysfunction shares similar risk factors with coronary artery disease (hypertension, hyperlipidemia, diabetes, smoking, obesity, and sedentary lifestyle). Erectile dysfunction is an early marker of coronary disease, with a lead time of 2–5 years [2–4]. Microvascular disease and endothelial dysfunction with decreased nitric oxide has been proposed as the most likely mechanism for erectile dysfunction in the majority of patients. Lifestyle interventions (Mediterranean diet, physical activity, smoking cessation) and pharmacotherapy for cardiac risk factors (including statin therapy) have been associated with improvement in sexual function [1, 5].

References
1. Gupta BP, Hassan Murad M, Clifton MM, et al. The effect of lifestyle modification and cardiovascular risk factor reduction on erectile dysfunction: a systematic review and meta-analysis. Arch Intern Med. 2011;171:1791–803.
2. Jackson G. Erectile dysfunction: a marker of silent coronary artery disease. Eur Heart J. 2006;27(22):2613–14.
3. Hodges LD, Kirby M, Solanki J, et al. The temporal relationship between erectile dysfunction and cardiovascular disease. Int J Clin Pract. 2007;61(12):2019–25.
4. Gazzaruso C, Giordanetti S, De Amici E, et al. Relationship between erectile dysfunction and silent myocardial ischemia in apparently uncomplicated type 2 diabetic patients. Circulation. 2004;110(1):22–6.
5. Esposito K, Ciotola M, Giugliano F, et al. Mediterranean diet improves erectile function in subjects with the metabolic syndrome. Int J Impot Res. 2006;18(4):405–10.

190. Correct Answer: A

Rationale
The Mediterranean diet has been associated with reduced risk of cardiovascular events, and the greater the intake of components of Mediterranean diet, the lower the incidence of cardiac events. In the Women's Health Study, a prospective cohort study of over 25,000 US women, the greatest benefit for cardiovascular risk reduction of the Mediterranean diet has been found to be due to its anti-inflammatory effect, which was greater than its lipid or glucose effects. The cardioprotective properties of extra-virgin olive oil, rich in mono-unsaturated fats, are attributed to the presence of its phenolic compounds. Multiple studies have shown that supplementation of diet with extra virgin olive oil leads to reduced systemic inflammation, improved endothelial function, and reduced oxidative stress.

References
1. Ahmad S, Moorthy MV, Demler OV, et al. Assessment of risk factors and biomarkers associated with risk of cardiovascular disease among women consuming a Mediterranean diet. JAMA Network Open. 2018;1(8):e185708.
2. Widmer RJ, Flammer AJ, Lerman LO, Lerman A. The Mediterranean diet, its components, and cardiovascular disease. Am J Med. 2015;128(3):229–38.
3. Covas MI, Nyyssonen K, Poulsen HE, et al. The effect of polyphenols in olive oil on heart disease risk factors: a randomized trial. Ann Intern Med. 2006;145(5):333–41.
4. Visioli F, Caruso D, Grande S, et al. Virgin Olive Oil Study (VOLOS): vasoprotective potential of extra virgin olive oil in mildly dyslipidemic patients. Eur J Nutr. 2005;44(2):121–7.

191. Correct Answer: E

Rationale

Although low-carbohydrate diets have increased popularity due to their short-term weight loss effect, their long-term effects could depend on whether the carbohydrate is replaced with animal-based fat and protein versus plant-based fat and protein. In a recent prospective cohort study and meta-analysis, which included adults enrolled in the Atherosclerosis Risk in Communities (ARIC) study and Prospective Urban Rural Epidemiology (PURE) cohort studies, there was a U-shaped curve between carbohydrate intake and all-cause mortality. The lowest mortality was observed when 50–55% of total energy intake came from unprocessed carbohydrates. Both low carbohydrate dietary intake (<40% of total energy from carbohydrates) and high carbohydrate intake (>70%) were associated with increased mortality. Mortality increased when carbohydrates were substituted with animal-derived fat and protein compared to plant-based fats and protein (such as whole grains, legumes, and nuts) which were associated with lower mortality.

References
1. Seidelmann SB, Claggett B, Cheng S, et al. Dietary carbohydrate intake and mortality: a prospective cohort study and meta-analysis. Lancet Public Health. 2018;3(9):e419–28.
2. Dehghan M, Mente A, Zhang X, et al. Associations of fats and carbohydrate intake with cardiovascular disease and mortality in 18 countries from five continents (PURE): a prospective cohort study. Lancet. 2017;390:2050–62.
3. The Atherosclerosis Risk in Communities (ARIC) Study: design and objectives. The ARIC investigators. Am J Epidemiol. 1989;129:687–702.

192. Correct Answer: B

Rationale

The Agatston CAC score is quantified per-lesion as the product of plaque area (mm^2) and a four-level categorical peak calcium density factor. A quantized calcium density weighting factor for the Agatston algorithm assigns a value of 1 through 4 based on the measured peak calcium density attenuation value of the lesion (1: 130–199 HU, 2: 200–299 HU, 3: 300–399 HU, 4: >400 HU). However, while the CAC score is weighted upward for higher peak calcium density on a per-plaque basis, it is well established that calcium density is inversely associated with lesion vulnerability and ASCVD risk in population-based cohorts when accounting for age and plaque area.

Answers

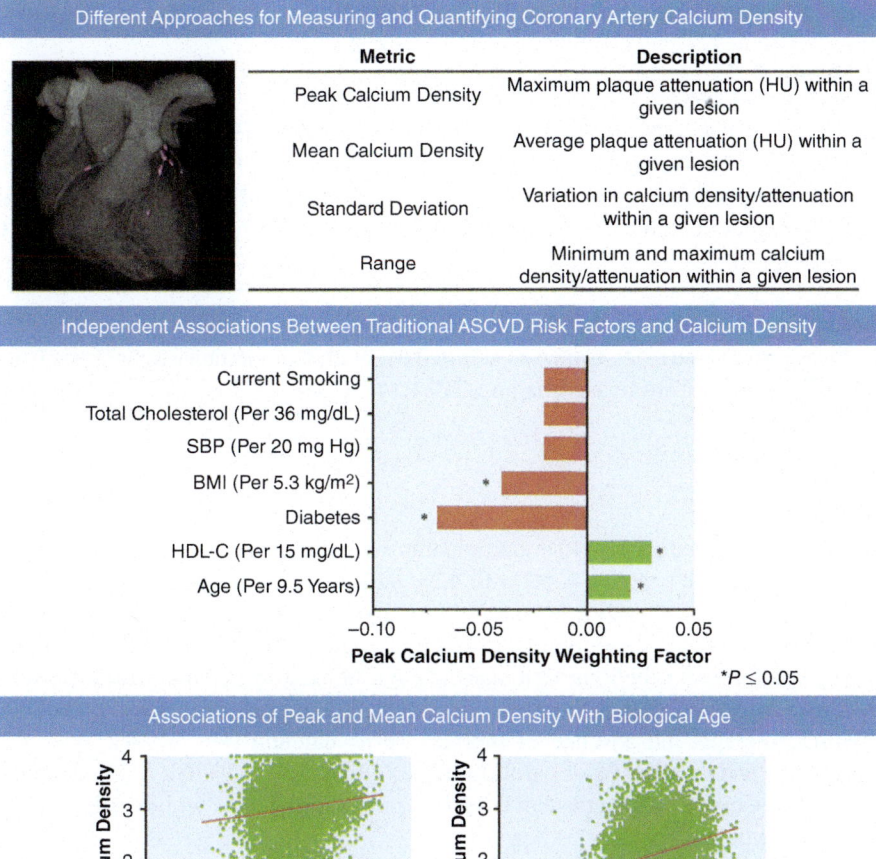

Figure reproduced with permission from JACC Cardiovasc Imaging. 2022 Sep;15(9):1648–1662

Reference

1. Razavi AC, Agatston AS, Shaw LJ, et al. Evolving role of calcium density in coronary artery calcium scoring and atherosclerotic cardiovascular disease risk. JACC Cardiovasc Imaging. 2022;15(9):1648–62.

193. Correct Answer: A

Rationale

It is suggested that evidence-based guidance should consider rescanning individuals with CAC = 0 in 3–7 years depending on individual demographics and their baseline risk profile. Beyond age, sex, and race/ethnicity, diabetes has a significant impact on the warranty period of a CAC score of 0. Contrastingly, family history of CHD and smoking have been found to have the smallest influences on the CAC = 0 warranty period.

Reference
1. Dzaye O, Dardari ZA, Cainzos-Achirica M, et al. Comprehensive analysis from MESA. JACC Cardiovasc Imaging. 2021;14(5):990–1002.

194. Correct Answer: C

Rationale

Among the approximately 40% participants with metabolic syndrome or Type 2 diabetes who have baseline CAC = 0. 42% have been observed to maintain long-term absence of CAC over a 10-year follow-up period. Younger age, a lower metabolic syndrome severity score, and absence of extra-coronary atherosclerosis serve as key predictors for the long-term absence of CAC among persons with metabolic syndrome or Type 2 diabetes. Independent of traditional risk factors and preventive pharmacotherapy, the absence of thoracic aortic calcium (OR = 2.72, 95% CI: 1.24–4.72) and/or absence of carotid plaque (OR = 1.81, 95% CI: 1.25–2.61) are strongly associated with persistent CAC = 0 among individuals with metabolic syndrome or Type 2 diabetes.

Reference
1. Razavi AC, Agatston AS, Shaw LJ, et al. Evolving role of calcium density in coronary artery calcium scoring and atherosclerotic cardiovascular disease risk. JACC Cardiovasc Imaging. 2022;15(9):1648–62.

195. Correct Answer: B

Rationale

Individuals with very high CAC (≥1000) are a unique population at substantially higher risk for ASCVD events, non-ASCVD outcomes, and mortality than those with lower CAC, with three-point major adverse cardiovascular event rates similar to those of a stable treated secondary prevention population. In particular, CAC ≥1000 corresponds to an annualized three-point major adverse cardiovascular event rate of 3.4 per 100 person-years, similar to that of the total FOURIER population (3.3) and higher than those of the lower-risk FOURIER subgroups.

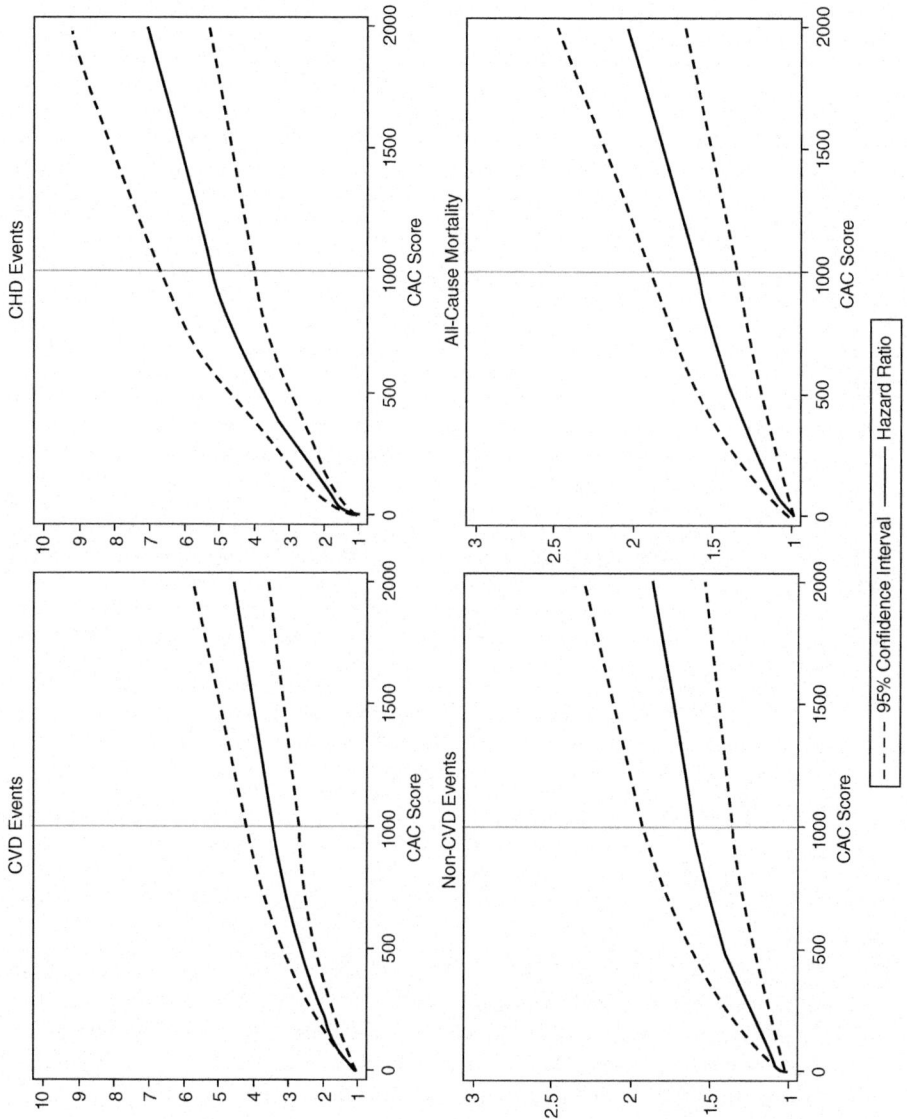

Multivariable-adjusted hazard ratios and 95% CIs for cardiovascular disease (CVD) events, coronary heart disease (CHD) events, non-CVD events, and all-cause mortality as a function of coronary artery calcium (CAC) score. Cubic splines were used in the multivariable model with knots placed at CAC 100 and CAC 1000. Hazard ratios were adjusted for age, sex, race/ethnicity, obesity, hypertension, total cholesterol, high-density lipoprotein cholesterol, triglycerides, smoking, diabetes, family history of myocardial infarction, antihypertensive medications, and cholesterol medications. (Figure and legend reproduced with permission from Circulation 2021 Apr 20;143(16):1571–1583)

Reference
1. Peng AW, Dardari ZA, Blumenthal RS, et al. Very high coronary artery calcium (≥1000) and association with cardiovascular disease events, non-cardiovascular disease outcomes, and mortality: results from MESA. Circulation. 2021;143(16):1571–83.

196. Correct Answer: D

Rationale
Individuals between 40 and 75 years of age with LDL-C (low-density lipoprotein cholesterol greater than 190 mg/dL (severe hypercholesterolemia) are candidates for high-intensity statin therapy (Class I) without the need for additional risk assessment according to the 2018 ACC/AHA Multisociety guidelines for the management of blood cholesterol. There is no recommended role for the use of the Pooled Cohort Equations or coronary artery calcium scoring to defer statin therapy in these individuals.

Reference
1. Grundy SM, Stone NJ, Bailey AL, et al. 2018 AHA/ACC/AACVPR/AAPA/ABC/ACPM/ADA/AGS/APhA/ASPC/NLA/PCNA guideline on the management of blood cholesterol: a report of the American College of Cardiology/American Heart Association task force on clinical practice guidelines. Circulation. 2019;139(25):e1082–143.

197. Correct Answer: B

Rationale
For primary prevention, patients whose ASCVD risk discussions remain uncertain may incorporate coronary artery calcium scoring into risk discussions according to the 2018 ACC/AHA Multisociety guidelines for the management of blood cholesterol. A calcium score between 0 and 99 favors consideration of statin therapy among those aged greater than 55 years. There is no recommended role for repeat calcium scoring or routine stress testing in this setting.

Reference
1. Grundy SM, Stone NJ, Bailey AL, et al. 2018 AHA/ACC/AACVPR/AAPA/ABC/ACPM/ADA/AGS/APhA/ASPC/NLA/PCNA guideline on the management of blood cholesterol: a report of the American College of Cardiology/American Heart Association task force on clinical practice guidelines. Circulation. 2019;139(25):e1082–143.

198. Correct Answer: C

Rationale
According to the 2018 ACC/AHA guideline for the management of blood cholesterol, statin therapy can be considered for individuals between 20 and 39 years of age with an LDL-C of 160 mg/dL or more AND a family history of premature ASCVD (atherosclerotic cardiovascular disease). The use of 10-year ASCVD risk to guide statin decisions is recommended for those between 40 and 75 years of age. There is no recommended role for garlic supplements in this setting.

Reference
1. Grundy SM, Stone NJ, Bailey AL, 2018 AHA/ACC/AACVPR/AAPA/ABC/ACPM/ADA/AGS/APhA/ASPC/NLA/PCNA guideline on the management of blood cholesterol: a report of the American College of Cardiology/American Heart Association task force on clinical practice guidelines. Circulation. 2019;139(25):e1082–143.

199. Correct Answer: A

Rationale
According to the 2018 ACC/AHA guideline for the management of blood cholesterol, statin therapy can be considered for individuals with borderline 10-year ASCVD risk (5% to <7.5%) in the presence of risk-enhancing factors which include South Asian ethnicity and preeclampsia (Class IIb). There is no role for routine stress testing in this setting.

Reference
1. Grundy SM, Stone NJ, Bailey AL, et al. 2018 AHA/ACC/AACVPR/AAPA/ABC/ACPM/ADA/AGS/APhA/ASPC/NLA/PCNA guideline on the management of blood cholesterol: a report of the American College of Cardiology/American Heart Association task force on clinical practice guidelines. Circulation. 2019;139(25):e1082–143.

200. Correct Answer: D

Rationale

The STOP-ACEi trial which randomized individuals with Stage 4–5 CKD to continuation versus discontinuation of RASi at a mean follow up of 3 years did not show any benefit to RASi use in this population, but there were no cardiorenal safety concerns either. Although a lack of cardiorenal efficacy data exists for individuals with GFR <30 mL/min/m^2, this study does not rule it out. However, it certainly does not support the use of potassium lowering drugs to continue RASi therapy in individuals with hyperkalemia and GFR (glomerular filtration rate) <60.

Reference
1. Bhandari S, Mehta S, Khwaja A, et al. Renin-angiotensin system inhibition in advanced chronic kidney disease. N Engl J Med. 2022;387(22):2021–32.

201. Correct Answer: D

Rationale

There are two independent predictors of CKD progression used to diagnose CKD, that is, GFR and albuminuria. A GFR of <60 mL/min/m^2 is used since this is where we see approximately a 50% increase in the hazard's ratio for CV mortality. The same is true for an ACR of 30 or greater. Microalbumin alone is not used to diagnose CKD since this value can be affected by the individual's hydration status, that ACR corrects for. ACRs are preferably done in the morning since activity/exercise can elevate albumin excretion.

References
1. Stevens PE, Levin A. Kidney Disease: Improving Global Outcomes Chronic Kidney Disease Guideline Development Work Group Members. Evaluation and management of chronic kidney disease: synopsis of the kidney disease: improving global outcomes 2012 clinical practice guideline. Ann Intern Med. 2013;158(11):825–30.
2. Lamb EJ, Levey AS, Stevens PE. The Kidney Disease Improving Global Outcomes (KDIGO) guideline update for chronic kidney disease: evolution not revolution. Clin Chem. 2013;59(3):462–5.

202. Correct Answer: C

Rationale

The SGLT2i as a class has been shown to do all of the above, except prevent DKA (diabetic ketoacidosis). SGLT2i have consistently shown a small but increased risk for ketoacidosis in patients with diabetes only. This usually occurs in patients with poor blood sugar control (A1c >10–12) on inadequate amounts of insulin.

Answers

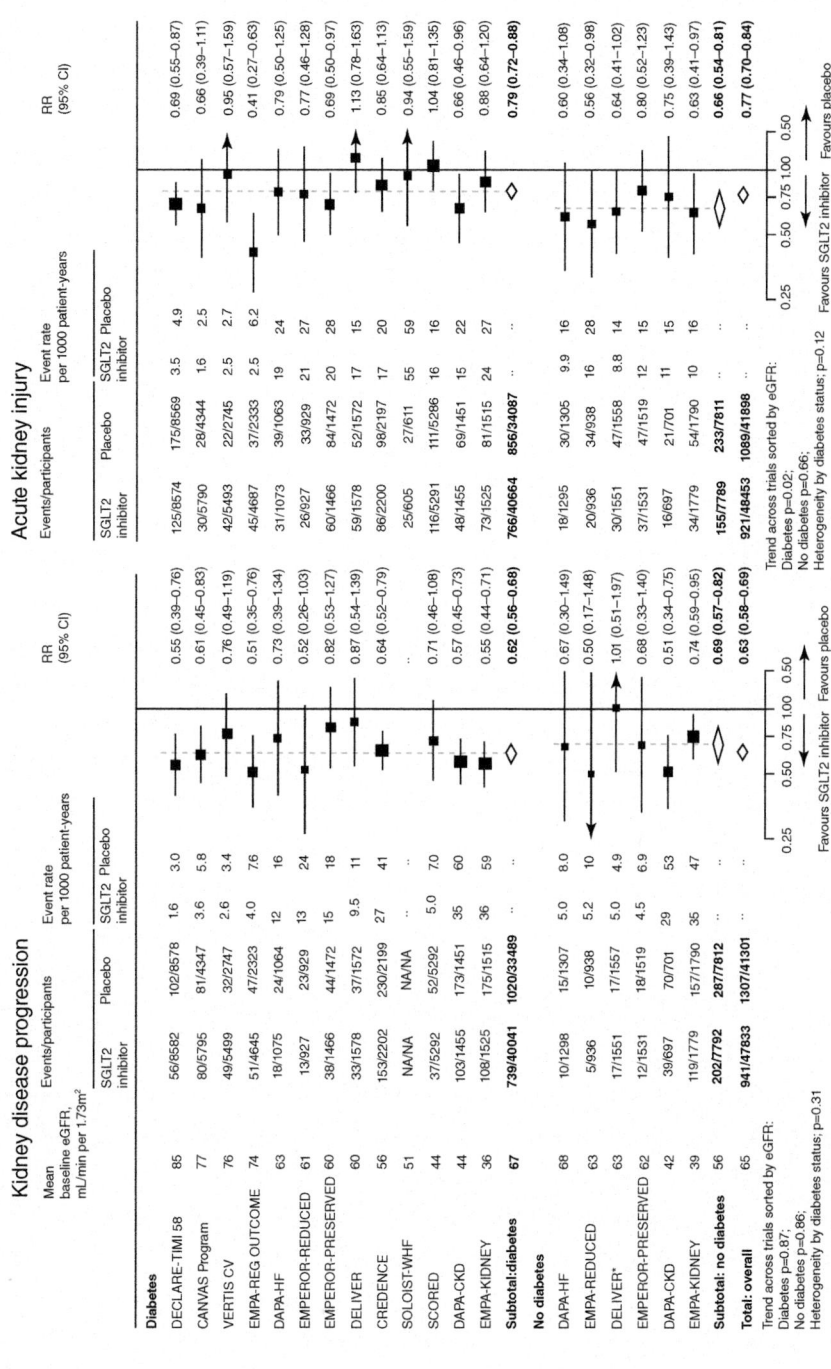

Effect of sodium glucose co-transporter-2 inhibition on kidney disease outcomes by diabetes status. (Figure reproduced with permission from Lancet. 2022 Nov 19;400(10365):1788–1801)

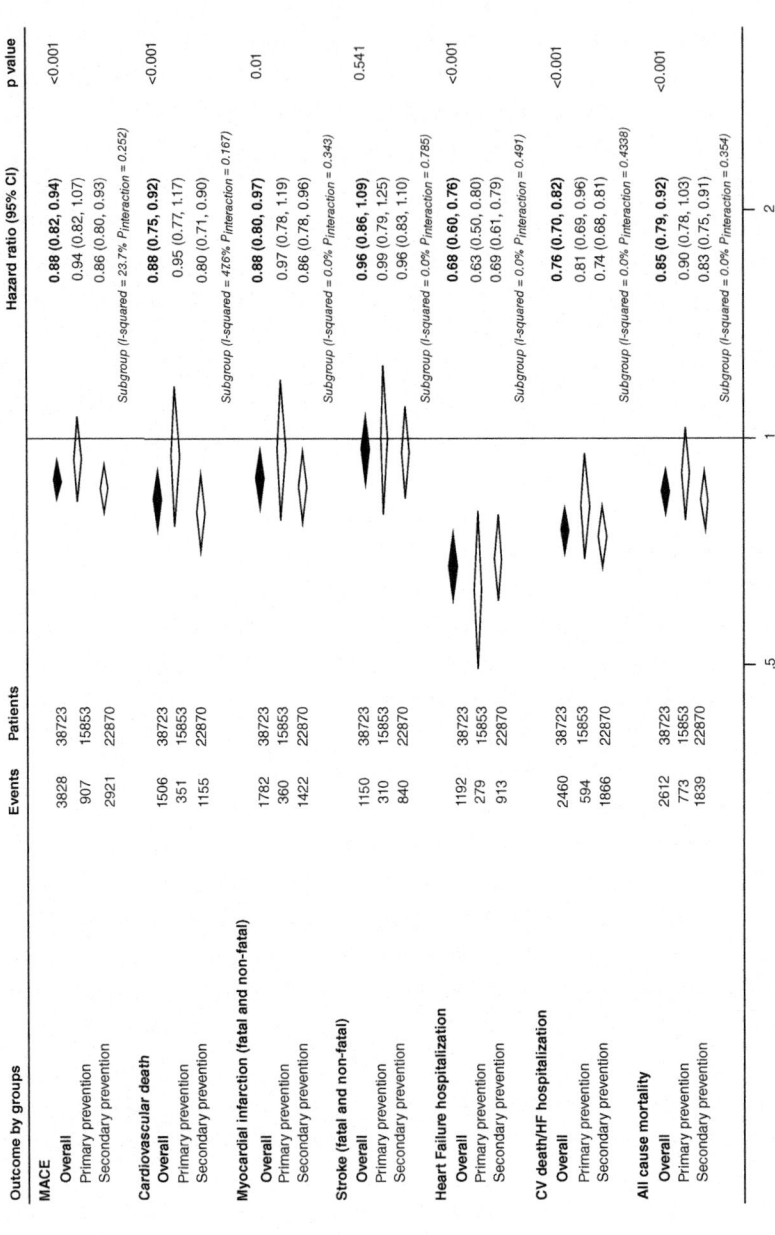

Effects of sodium-glucose cotransporter 2 inhibition on death and cause-specific cardiovascular (CV) events for patients with (secondary prevention) and without (primary prevention) CV disease at baseline. *HF* heart failure, *MACE* major adverse cardiac events. (Figure and legend reproduced with permission from Arnott et al. J Am Heart Assoc. 2020 Feb 4;9(3):e014908)

References

1. Nuffield Department of Population Health Renal Studies Group; SGLT2 inhibitor Meta-Analysis Cardio-Renal Trialists' Consortium. Impact of diabetes on the effects of sodium glucose co-transporter-2 inhibitors on kidney outcomes: collaborative meta-analysis of large placebo-controlled trials. Lancet. 2022;400(10365):1788–801.
2. The EMPA-KIDNEY Collaborative Group; Herrington WG, Staplin N, Wanner C, et al. Empagliflozin in patients with chronic kidney disease. N Engl J Med. 2023;388(2):117–27.
3. Solomon SD, McMurray JJV, Claggett B, et al. DELIVER Trial Committees and Investigators. Dapagliflozin in heart failure with mildly reduced or preserved ejection fraction. N Engl J Med. 2022;387(12):1089–98.
4. Vaduganathan M, Docherty KF, Claggett BL, et al. SGLT-2 inhibitors in patients with heart failure: a comprehensive meta-analysis of five randomised controlled trials. Lancet. 2022;400(10354):757–67.
5. Arnott C, Li Q, Kang A, Neuen BL, et al. Sodium-glucose cotransporter 2 inhibition for the prevention of cardiovascular events in patients with type 2 diabetes mellitus: a systematic review and meta-analysis. J Am Heart Assoc. 2020;9(3):e014908.

203. Correct Answer: E

Rationale
All of the above have been observed.

References
1. Palaka E, Grandy S, van Haalen H, et al. The impact of CKD anaemia on patients: incidence, risk factors, and clinical outcomes—a systematic literature review. Int J Nephrol. 2020;2020:7692376.
2. Karaboyas A, Morgenstern H, Waechter S, et al. Low hemoglobin at hemodialysis initiation: an international study of anemia management and mortality in the early dialysis period. Clin Kidney J. 2019;13(3):425–33.
3. Farrington DK, Sang Y, Grams ME, et al. Anemia prevalence, type, and associated risks in a cohort of 5.0 million insured patients in the United States by level of kidney function. Am J Kidney Dis. 2023; 81(2):201–9.e1.

204. Correct Answer: B

Rationale
The human bacterial microbiome is highly diverse and comprised of over 1000 species. These bacteria are metabolically highly active and produce chemical moieties

that impact systemic inflammatory tone and risk for ASCVD. Trimethylamine is a gas produced from the dietary quaternary amines choline and carnitine. Trimethylamine is absorbed and converted into trimethylamine-N-oxide (TMAO) by hepatic flavin monooxygenases. TMAO is highly bioactive, and its serum levels correlate with risk for ASCVD, myocardial infarction, peripheral arterial disease, macrophage-derived foam cell formation, and reduced reverse cholesterol transport. Histidine is converted into imidazole propionate by gut bacteria and induces both insulin resistance and systemic inflammation. Lipopolysaccharide (LPS) is a toxin produced by gram negative bacteria. Dysfunctional gut epithelial cells can allow for chronic LPS leakage into the central circulation. LPS binds to toll-like 4 receptors and potentiates an inflammatory response by activating macrophages. The short chain fatty acids (SCFAs) include acetic, propionic, and butyric acids which are produced by bacterial fermentation of starches and dietary fibers not hydrolyzed by gut enzymes. The SCFAs can be absorbed across the gut epithelium and bind to G-coupled receptors on the surface of inflammatory white cells. The SCFAs attenuate the activation of neutrophils, T cells, and monocytes/macrophages.

References
1. Tilg H, Zmora N, Adolph TE, Elinav E. The intestinal microbiota fuelling metabolic inflammation. Nat Rev Immunol. 2020;20;40–54.
2. Hajishengallis G. Periodontitis: from microbial immune subversion to systemic inflammation. Nat Rev Immunol. 2015;15:30–44.
3. Emoto T, Yamashita T, Sasaki N, et al. Analysis of gut microbiota in coronary artery disease patients: a possible link between gut microbiota and coronary artery disease. J Atheroscler Thromb. 2016;23:908–21.
4. Rath S, Heidrich B, Pieper DH, Vital M. Uncovering the trimethylamine-producing bacteria of the human gut microbiota. Microbiome. 2017;5:54.
5. Koeth RA, Wang Z, Levison BS, et al. Intestinal microbiota metabolism of l-carnitine, a nutrient in red meat, promotes atherosclerosis. Nat Med. 2013;19:576–85.
6. Senthong V, Li XS, Hudec T, et al. Plasma trimethylamine N-oxide, a gut microbe–generated phosphatidylcholine metabolite, is associated with atherosclerotic burden. J Am Coll Cardiol. 2016;67:2620–8.
7. Ohira H, Tsutsui W, Fujioka Y. Are short chain fatty acids in gut microbiota defensive players for inflammation and atherosclerosis? J Atheroscler Thromb. 2017;24:660–72.
8. Le Poul E, Loison C, Struyf S, et al. Functional characterization of human receptors for short chain fatty acids and their role in polymorphonuclear cell activation. J Biol Chem. 2003;278:25481–9.

205. Correct Answer: C

Rationale

The resolution of inflammation is highly conserved and carefully orchestrated (see figure). The resolution of inflammation does not consist of a system of inflammatory inputs suddenly shutting down; the process of inflammation is actively controlled by a wide-ranging array of molecular and cellular machinery designed to put the "fire out" in an orderly and noninjurious manner. Leukotrienes and prostaglandins are metabolites of arachidonic acid (AA) that potentiate inflammation. Specialized pro-resolving molecules (SPMs) are formed from such omega-3 fatty acids as eicosapentaenoic acid (EPA), docosapentaenoic acid (DPA), and docosahexaenoic acid (DHA). The SPMs do not increase the production of prostaglandins and leukotrienes. Efferocytosis is the process by which apoptotic cells and apoptotic bodies are removed by macrophages in a manner that does not activate inflammation. Atherosclerotic plaques with expanding necrotic cores have impaired efferocytosis, resulting in cellular debris continuing to accumulate. This is highly pro-inflammatory and contributes to plaque vulnerability and instability. The SPMs promote orderly efferocytosis, reduce neutrophil density in plaque, attenuate pro-inflammatory interleukin and cytokine production, and reduce the binding of inflammatory white blood cells to endothelium. The SPMs include the maresins, protectins, resolvins, and lipoxins. Lipoxins (A4 and B4) are synthesized by platelets and neutrophils and regulate the activity of NF-κB (a nuclear transcription factor regulating many genes in the inflammatory cascade), macrophages, T cells and neutrophils. The maresins are 12′-lipoxygenase-derived metabolites of DHA and ae produced by macrophages. The resolvin E and D series of mediators are derived from EPA and DHA, respectively, via the action of 15′-lipoxygenase. The protectins are also produced from DHA.

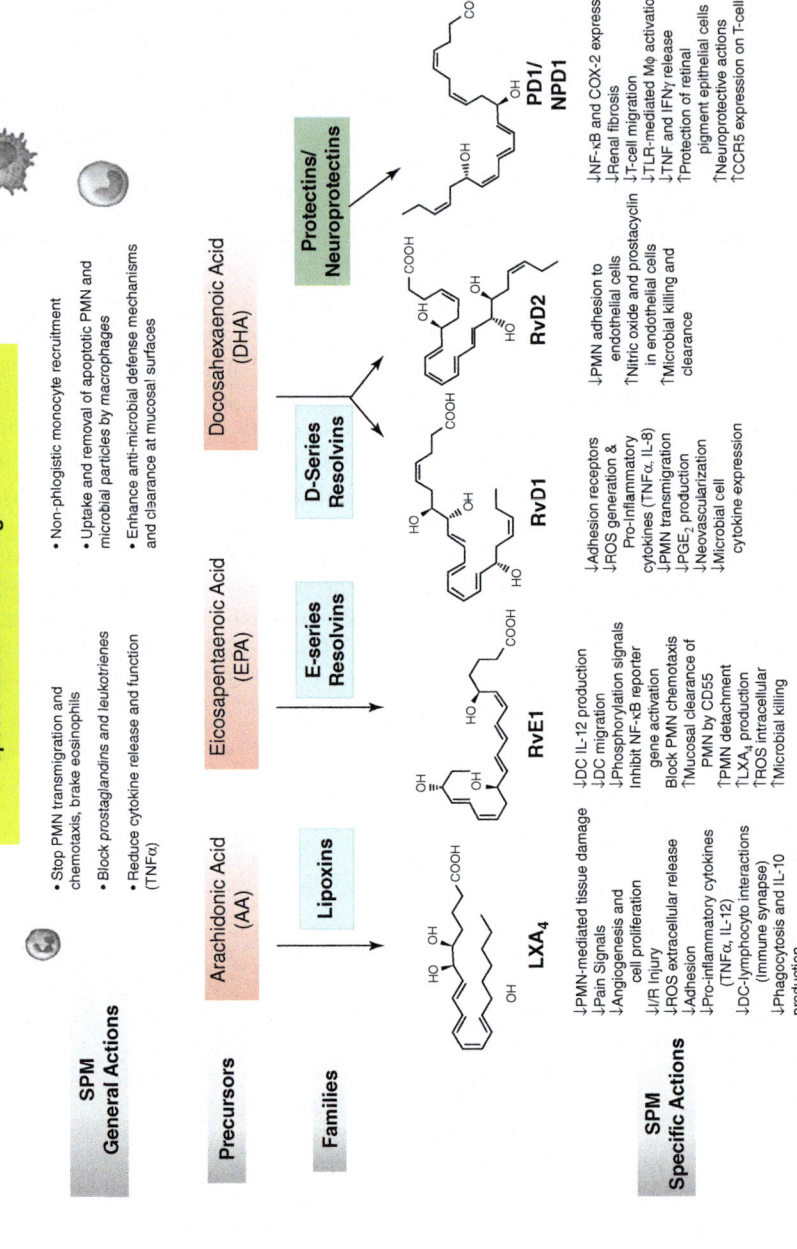

Reproduced with permission from *The American Journal of Pathology* 2010 177:1576–1591. https://doi.org/10.2353/ajpath.2010.100322

References

1. Jala VR, Haribabu B. Leukotrienes and atherosclerosis: new roles for old mediators. Trends Immunol. 2004;25:315–22.
2. Ricciotti E, FitzGerald GA. Prostaglandins and inflammation. Arterioscler Thromb Vasc Biol. 2011;31:986–1000.
3. Chandrasekharan JA, Sharma-Walia N. Lipoxins: nature's way to resolve inflammation. J Inflamm Res. 2015;8:181–92.
4. Prieto P, Cuenca J, Traves PG, Fernandez-Velasco M, Martin-Sanz P, Bosca L. Lipoxin A4 impairment of apoptotic signaling in macrophages: implication of the PI3K/Akt and the ERK/Nrf-2 defense pathways. Cell Death Differ. 2010;17:1179–88.
5. Tang S, Wan M, Huang W, Stanton RC, Xu Y. Maresins: specialized proresolving lipid mediators and their potential role in inflammatory-related diseases. Mediators Inflamm. 2018;2018:2380319.
6. Serhan CN, Levy BD. Resolvins in inflammation: emergence of the pro-resolving superfamily of mediators. J Clin Invest. 2018;128:2657–69.
7. Hansen TV, Vik A, Serhan CN. The protectin family of specialized pro-resolving mediators: potent immunoresolvents enabling innovative approaches to target obesity and diabetes. Front Pharmacol. 2019;9.
8. Kasikara C, Doran AC, Cai B, Tabas I. The role of non-resolving inflammation in atherosclerosis. J Clin Invest. 2018;128:2713–23.

206. Correct Answer: D

Rationale

CRP is a pentraxin molecule; it is a closed pentamer of CRP monomers. It is an important acute phase reactant produced by the liver subsequent to activation of the inflammasome by IL-1. It does participate in the opsonization and phagocytosis of infectious agents through the classical complement pathway. A large number of prospective longitudinal cohorts from around the world have demonstrated that hsCRP is highly predictive of risk for future cardiovascular events and new-onset diabetes mellitus in both men and women. Both experimental infusions of CRP and Mendelian inheritance studies of this molecule fail to demonstrate that it is causal for atherosclerosis. In a series of post-hoc analyses of major secondary prevention statin trials, the concept of "dual targets" (both LDL-C and hsCRP) was tested and affirmed. In the Aggrastsat to Zocor trial (A to Z), Pravastatin or Atorvastatin Evaluation and Infection Therapy trial (PROVE-IT), and the IMProved Reduction of Outcomes: Vytorin Efficacy International Trial (IMPROVE-IT) the participants with the lowest rates of CVD (cardiovascular disease) events had the lowest LDL-C and hsCRP; those with the highest rates had the highest levels of these two risk factors (see figure). Similarly, in two primary prevention statin trials (The Air Force/Texas Coronary Atherosclerosis Prevention Study [AFCAPS/TexCAPS] and Justification for the Use of Statins in Prevention: An Intervention Trial Evaluating Rosuvastatin [JUPITER]), this relationship was again observed. The JUPITER trial also showed that hsCRP (>2.0 mg/L) helped to identify a group of patients with "average" LDL-C (<130 mg/dL) who derived benefit for CVD event reduction from statin therapy. An individual level meta-analysis of 160,309 persons without CVD by the Emerging Risk Factors Collaboration demonstrated that CRP levels have a continuous relationship with risk for CAD, ischemic stroke, and cardiovascular mortality.

References
1. Lane T, Wassef N, Poole S, et al. Infusion of pharmaceutical-grade natural human C-reactive protein is not proinflammatory in healthy adult human volunteers. Circ Res. 2014;114:672–6.
2. Noveck R, Stroes ES, Flaim JD, et al. Effects of an antisense oligonucleotide inhibitor of C-reactive protein synthesis on the endotoxin challenge response in healthy human male volunteers. J Am Heart Assoc. 2014;3.
3. Ridker PM. A test in context: high-sensitivity C-reactive protein. J Am Coll Cardiol. 2016;67:712–23.
4. Ridker PM, Rifai N, Rose L, Buring JE, Cook NR. Comparison of C-reactive protein and low-density lipoprotein cholesterol levels in the prediction of first cardiovascular events. N Engl J Med. 2002;347:1557–65.
5. Morrow DA, Lemos JAd, Sabatine MS, et al. Clinical relevance of C-reactive protein during follow-up of patients with acute coronary syndromes in the aggrastat-to-zocor trial. Circulation. 2006;114:281–8.
6. Ridker PM, Cannon CP, Morrow D, et al. C-Reactive protein levels and outcomes after statin therapy. N Engl J Med. 2005;352:20–8.
7. Bohula EA, Giugliano RP, Cannon CP, et al. Achievement of dual low-density lipoprotein cholesterol and high-sensitivity C-reactive protein targets more frequent with the addition of ezetimibe to simvastatin and associated with better outcomes in IMPROVE-IT. Circulation. 2015;132:1224–33.

207. Correct Answer: A

Rationale
In the CANTOS trial, both IL-6 and CRP decreased in a dose-dependent manner among those randomized to the Canakinumab treatment arm. There were no changes in serum lipoprotein levels in response to Canakinumab. Hence, it was assumed that the bulk of cardiovascular benefit in this trial was attributable to the attenuation of systemic inflammatory tone. This was a proof-of-concept study, that is, reducing inflammation decreases risk of cardiovascular events. Because Canakinumab is an interleukin (IL)-1β neutralizing monoclonal antibody, risk for infection and sepsis did increase, but risk for cancer, particularly lung cancer, was reduced. Achieving a CRP <2.0 did confer a mortality benefit compared to not achieving this level in a *post hoc* analysis. The CANTOS trial demonstrated that inflammation is an important etiologic factor in CVD.

References
1. Ridker PM, Everett BM, Thuren T, et al. Antiinflammatory therapy with canakinumab for atherosclerotic disease. N Engl J Med. 2017;377:1119–31.
2. Ridker PM. Mortality differences associated with treatment responses in CANTOS and FOURIER: insights and implications. Circulation. 2018;137:1763–6.

208. Correct Answer: A

Rationale

LpPLA$_2$ does promote inflammation of hydrolyzing phospholipids at the sn-2 position into an oxidized fatty acid and a lysophospholipid. Both of these catabolites stimulate inflammation. LpPLA2 is transported in serum on LDL and HDL particles. It can also be produced locally within plaque by activated macrophages and foam cells. Although LpPLA2 is highly predictive of CVD when expressed either as activity or mass in serum independent of other risk factor covariates, it is not a target for treatment. Studies in patients with either stable CHD using the LpPLA2 inhibitor darapladib (Stabilization of Atherosclerotic Plaque by Initiation of Darapladib Therapy) or recent non-ST segment elevating or ST-segment elevating MI (Stabilization of Plaques using Darapladib–Thrombolysis in Myocardial Infarction 52) failed to demonstrate any benefit on acute CV events compared to placebo.

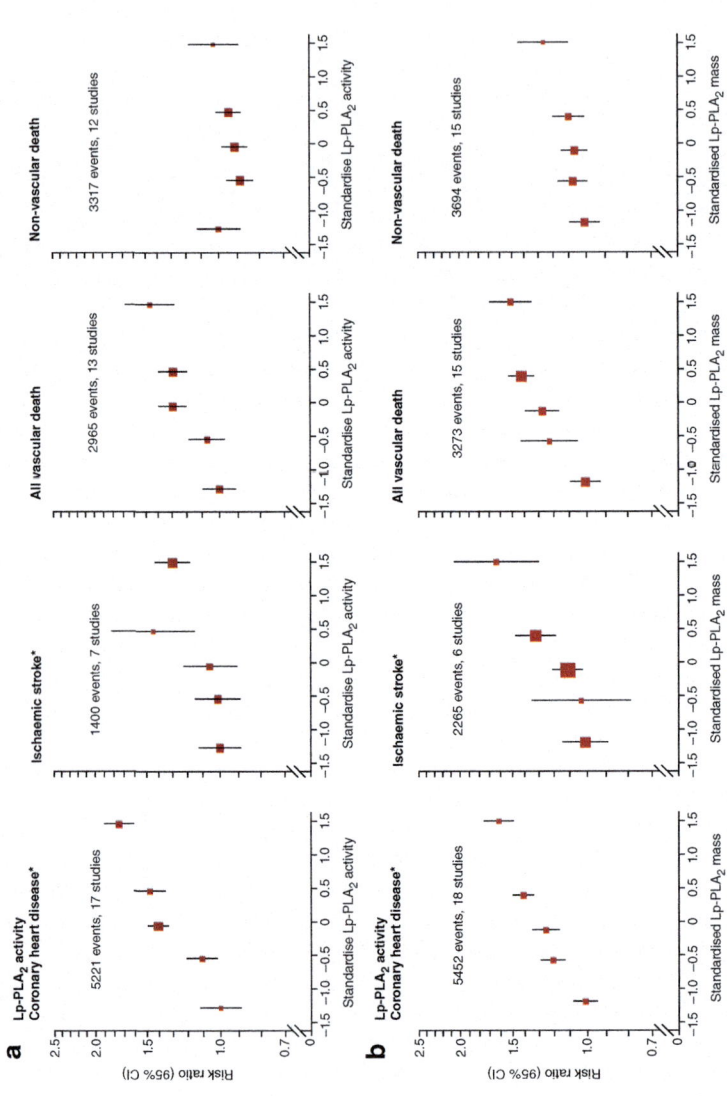

Risk ratios were adjusted for age, sex, baseline history of vascular disease, history of diabetes, and trial group (as appropriate). Data are shown for the 71,439 participants who were initially healthy or had a history of stable vascular disease at baseline only. One unit on the standardized scale is equal to 1 SD on the untransformed scale. Error bars represent 95% confidence intervals. The sizes of the boxes are proportional to the inverse of the variance of the risk ratios. $Lp\text{-}PLA_2$ lipoprotein-associated phospholipase A_2. *Fatal and nonfatal events. (Figure and legend reproduced with permission from The Lp-PLA$_2$ Studies Collaboration. *Lancet.* 2010;375:1536–1544)

References
1. Gonçalves I, Edsfeldt A, Ko NY, et al. Evidence supporting a key role of Lp-PLA2-generated lysophosphatidylcholine in human atherosclerotic plaque inflammation. Arterioscler Thromb Vasc Biol. 2012;32:1505–12.
2. Kolodgie FD, Burke AP, Skorija KS, et al. Lipoprotein-associated phospholipase A2 protein expression in the natural progression of human coronary atherosclerosis. Arterioscler Thromb Vasc Biol. 2006;26:2523–9.
3. Silva IT, Mello AP, Damasceno NR. Antioxidant and inflammatory aspects of lipoprotein-associated phospholipase A(2) (Lp-PLA(2)): a review. Lipids Health Dis. 2011;10:170.
4. Garza CA, Montori VM, McConnell JP, Somers VK, Kullo IJ, Lopez-Jimenez F. Association between lipoprotein-associated phospholipase A2 and cardiovascular disease: a systematic review. Mayo Clin Proc. 2007;82:159–65.
5. O'Donoghue ML, Braunwald E, White HD, et al. Effect of darapladib on major coronary events after an acute coronary syndrome: the SOLID-TIMI 52 randomized clinical trial. JAMA. 2014;312:1006–15.
6. White HD, Held C, Stewart R, et al. Darapladib for preventing ischemic events in stable coronary heart disease. N Engl J Med. 2014;370:1702–11.

209. Correct Answer: C

Rationale
When visceral adipose tissue becomes insulin resistant, a variety of biochemical and physiological changes ensue. The following transitions occur: (1) JNK expression increases; (2) there is a switch from tyrosine phosphorylation to serine phosphorylation of insulin receptor substrate- 1 (IRS-1) which reduces cell surface expression of glucose transport proteins and capacity to internalize extracellular glucose; (3) there is increased influx of inflammatory white cells such as macrophages, T cells, mast cells, and neutrophils which become activated and release inflammatory mediators; (4) hormone sensitive lipase is no longer inhibited by insulin and there is constitutive release of free fatty acid from adipose tissue secondary to increased hydrolysis of triglycerides; the large increase in free fatty acid availability worsens insulin resistance and supports ectopic fat deposition in skeletal muscle, the pancreas, liver, and epicardial fat pads resulting in insulin resistance in these organs; (5) there is decreased production of adiponectin and increased production of TNF-alpha and retinol binding protein 4, changes which potentiate insulin resistance. Up to 50 different adipokines can be produced and secreted by visceral aipose tissue and these moieties augment both local and systemic inflammation. Among the inflammatory mediators expressed by insulin resistant adipocytes are IL-1, IL-6, IL-8, CRP, TGF-beta, and macrophage chemotactic protein-1, among many others.

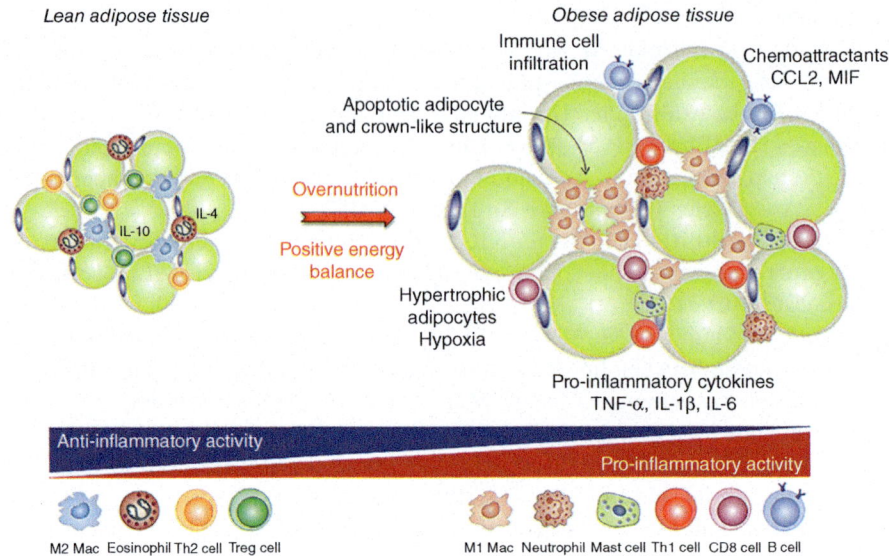

Visceral adipose tissue in obese, insulin-resistant individuals is a proinflammatory organ. (Reproduced with permission from Francisco et al. British J Pharmacology, Volume: 175, Issue: 10, Pages: 1569–1579)

References

1. Yang Q, Graham TE, Mody N, et al. Serum retinol binding protein 4 contributes to insulin resistance in obesity and type 2 diabetes. Nature. 2005;436:356–62.
2. Farjo KM, Farjo RA, Halsey S, Moiseyev G, Ma JX. Retinol-binding protein 4 induces inflammation in human endothelial cells by an NADPH oxidase- and nuclear factor kappa B-dependent and retinol-independent mechanism. Mol Cell Biol. 2012;32:5103–15.
3. Tabata M, Kadomatsu T, Fukuhara S, et al. Angiopoietin-like protein 2 promotes chronic adipose tissue inflammation and obesity-related systemic insulin resistance. Cell Metab. 2009;10:178–88.
4. Kwon H, Pessin JE. Adipokines mediate inflammation and insulin resistance. Front Endocrinol (Lausanne). 2013;4:71.
5. Lettner A, Roden M. Ectopic fat and insulin resistance. Curr Diab Rep. 2008;8:185–91.
6. Iacobellis G, Sharma AM. Epicardial adipose tissue as new cardio-metabolic risk marker and potential therapeutic target in the metabolic syndrome. Curr Pharm Des. 2007;13:2180–4.
7. Rabkin SW. Epicardial fat: properties, function and relationship to obesity. Obes Rev. 2007;8:253–61.

210. Correct Answer: C

Rationale

Macrophages scavenge lipoproteins in the extracellular milieu via the scavenger receptor A family of cell surface proteins. The macrophage has evolved multiple safety mechanisms that allow it to also externalize cholesterol and transfer it to HDL (high-density lipoprotein cholesterol) species for reverse cholesterol transport back to the liver. ABCA1 and SR-BI can lipidate nascent discoidal HDL; ABCG1 lipidates spherical HDL particles. The macrophage can also produce and secrete apo E which can then function as a receiving platform for excess cholesterol. ABCG5/8 is not expressed by macrophages. It is the membrane cassette transport protein in jejunal enterocytes that allows these cells to pump dietary and biliary sources of cholesterol back into the gut lumen for elimination.

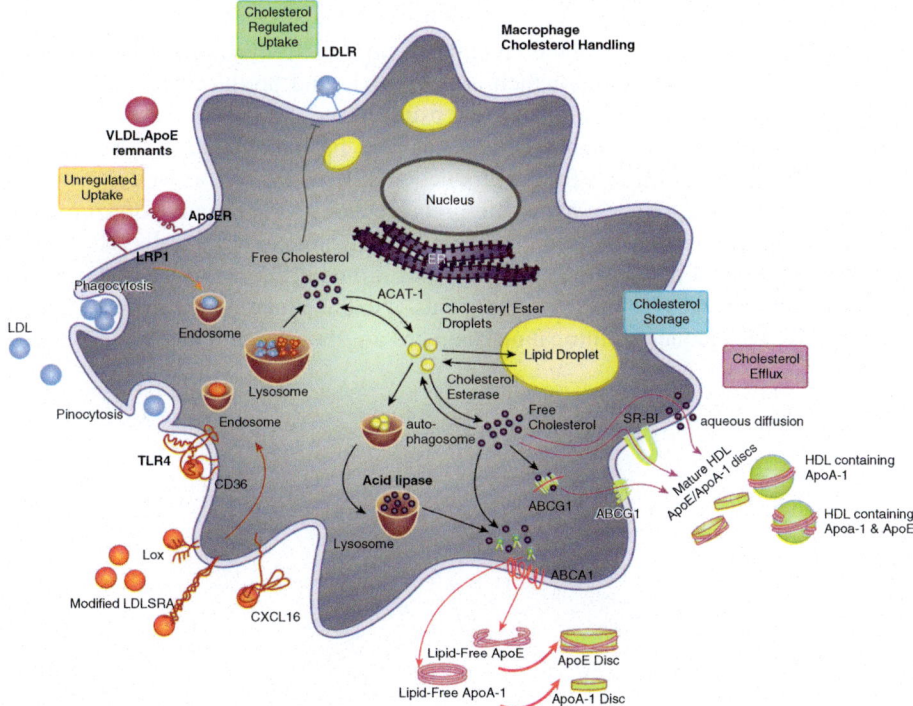

ABCG1 may also play a role in the intracellular trafficking of cholesterol. (Figure and legend reproduced from Linton MRF, Yancey PG, Davies SS, et al. The Role of Lipids and Lipoproteins in Atherosclerosis. [Updated 2019 Jan 3]. In: Feingold KR, Anawalt B, Boyce A, et al., editors. Endotext [Internet]. South Dartmouth (MA): MDText.com, Inc.; 2000. [Macrophage Cholesterol Metabolism. Native LDL is recognized by the LDL receptor (LDLR). The LDL is endocytosed and trafficked to lysosomes, where the cholesteryl ester (CE) is hydrolyzed to free cholesterol (FC) by the acid lipase. ABCG1 may also play a role in the intracellular trafficking of cholesterol]. Available from: https://www.ncbi.nlm.nih.gov/sites/books/NBK343489/figure/lipid_athero. http://creativecommons.org/licenses/by-nc-nd/2.0/)

References
1. Sukhorukov VN, Khotina VA, Chegodaev YS, et al. Lipid metabolism in macrophages: focus on atherosclerosis. Biomedicines. 2020;8(8):262.
2. Pennings M, Meurs I, Ye D, et al. Regulation of cholesterol homeostasis in macrophages and consequences for atherosclerotic lesion development. FEBS Lett. 2006;580:5588–96.
3. Juhl AD, Wüstner D. Pathways and mechanisms of cellular cholesterol efflux—insight from imaging. Front Cell Dev Biol. 2022;10.
4. Matsuura F, Wang N, Chen W, et al. HDL from CETP-deficient subjects shows enhanced ability to promote cholesterol efflux from macrophages in an apoE- and ABCG1-dependent pathway. J Clin Invest. 2006;116(5):1435–42.

211. Correct Answer: E

Rationale
Neutrophils can precipitate acute enodthelial injury and dysfunction by releasing neutrophil extracellular traps, which are cytotoxic and prothrombotic. NETs are comprised of histones, lysosomal cathepsins, proteases, myeloperoxidase, and alpha-defensins, all of which are injurious and pro-inflammatory. The NLR3P inflammasome is responsible for the production of IL-1 and Il-6, as well as caspases which trigger cellular apoptosis. Neutrophils are an important source of azurocidin and helicidin, both of which promote monocyte influx into arterial walls. The matrix metalloproteinases are pro-inflammatory and promote the hydrolysis of proteins such as collagen and elastin, key components of extracellular matrix material and of atherosclerotic plaque. Additional mechanisms are shown in the figure.

Answers

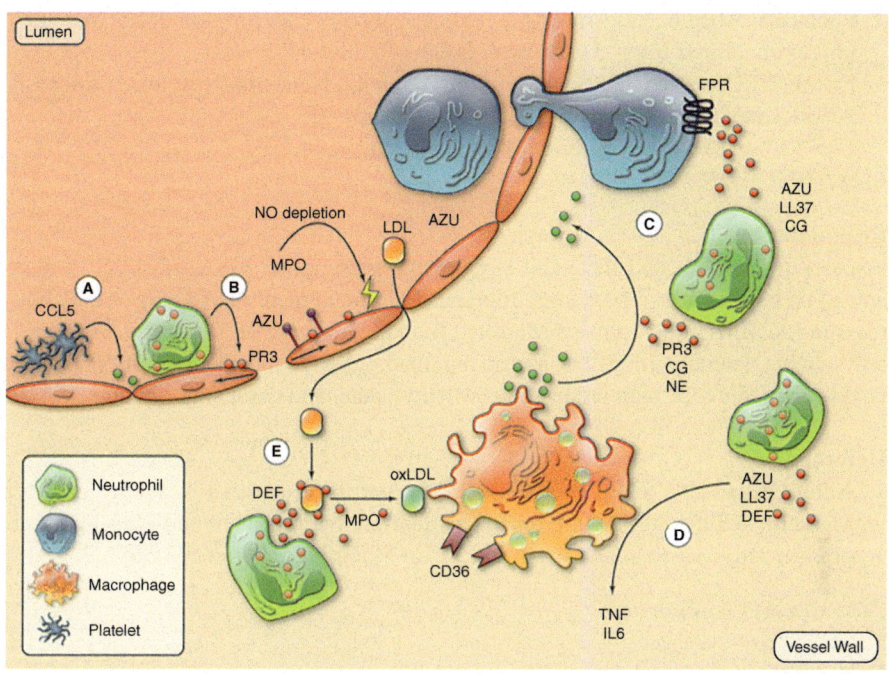

Neutrophils feed mechanisms of atherogenesis. (**a**) Neutrophils are recruited to the atherosclerotic lesion in a partially platelet-dependent manner. These deposit C-C motif chemokine ligand (CCL)5, which activates neutrophils via CCR1 and CCR5, thereby promoting firm adhesion. (**b**) Activated neutrophils secrete granule proteins such as myeloperoxidase, azurocidin, and proteinase-3, which induce expression of adhesion molecules and permeability changes and limit the bioavailability of nitric oxide, altogether aggravating endothelial dysfunction. (**c**) Granule proteins deposited on the endothelium and secreted at the site of inflammation induce adhesion and recruitment of inflammatory monocytes involving formyl-peptide receptors. Proteolytic modification of chemokines enhances their ability to attract monocytes. (**d**) Neutrophil granule proteins promote macrophage polarization toward a proinflammatory M1 phenotype and induce expression of scavenger receptors (eg, CD36). (**e**) Binding of α-defensins to low-density lipoprotein (LDL) traps LDL in the vessel wall. Oxidation of LDL through myeloperoxidase-dependent mechanisms enhances foam cell formation. *AZU* azurocidin, *CG* cathepsin G, *DEF* α-defensins, *FPR* formyl-peptide receptor, *MPO* myeloperoxidase, *NE* neutrophil elastase, *PR3* proteinase-3. (Figure and legend reproduced with permission from Soehnlein O. Multiple Roles for Neutrophils in Atherosclerosis. Circulation Research. 2012;110(6):875–88)

References

1. Münzer P, Negro R, Fukui S, et al. NLRP3 inflammasome assembly in neutrophils is supported by PAD4 and promotes NETosis under sterile conditions. Front Immunol. 2021;12.
2. Döring Y, Drechsler M, Soehnlein O, Weber C. Neutrophils in atherosclerosis. Arterioscler Thromb Vasc Biol. 2015;35:288–95.
3. Pende A, Artom N, Bertolotto M, et al. Role of neutrophils in atherogenesis: an update. Eur J Clin Invest. 2016;46:252–63.
4. Doring Y, Soehnlein O, Weber C. Neutrophil extracellular traps in atherosclerosis and atherothrombosis. Circ Res. 2017;120:736–43.

5. Fuchs TA, Abed U, Goosmann C, et al. Novel cell death program leads to neutrophil extracellular traps. J Cell Biol. 2007;176:231–41.
6. Döring Y, Drechsler M, Soehnlein O, Weber C. Neutrophils in atherosclerosis. Arterioscler Thromb Vasc Biol. 2015;35(2):288–95.

212. Correct Answer: C

Rationale

Features to be evaluated that may suggest the presence of OSA (obstructive sleep apnea) include increased neck circumference (>17 in. in men, >16 in. in women), body mass index (BMI) ≥30 kg/m^2, a Modified Mallampati score of 3 or 4, the presence of retrognathia, lateral peritonsillar narrowing, macroglossia, tonsillar hypertrophy, elongated/enlarged uvula, high arched/narrow hard palate, and nasal abnormalities.

Reference

1. Adult Obstructive Sleep Apnea Task Force of the American Academy of Sleep Medicine. Clinical guideline for the evaluation, management and long-term care of obstructive sleep apnea in adults. J Clin Sleep Med. 2009; 5(3):263–7.

213. Correct Answer: C

Rationale

The 2013 AHA/ACC/TOS Obesity Treatment guidelines recommend that patients increase aerobic exercise to approximately 30 min per day or ≥150 min per week as part of a comprehensive weight loss management program.

Reference

1. Jensen MD, Ryan DH, Apovian CM, et al. American College of Cardiology/American Heart Association Task Force on Practice Guidelines; Obesity Society. 2013 AHA/ACC/TOS guideline for the management of overweight and obesity in adults: a report of the American College of Cardiology/American Heart Association task force on practice guidelines and the Obesity Society. J Am Coll Cardiol. 2014;63(25 Pt B):2985–3023.

214. Correct Answer: A

Rationale

Among non-Hispanic Whites, the age-adjusted prevalence for metabolic syndrome is 35% among men and 36% among women. Minority populations are disproportionately affected; however, the prevalence of metabolic syndrome varies for men and women. Prevalence in non-Hispanic Black women is 34%; prevalence in non-Hispanic black men is 27%. Mexican American women have a prevalence that is slightly higher (31%) than in Mexican American men (27.5%).

Reference

1. Deboer MD. Ethnicity, obesity, and the metabolic syndrome: implications on assessing risk and targeting intervention. Expert Rev Endocrinol Metab. 2011;6(2):279–89.

Answers

215. Correct Answer: C

Rationale

Stimulus (cue) control involves learning what social or environmental cues seem to encourage undesired eating and subsequently changing those cues.

Reference
1. Watson P, Wiers RW, Hommel B, et al. Stimulus control over action for food in obese versus healthy-weight individuals. Front Psychol. 2017;8:580.

216. Correct Answer: D

Rationale

This patient with multiple cardiovascular risk factors, diabetes mellitus, known CAD, and symptoms of Class III angina warrants revascularization. The BARI-2D trial investigated revascularization (either PCI [percutaneous coronary intervention] or CABG [coronary artery bypass surgery]) versus optimal medical therapy in diabetic patients and found a significant benefit of coronary bypass grafting (CABG) in the presence of multivessel disease. Similarly, a SYNTAX score of 30 (intermediate complexity) indicated that CABG would be preferred. In subgroup analyses, SYNTAX scores of 22 or more had the greatest benefit of CABG.

Reference
1. BARI 2D Study Group, Frye RL, August P, Brooks MM, et al. A randomized trial of therapies for type 2 diabetes and coronary artery disease. N Engl J Med. 2009;360(24):2503–15.

217. Correct Answer: A

Rationale

This patient presents with likely cardiac chest pain and a notable family history of early CAC in her brother as well as a markedly elevated Lp(a) [lipoprotein(a)]. The presence of these additional risk factors increases the likelihood of a coronary etiology in this patient. Her young age, the intermediate pretest probability for disease indicate that anatomic testing would be preferred. According to the 2021 Chest Pain guidelines, a patient with intermediate risk who is younger or is less likely to have obstructive CAD (coronary artery disease), should proceed with a CCTA (coronary computed tomography angiography)as the first test (i.e., exercise ECG, stress echocardiogram would not be the preferred next tests). As the patient is not symptomatic at present, a troponin would not be expected to yield a diagnosis. Lastly, in symptomatic young patients, there is no indication for CAC (coronary artery calcium) testing given (1) the body of evidence for CAC testing is largely in asymptomatic patients and (2) Mortensen and colleagues found that the presence of CAC = 0 in patients with documented obstructive disease on CCTA <40 years old was 58%, indicating that a CAC of 0 is not reassuring in a young symptomatic patient.

Pretest likelihood of CAD	Low	→	No testing necessary		Option for CAC for ASCVD risk stratification
	Intermediate-high	→	Younger patient (<65 y of age)	OR	Less obstructive CAD suspected → CCTA favored
	Intermediate-high	→	Older patient (≥65 y of age)		More obstructive CAD suspected → Stress testing favored

	Favors use of CCTA	Favors use of stress imaging
Goal	• Rule out obstructive CAD • Detect nonobstructive CAD	• Ischemia-guided management
Availability and expertise	• High-quality imaging and expert interpretation routinely available	• High-quality imaging and expert interpretation routinely available
Likelihood of obstructive CAD	• Age <65 y	• Age ≥65y
Prior test results	• Prior functional study inconclusive	• Prior CCTA inconclusive
Other compelling indications	• Anomalous coronary arteries • Require evaluation of aorta or pulmonary arteries	• Suspect scar (especially if PET or stress CMR available) • Suspect coronary microvascular dysfunction (when PET or CMR available)

Figure reproduced with permission from Gulati et al. Circulation. 2021 Nov 30;144(22):e368–e454

References
1. Gulati M, Levy PD, Mukherjee D, et al. 2021 AHA/ACC/ASE/CHEST/SAEM/SCCT/SCMR guideline for the evaluation and diagnosis of chest pain: a report of the American College of Cardiology/American Heart Association Joint Committee on clinical practice guidelines. Circulation. 2021;144(22):e368–454.
2. Mortensen MB, Gaur S, Frimmer A, et al. Association of age with the diagnostic value of coronary artery calcium score for ruling out coronary stenosis in symptomatic patients. JAMA Cardiol. 2022;7(1):36–44.

218. Correct Answer: C

Rationale

The ACC/AHA Guidelines recommend at least 150 min/week of moderate/vigorous PA, so A is wrong. Some activities, even less than recommended, is beneficial, so B is wrong. Sedentary behavior confers risk even among those who are active (although attenuated) so D is wrong. Counseling is effective in increasing physical activity behavior in RCTs (randomized controlled trials) so E is wrong. C is correct answer—fitness is associated with survival even in older adults.

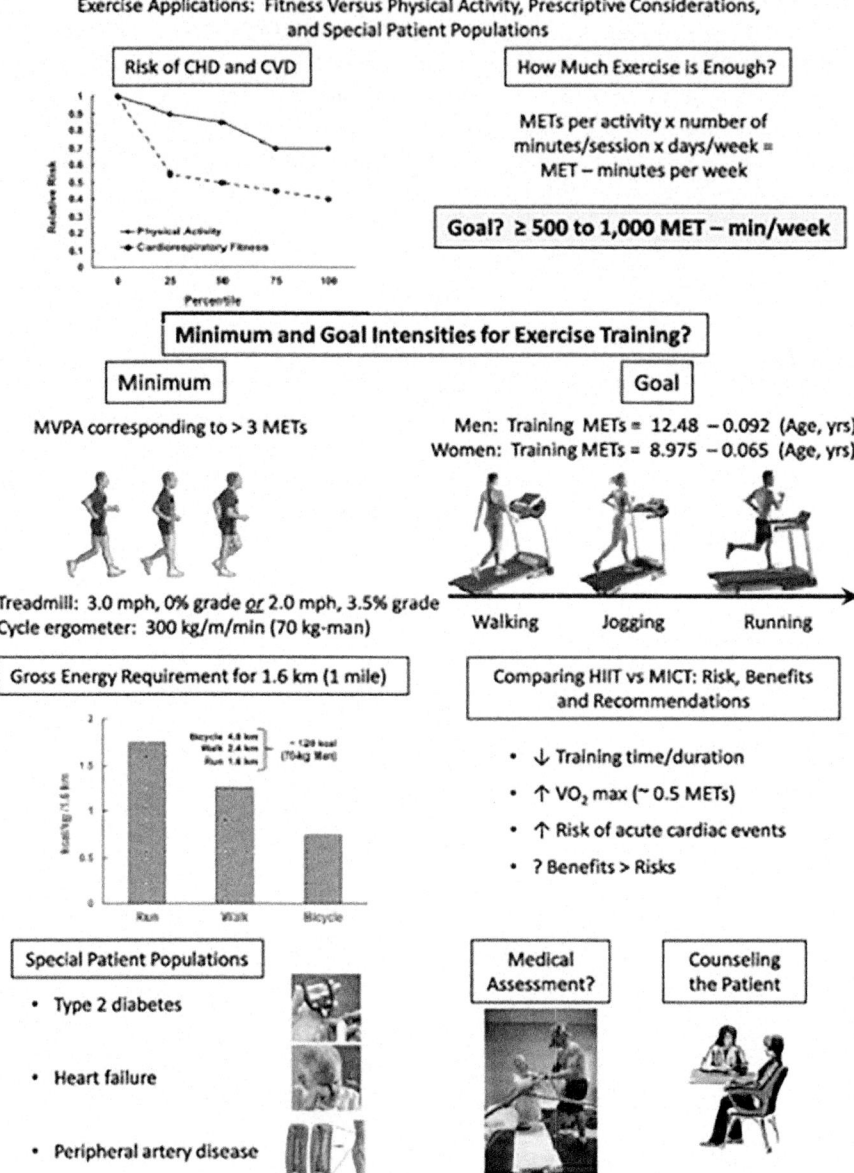

Figure reproduced with permission from Franklin et al. Am J Prev Cardiol. 2022 Oct 13;12:100425

References

1. Franklin BA, Eijsvogels TMH, Pandey A, Quindry J, Toth PP. Physical activity, cardiorespiratory fitness, and cardiovascular health: a clinical practice statement of the American Society for Preventive Cardiology Part II: physical activity, cardiorespiratory fitness, minimum and goal intensities for exercise training, prescriptive methods, and special patient populations. Am J Prev Cardiol. 2022;12:100425.
2. Franklin BA, Eijsvogels TMH, Pandey A, Quindry J, Toth PP. Physical activity, cardiorespiratory fitness, and cardiovascular health: A clinical practice statement of the ASPC Part I: bioenergetics, contemporary physical activity recommendations, benefits, risks, extreme exercise regimens, potential maladaptations. Am J Prev Cardiol. 2022;12:100424.

219. Correct Answer: A

Rationale

The Dept of HHS recommended muscle strengthening activities in addition to PA. B is wrong because moderate intensity activity achieves cardiovascular benefit, PA does not have to be vigorous to have benefit. C is wrong, as moderate intensity is defined as 3–5.9 METS with vigorous being ≥6 METS. Healthy adults do not need medical screening before starting exercise, only those with cardiovascular symptoms, so D is wrong. E is wrong, because even trading sedentary behavior for light activity is associated with lower mortality risk—*all steps count*.

Reference

1. https://health.gov/sites/default/files/2019-09/Physical_Activity_Guidelines_2nd_edition.pdf

220. Correct Answer: C

Rationale

Semaglutide is the most recently (June 2021) approved GLP-1 RA for obesity treatment in those with BMI ≥30 kg/m² or 27–29 kg/m² with one weight-related comorbidity. Liraglutide was approved for obesity treatment in 2014. Cagrilintide is a long-acting amylin analog that is under evaluation as an anti-obesity medication. Tirzepitide is a dual GLP-1 and GIP receptor agonist that is undergoing evaluation for Type 2 diabetes and obesity treatment. Dulaglutide is a GLP-1 receptor agonist that is approved for treating Type 2 diabetes.

Reference

1. Wilding JPH, Batterham RL, Calanna S, et al. STEP 1 Study Group. Once-weekly semaglutide in adults with overweight or obesity. N Engl J Med. 2021;384(11):989–1002.

221. Correct Answer: E

Rationale

Compared to performance art controls, standup comics have a higher rate of premature death, largely due to suicide, drug overdose, and premature cardiovascular disease.

Humor improves capability to manage life stressors (i.e., coping), decreases post-encounter stress hormones (epinephrine and cortisol), and favorably affects the immune system. Humor may favorably affect endothelial function (enhances vasodilation and blood flow). Laughter and humor orientation may help prevent stress-related endothelial dysfunction, and potentially reduce the risk of cardiovascular disease.

References
1. Savage BM, Lujan HL, Thipparthi RR, DiCarlo SE. Humor, laughter, learning, and health! A brief review. Adv Physiol Educ. 2017;41(3):341–7.
2. Toda N, Nakanishi-Toda M. How mental stress affects endothelial function. Pflugers Arch. 2011;462(6):779–94.

222. Correct Answer: B

Rationale

With decreased kidney function patients on metformin are at increasing risk for lactic acidosis.

Reference
1. American Diabetes Association. Pharmacologic approaches to glycemic treatment: standards of medical care in diabetes-2021. Diabetes Care. 2021; 44(Suppl 1):S111–24.

223. Correct Answer: D

Rationale

Increased urinary glucose associated with SGLT2 therapy can lead to severe infections in the perineal area.

Reference
1. American Diabetes Association. Pharmacologic approaches to glycemic treatment: standards of medical care in diabetes-2021. Diabetes Care. 2021;44(Suppl 1):S111–24.

224. Correct Answer: C

Rationale

Women have worse outcomes compared with men after acute myocardial infarction (AMI) [1]. Women are less likely after AMI to receive guideline directed medical therapy (GDMT) [2]. Women are equally likely to experience chest pain with AMI, but more likely to have other associated symptoms [3]. Young women with an AMI who sought care in the VIRGO study were less likely to be told that their symptoms were heart related, when compared with young men (<age 55). Women remain under-enrolled in cardiovascular trials of device therapies, drug trials, procedures and lifestyle interventions [4].

References
1. Izadnegahdar M, Mackay M, Lee MK, Sedlak TL, Gao M, Bairey Merz CN, Humphries KH. Sex and ethnic differences in outcomes of acute coronary syndrome and stable angina patients with obstructive coronary artery disease. Circ Cardiovasc Qual Outcomes. 2016;9 (2 Suppl 1):S26–35.
2. Alabas OA, Gale CP, Hall M, Rutherford MJ, Szummer K, Lawesson SS, Alfredsson J, Lindahl B, Jernberg T. Sex differences in treatments, relative survival, and excess mortality following acute myocardial infarction: National Cohort Study Using the SWEDEHEART Registry. J Am Heart Assoc. 2017;6(12):e007123.
3. Ferry AV, Anand A, Strachan FE, Mooney L, Stewart SD, Marshall L, Chapman AR, Lee KK, Jones S, Orme K, Shah ASV, Mills NL. Presenting symptoms in men and women diagnosed with myocardial infarction using sex-specific criteria. J Am Heart Assoc. 2019;8(17):e012307.
4. Jin X, Chandramouli C, Allocco B, Gong E, Lam CSP, Yan LL. Women's participation in cardiovascular clinical trials from 2010 to 2017. Circulation. 2020;141(7):540–8.

225. Correct Answer: D

Rationale

High sensitivity troponins improve the sensitivity for the diagnosis of AMI in women but not in men.

References
1. Mills NL, Churchhouse AM, Lee KK, et al. Implementation of a sensitive troponin I assay and risk of recurrent myocardial infarction and death in patients with suspected acute coronary syndrome. JAMA. 2011;305(12):1210–6.
2. Shah AS, Griffiths M, Lee KK, et al. High sensitivity cardiac troponin and the under-diagnosis of myocardial infarction in women: prospective cohort study. BMJ. 2015;350:g7873.

3. Roffi M, Patrono C, Collet JP, et al. ESC Scientific Document Group. 2015 ESC Guidelines for the management of acute coronary syndromes in patients presenting without persistent ST-segment elevation: task force for the management of acute coronary syndromes in patients presenting without persistent ST-segment elevation of the European Society of Cardiology (ESC). Eur Heart J. 2016;37(3):267–315.

226. Correct Answer: C

Rationale

There has been some controversy over what the lower level of total testosterone (range from 240 to 400 ng/dL) should be since the diagnosis of testosterone deficiency requires both chemical hypogonadism and symptoms. Guidelines for Testosterone Deficiency by the Endocrine Society and the Am Urologic Assoc in 2018 both chose TT <300 ng/dL as the criteria, hence, setting the standard.

Reference
1. Park HJ, Ahn ST, Moon DG. Evolution of guidelines for testosterone replacement therapy. J Clin Med. 2019;8(3):410.

227. Correct Answer: E

Rationale

Proven Clinical TRT Benefits
- Erectile Dysfunction
- Low sex drive
- Anemia
- Bone mineral density
- Lean body mass
- Depressive symptoms

There also has been controversy over what symptoms may both be consistently caused by testosterone deficiency and improved with TRT. The FDA, after reviewing multiple studies evaluating symptom improvement with TRT, has concluded that erectile dysfunction, decreased libido, anemia, reduced bone mineral density, low lean body mass, and depressive symptoms are consistently associated with Low T and improved by TRT.

Reference
1. Pastuszak AW, Mittakanti H, Liu JS, et al. Pharmacokinetic evaluation and dosing of subcutaneous testosterone pellets. J Androl. 2012;33(5):927–37.

228. Correct Answer: B

Rationale

Per the AHA/ACC 2018 Cholesterol Management Guideline, elevated lipoprotein(a) ≥50 mg/dL is a risk enhancing feature. ApoB ≥130 mg/dL and HsCRP >2 mg/L and triglycerides ≥175 mg/dL, non-HDL-C ≥190 are also risk-enhancing features.

Reference
1. Grundy SM, Stone NJ, Bailey AL, et al. 2018 AHA/ACC/AACVPR/AAPA/ABC ACPM/ADA/AGS/APhA/ASPC/NLA/PCNA guideline on the management of blood cholesterol: executive summary: a report of the American College of Cardiology/American Heart Association task force on clinical practice guidelines. Circulation. 2019;139(25):e1046–81.

229. Correct Answer: E

Rationale

In patients with elevated triglycerides, the calculated LDL may be inaccurate when estimated by the Friedewald equation. Better assessment of atherogenic lipids are direct LDL, non-HDL-C, ApoB, and LDL-P.

References
1. Martin SS, Blaha MJ, Elshazly MB, et al. Friedewald-estimated versus directly measured low-density lipoprotein cholesterol and treatment implications. J Am Coll Cardiol. 2013;62(8):732–9.
2. Martin SS, Blaha MJ, Elshazly MB, et al. Comparison of a novel method vs the Friedewald equation for estimating low-density lipoprotein cholesterol levels from the standard lipid profile. JAMA. 2013;310(19):2061–8.

230. Correct Answer: E

Rationale

Pericytes and astrocytes reinforce the endothelium to create the blood brain barrier. Endothelial cells of the central nervous system exhibit low rates of pinocytosis and passive diffusion. Brain entry of blood-derived substances is restricted by the presence of tight junctions that connect endothelial cells. The blood brain barrier does not express lipoprotein receptors and is resistant to lipoprotein influx.

Reference
1. Storck SE, Pietrzik CU. Neuroforum. 2018;24(4):A197–205.

231. Correct Answer: E

Rationale

To date, no prospective randomized clinical trial with lipid-lowering agents has demonstrated an increased risk for neurocognitive impairment, even at ultra-low levels of LDL-C (low density lipoprotein-cholesterol) (<20 mg/dL). In the Heart Protection Study and PROSPER trials, no between group differences were found in the statin and placebo treated groups. In the Ebbinghaus trial, neither patients nor the clinical investigators conducting the trial were able to detect any between group differences when comparing treatments that included statin monotherapy or combination therapy with a statin and evolocumab.

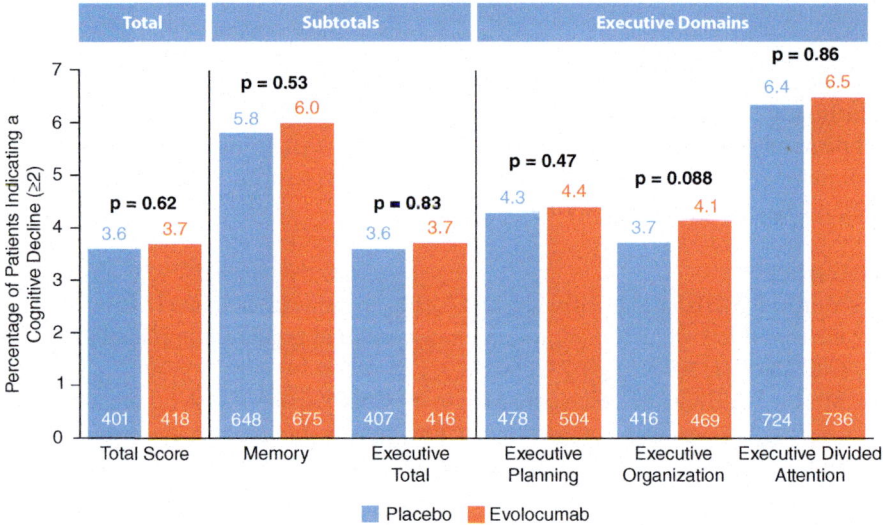

Baris *Gencer et al. J Am Coll Cardiol* 2020; 75:22832293.

Figure reproduced with permission from J Am Coll Cardiol. 2020 May 12;75(18):2283–2293

References
1. Rojas-Fernandez CH, Goldstein LB, et al. The National Lipid Association's Safety Task Force. An assessment by the Statin Cognitive Safety Task Force: 2014 update. J Clin Lipidol. 2014;8(3 Suppl):S5–16.
2. Trompet S, van Vliet P, de Craen AJ, et al. Pravastatin and cognitive function in the elderly. Results of the PROSPER study. J Neurol. 2010;257(1):85–90.
3. Gencer B, Mach F, Guo J, et al. FOURIER Investigators. Cognition after lowering LDL-cholesterol with evolocumab. J Am Coll Cardiol. 2020;75(18):2283–93.
4. Giugliano RP, Mach F, Zavitz K, et al. EBBINGHAUS Investigators. Cognitive function in a randomized trial of evolocumab. N Engl J Med. 2017;377(7):633–43.

232. Correct Answer: D

Rationale
In the CANTOS trial, the use of canakinumab in patients with a history of myocardial infarction and elevated hs-CRP levels (≥ 2 mg/L) was associated with a reduction in the primary efficacy end point of nonfatal myocardial infarction, nonfatal stroke, or cardiovascular death. Although hs-CRP levels decreased significantly in the group receiving canakinumab, there was no significant reduction in LDL-C levels in the group receiving canakinumab compared to placebo.

Reference
1. Ridker PM, Everett BM, Thuren T, et al. Anti-inflammatory therapy with canakinumab for atherosclerotic disease. N Engl J Med. 2017;377(12):1119–31.

233. Correct Answer: D

Rationale
JUPITER trial was a primary prevention trial performed in patients without history of cardiovascular disease (including prior myocardial infarction). To be included, participants needed to have LDL-C levels of 130 mg/dL or lower and hs-CRP levels of 2 mg/L or higher. In JUPITER trial, rosuvastatin was associated with a 50% reduction in LDL-C levels and 37% reduction in hs-CRP levels. The relative risk reduction in the primary end point (occurrence of a first major cardiovascular event, defined as nonfatal myocardial infarction, nonfatal stroke, hospitalization for unstable angina, an arterial revascularization procedure, or confirmed death from cardiovascular causes) was 44% in the rosuvastatin group compared to the group receiving placebo.

Reference
1. Ridker PM, Danielson E, Fonseca FAH, et al. Rosuvastatin to prevent vascular events in men and women with elevated C-reactive protein. N Engl J Med. 2008;359(21):2195–207.

234. Correct Answer: D

Rationale
Although approximately 80% of olive oil is comprised of monounsaturated fat, about 10% of the oil is polyunsaturated and 10% is saturated. It is a common misconception that oils are purely one type of fat or another. For example, although coconut oil is about 90% saturated fat, 10% of the oil is comprised of a combination of polyunsaturated and monounsaturated fat. Likewise, although sunflower oil is approximately 70% polyunsaturated fat, 30% is a combination of saturated and monounsaturated fat.

Reference

1. U.S. Department of Agriculture, Agricultural Research Service, Nutrient Data Laboratory. USDA National Nutrient Database for Standard Reference, Release 22. http://www.ars.usda.gov/ba/bhnrc/ndl.

235. Correct Answer: B

Rationale

The use of CPAP in patients with OSA reduces the risk of recurrent AF after radiofrequency ablation.

Reference

1. Nalliah CJ, Wong GR, Lee G, et al. Impact of CPAP on the atrial fibrillation substrate in obstructive sleep apnea: the SLEEP-AF Study. JACC Clin Electrophysiol. 2022;8(7):869–77.

236. Correct Answer: C

Rationale

It appears that some exercise is beneficial, while sustained vigorous exercise (such as cross-country skiing) may increase the risk of AF.

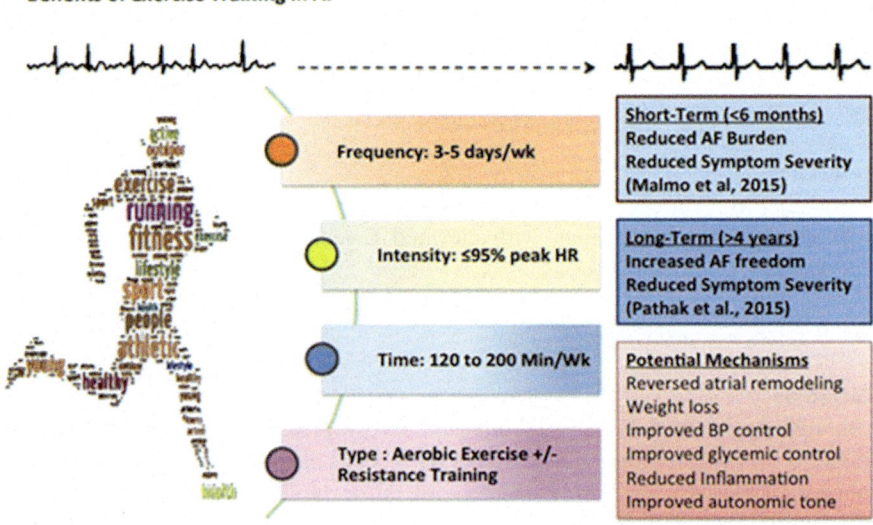

Figure reproduced with permission from Elliott et al. Circulation 2016; 133(5) 457–9

References
1. Sepehri Shamloo A, Arya A, Dagres N, Hindricks G. Exercise and atrial fibrillation: some good news and some bad news. Galen Med J. 2018;7:e1401.
2. Elliott AD, Mahajan R, Pathak RK, Lau DH, Sanders P. Exercise training and atrial fibrillation: further evidence for the importance of lifestyle change. Circulation. 2016;133(5):457–9.

237. Correct Answer: E

Rationale
Digoxin therapy in patients with HFrEF has been associated with a reduction in the risk for hospitalization but not mortality.

Reference
1. Yancy CW, Jessup M, Bozkurt B, et al. 2017 ACC/AHA/HFSA focused update of the 2013 ACCF/AHA guideline for the management of heart failure: a report of the American College of Cardiology/American Heart Association task force on clinical practice guidelines and the Heart Failure Society of America. J Am Coll Cardiol. 2017;70(6):776–803.

238. Correct Answer: D

Rationale
While secondary analysis of trials with multiple agents have shown reduction in heart failure hospitalization risk, no therapy has shown reduction in cardiovascular mortality in patients with heart failure and preserved ejection fraction.

Reference
1. Yancy CW, Jessup M, Bozkurt B, et al. 2017 ACC/AHA/HFSA focused update of the 2013 ACCF/AHA guideline for the management of heart failure: a report of the American College of Cardiology/American Heart Association task force on clinical practice guidelines and the Heart Failure Society of America. J Am Coll Cardiol. 2017;70(6):776–803.

239. Correct Answer: C

Rationale
Use of BP-lowering medication is recommended for primary prevention of CVD in adults with no history of CVD and with an estimated 10-year ASCVD risk <10% and an SBP of 140 mmHg or higher or a DBP (diastolic blood pressure) of 90 mmHg or higher.

References
1. J. Sundstrom, H. Arima, M. Woodward, et al. Blood Pressure Lowering Treatment Trialists' Collaboration. Blood pressure-lowering treatment based on cardiovascular risk: a meta-analysis of individual patient data. Lancet. 2014;384:591–8.

2. Lewington S, Clarke R, Qizilbash N, et al. Age-specific relevance of usual blood pressure to vascular mortality: a meta-analysis of individual data for one million adults in 61 prospective studies. Lancet. 2002;360:1903–3.
3. van Dieren S, Kengne AP, Chalmers J, et al. Effects of blood pressure lowering on cardiovascular outcomes in different cardiovascular risk groups among participants with type 2 diabetes. Diabetes Res Clin Pract. 2012;98:83–90.
4. Montgomery AA, Fahey T, Ben-Shlomo Y, et al. The influence of absolute cardiovascular risk, patient utilities, and costs on the decision to treat hypertension: a Markov decision analysis. J Hypertens. 2003;21:1753–9.
5. Kassai B, Boissel J-P, Cucherat M, et al. Treatment of high blood pressure and gain in event-free life expectancy. Vasc Health Risk Manag. 2005;1:163–9.
6. Whelton PK, Carey RM, Aronow WS, Casey DE Jr, Collins KJ, Dennison Himmelfarb C, DePalma SM, Gidding S, Jamerson KA, Jones DW, MacLaughlin EJ, Muntner P, Ovbiagele B, Smith SC Jr, Spencer CC, Stafford RS, Taler SJ, Thomas RJ, Williams KA Sr, Williamson JD, Wright JT Jr. 2017 ACC/AHA/AAPA/ABC/ACPM/AGS/APhA/ASH/ASPC/NMA/PCNA guideline for the prevention, detection, evaluation, and management of high blood pressure in adults: a report of the American College of Cardiology/American Heart Association task force on clinical practice guidelines. J Am Coll Cardiol. 2018;71(19):e127–248.

240. Correct Answer: D

Rationale
The 2017 ACC/AHA hypertension guideline recommends starting with either two separate agents or a fixed dose combination of two different classes when the blood pressure is at least 20 mmHg systolic or 10 mmHg diastolic above target.

COR	LOE	Recommendations for choice of initial monotherapy versus initial combination drug therapy
I	C-EO	Initiation of antihypertensive drug therapy with *two first-line agents of different classes*, either as separate agents or in a fixed-dose combination, is recommended in adults with *Stage 2 HTN* and an average BP more than **20/10 mmHg** above their BP target
IIa	C-EO	Initiation of antihypertensive drug therapy with *a single antihypertensive drug* is reasonable in adults with *Stage 1 HTN* with dosage titration and sequential addition of other agents to achieve the BP target

Answers

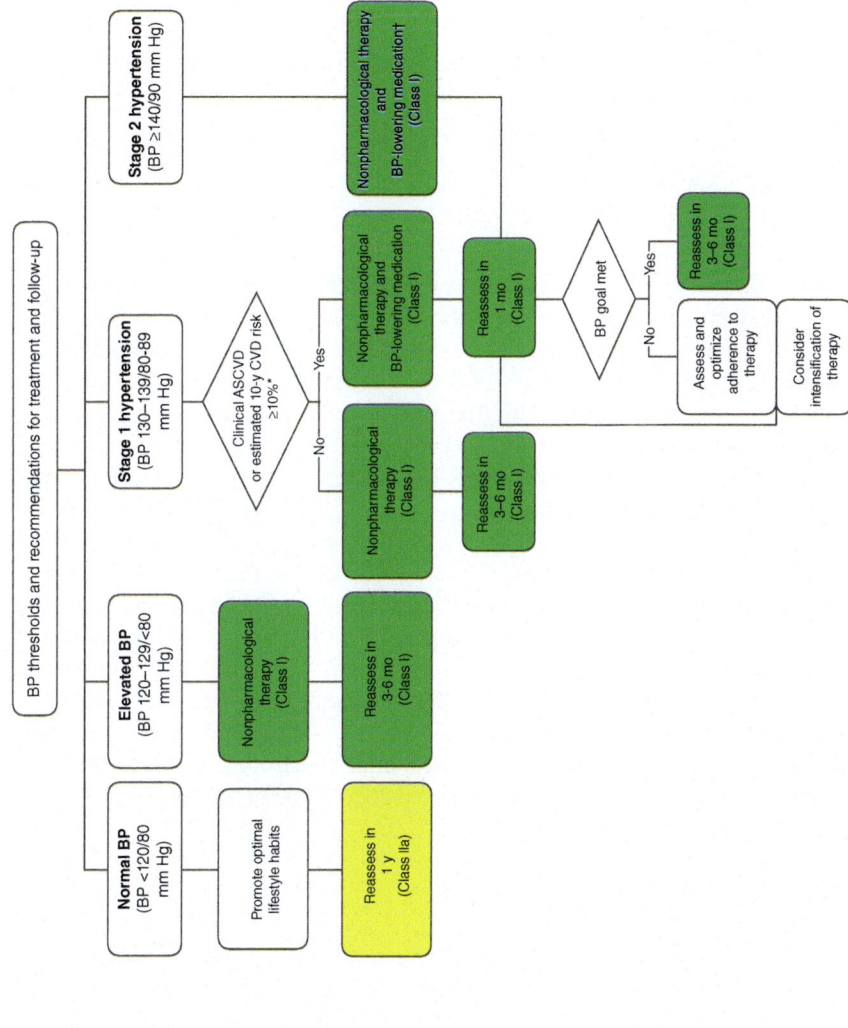

Figures reproduced with permission from J Am Coll Cardiol. 2018 May 15;71(19):e127–e248

References
1. Ambrosius WT, Sink KM, Foy CG, et al. The design and rationale of a multicenter clinical trial comparing two strategies for control of systolic blood pressure: the Systolic Blood Pressure Intervention Trial (SPRINT). Clin Trials. 2014;11:532–46.
2. Cushman WC, Grimm RH Jr, Cutler JA, et al. Rationale and design for the blood pressure intervention of the Action to Control Cardiovascular Risk in Diabetes (ACCORD) trial. Am J Cardiol. 2007;99:44i–55i.
3. ACC/AHA/AAPA/ABC/ACPM/AGS/APhA/ASH/ASPC/NMA/PCNA guideline for the prevention, detection, evaluation, and management of high blood pressure in adults: a report of the American College of Cardiology/American Heart Association task force on clinical practice guidelines. J Am Coll Cardiol. 2018;71(19):e127–248.

241. Correct Answer: C

Rationale
Although the vast majority of FH cases are caused by mutations in the LDL receptor gene (LDLR) gene, there are etiologic polymorphisms in other genes, such as apolipoprotein B (APOB) that codes for the natural ligand of the LDL-R protein. Mutations in proprotein convertase subtilisin/kexin type 9 (PCSK9) has been more recently identified as a cause of FH; however, mutations in this latter gene seems to be rare in the populations studied so far. Mutations have also been identified in the gene for adaptor protein-1, which facilitates the alignment of the LDL-R-LDL particle complex within coated pits of the hepatocyte cell membrane, facilitating endosomal uptake and clearance.

References
1. Gratton J, Humphries SE, Futema M. Prevalence of FH-causing variants and impact on LDL-C concentration in European, South Asian, and African Ancestry Groups of the UK Biobank. Arterioscler Thromb Vasc Biol. 2023. https://doi.org/10.1161/ATVBAHA.123.319438. Epub ahead of print. PMID: 37409534.
2. Gidding SS, Kirchner HL, Brangan A, et al. Yield of familial hypercholesterolemia genetic and phenotypic diagnoses after electronic health record and genomic data screening. J Am Heart Assoc. 2023;12(13):e030073.

242. Correct Answer: B

Rationale
PCSK9 binds specifically to the epidermal growth factor-A (EGF-A) domain of the LDL receptor (LDLR) in a calcium-dependent manner. Other regions of the LDLR that do not contact PCSK9 are required for PCSK9-mediated degradation, including the b-propeller domain and at least three ligand binding repeats. The reason for these structural requirements is not known. The C-terminal domain of PCSK9 does not bind to the LDLR, but this region is required for LDLR degradation. Thus, the C terminus may bind another protein that directs LDLRs to lysosomes, or the domain may prevent the binding of a protein required for recycling of the LDLR from endosomes to the cell surface.

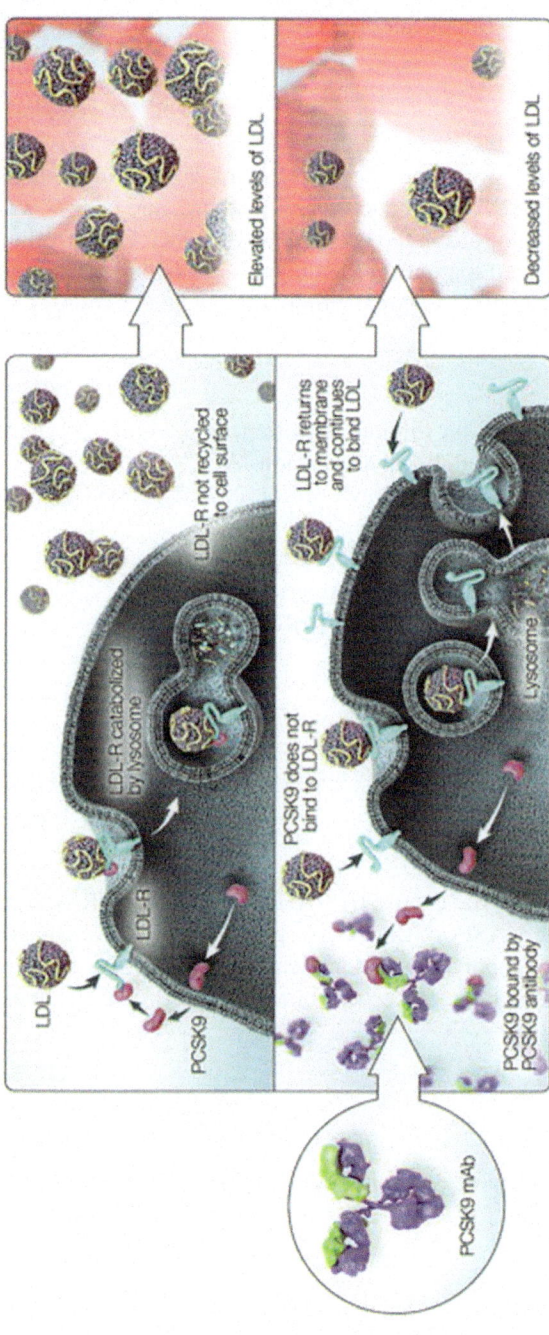

Top panel: PCSK9 secreted by hepatocytes binds to LDL-R on the hepatocyte surface. Upon subsequent binding of the receptor by LDL, the PCSK9/LDL/LDL-R complex is internalized within an endosomal vesicle. The endosome fuses with a lysosome, and the PCSK9 chaperones the LDL/LDL-R complex into the lysosome for destruction. As a result, the number of LDL-Rs is decreased, resulting in less clearance of LDL from the circulation and elevated LDL concentration. *Bottom panel*: Monoclonal antibody binds to PCSK9 and prevents it from engaging the LDL-R. In the absence of PCSK9, the LDL-R is not routed to the lysosome for degradation and is returned instead to the hepatocyte surface. The recycled LDL-R is available for additional LDL binding and clearance, resulting in decreased levels of LDL. *LDL* low-density lipoprotein, *LDL-R* low-density lipoprotein receptor. (Figure and legend reproduced from Toth PP. Novel Therapies for Low-Density Lipoprotein Cholesterol Reduction. Am J Cardiol. 2016 Sep 15;118(6 Suppl):19A–32A)

Reference
1. Horton JD, Cohen JC, Hobbs HH. PCSK9: a convertase that coordinates LDL catabolism. J Lipid Res. 2009;50 Suppl(Suppl):S172–7.

243. Correct Answer: C

Rationale
Awareness was equal among African American and Hispanic/Latinx individuals compared to Non-Hispanic White individuals; however, blood pressure control was less across multiple minority populations in the latest NHANES data. Out-of-office BP measurements are recommended to confirm the diagnosis of hypertension and for titration of BP-lowering medication, in conjunction with telehealth counseling or clinical interventions.

References
1. 2017 ACC-AHA guideline for the prevention, detection, evaluation, and management of high blood pressure in adults. Hypertension JACC. 2017.
2. Ferdinand KC, Vo TN, Echols MR. Am J Prev Cardiol. 2020;2:100038. https://doi.org/10.1016/j.ajpc.2020.100038.
3. Shimbo D, Artinian NT, Basile JN, et al. Self-Measured blood pressure monitoring at home: a joint policy statement from the American Heart Association and American Medical Association. Circulation. 2020;142(4).

244. Correct Answer: D

Rationale
Black adults have higher levels of HDL-C, lower levels of triglycerides, and lower severity of coronary artery calcification.

Reference:
1. Grundy SM, Stone NJ, Bailey AL, et al. 2018 AHA/ACC/AACVPR/AAPA/ABC/ACPM/ADA/AGS/APhA/ASPC/NLA/PCNA guideline on the management of blood cholesterol: a report of the American College of Cardiology/American Heart Association task force on clinical practice guidelines. Circulation. 2019;139(25):e1082–143.

245. Correct Answer: A

Rationale
Deaths attributable to CVD have increased, although higher than 1940 as it has shown significant upward trend.

Reference
1. Virani SS, Alonso A, Aparicio HJ, et al. American Heart Association Council on Epidemiology and Prevention Statistics Committee and Stroke Statistics Subcommittee. Heart disease and stroke statistics-2021 update: a report from the American Heart Association. Circulation. 2021;143(8):e254–743.

246. Correct Answer: B

Rationale

The CORAL trial was designed to test whether renal-artery stenting, when added to protocol-driven contemporary medical therapy, improves clinical outcomes in persons with atherosclerotic renal-artery stenosis. The investigators found no benefit of stenting with respect to the rate of the composite primary end point or any of its individual components, including death from cardiovascular or renal causes, stroke, myocardial infarction, congestive heart failure, progressive renal insufficiency, and the need for renal-replacement therapy. This result was consistent across all pre-specified subgroups, including patients with global renal ischemia and patients with other high-risk characteristics. We did observe a modest, but statistically significant, reduction of 2 mmHg in systolic blood pressure with stenting, but this reduction did not translate into a reduction in clinical events.

Reference
1. Cooper CJ, Murphy TP, Cutlip DE, Jamerson K, Henrich W, Reid DM, Cohen DJ, Matsumoto AH, Steffes M, Jaff MR, Prince MR, Lewis EF, Tuttle KR, Shapiro JI, Rundback JH, Massaro JM, D'Agostino RB Sr, Dworkin LD; CORAL Investigators. Stenting and medical therapy for atherosclerotic renal-artery stenosis. N Engl J Med. 2014;370(1):13–22.

247. Correct Answer: D

Rationale

Individual studies have shown a wide variation in the magnitude of the BP reduction with CPAP (continuous positive airway pressure). Overall, several meta-analyses suggest that only a modest fall is evident. It is likely that factors such as sleepiness, severity of hypoxemia, and adherence to CPAP contribute to the efficacy of the antihypertensive effects of treating OSA.

Reference
1. Hu X, Fan J, Chen S, Yin Y, Zrenner B. The role of continuous positive airway pressure in blood pressure control for patients with obstructive sleep apnea and hypertension: a meta-analysis of randomized controlled trials. J Clin Hypertens (Greenwich). 2015;17(3):215–22.

248. Correct Answer: E

Rationale

Despite compelling observational data implicating OSA (obstructive sleep apnea) in heightened risk of CV events and showing that CPAP (continuous positive airway pressure) reduces these events, several randomized controlled trials have not been able to show any benefit. This may possibly be due to patient selection and/or level of CPAP adherence.

Reference
1. Yeghiazarians Y, Jneid H, Tietjens JR, et al. Obstructive sleep apnea and cardiovascular disease: a scientific statement from the American Heart Association. Circulation. 2021;144(3):e56–67.

249. Correct Answer: D

Rationale
The patient is asymptomatic. CTA parameters have not been found to improve ASCVD prediction on top of CAC scoring in asymptomatic individuals. Further, his high CAC score would make interpretation of the CTA more challenging. Per the ESC (European Society of Cardiology) Guidelines, one generally would not pursue functional imaging testing in this situation, let alone functional testing such as an ETT without imaging. He is already at high ASCVD (atherosclerotic cardiovascular disease) risk, so carotid IMT testing would not change his clinical management.

Reference
1. Knuuti J, Wijns W, Saraste A, et al. ESC Scientific Document Group. 2019 ESC guidelines for the diagnosis and management of chronic coronary syndromes. Eur Heart J. 2020;41(3):407–77.

250. Correct Answer: A

Rationale
The patient has a high-risk stress test due to her reduced functional capacity, higher Duke treadmill score, large territory of ischemia, and decrement in ejection fraction. This is in addition to her risk factor of diabetes. Per the SIHD guidelines, coronary angiography is recommended given the high likelihood of severe ischemic heart disease. Given the higher pretest probability and potential for severe disease (i.e., three vessel CAD or left main disease), invasive angiography is preferred over coronary CT angiography, as is recommended by the 2019 ESC (European Society of Cardiology) CAD guidelines. Stress perfusion imaging will add little clinical value to the stress echo findings.

References
1. Fihn SD, Blankenship JC, Alexander KP, et al. 2014 ACC/AHA/AATS/PCNA/SCAI/STS focused update of the guideline for the diagnosis and management of patients with stable ischemic heart disease: a report of the American College of Cardiology/American Heart Association Task Force on Practice Guidelines, and the American Association for Thoracic Surgery, Preventive Cardiovascular Nurses Association, Society for Cardiovascular Angiography and Interventions, and Society of Thoracic Surgeons. J Am Coll Cardiol. 2014;64(18):1929–49.
2. Fihn SD, Gardin JM, Abrams J, et al. American College of Cardiology Foundation; American Heart Association Task Force on Practice Guidelines; American College of Physicians; American Association for Thoracic Surgery;

Preventive Cardiovascular Nurses Association; Society for Cardiovascular Angiography and Interventions; Society of Thoracic Surgeons. 2012 ACCF/AHA/ACP/AATS/PCNA/SCAI/STS Guideline for the diagnosis and management of patients with stable ischemic heart disease: a report of the American College of Cardiology Foundation/American Heart Association Task Force on Practice Guidelines, and the American College of Physicians, American Association for Thoracic Surgery, Preventive Cardiovascular Nurses Association, Society for Cardiovascular Angiography and Interventions, and Society of Thoracic Surgeons. J Am Coll Cardiol. 2012;60(24):e44–164.

251. Correct Answer: F

Rationale
The Pooled Cohort Equation estimating 10-year ASCVD risk is intended to be used in primary prevention among those without diabetes and no prior clinically significant ASCVD. Moreover, the equation only applies to those aged 40–79 years of age given the longitudinal studies it was derived from; there was inadequate data in younger or older persons. Finally, those whose LDL-C is ≥190 mg/dL have a high lifetime burden of hypercholesterolemia, such as from familial hypercholesterolemia, and hence, use of the pooled cohort equation could underestimate risk. Such persons are also indicated for at least high intensity statin to lower LDL-C by at least 50%, so the risk calculation would not influence the decision regarding initiation or intensification of statin therapy.

Reference
1. Grundy SM, Stone NJ, Bailey AL, 2018 AHA/ACC/AACVPR/AAPA/ABC/ACPM/ADA/AGS/APhA/ASPC/NLA/PCNA guideline on the management of blood cholesterol: a report of the American College of Cardiology/American Heart Association task force on clinical practice guidelines. Circulation. 2019;139(25):e1082–143.

252. Correct Answer: A

Rationale
The 2018 cholesterol management guidelines note that if there is still uncertainty about the treatment decision after consideration of risk enhancement factors in those at borderline or intermediate ASCVD risk that one may consider the use of CAC scoring, with a score of 0 (as long as the patient is not diabetic, does not smoke, and does not have a history of premature onset ASCVD) to consider withholding or delaying statin therapy. The current guidelines do not recommend using the CAC score for those with known ASCVD or diabetes where statin treatment is already recommended.

Reference
1. Grundy SM, Stone NJ, Bailey AL, 2018 AHA/ACC/AACVPR/AAPA/ABC/ACPM/ADA/AGS/APhA/ASPC/NLA/PCNA guideline on the management of blood cholesterol: a report of the American College of Cardiology/American Heart Association task force on clinical practice guidelines. Circulation. 2019;139(25):e1082–143.

253. Correct Answer: B

Rationale
About 2% of individuals who present to the hospital with a myocardial infarction at age less than 55 years harbor a familial hypercholesterolemia mutation that confers significantly increased risk. The prevalence of these mutations in the general population is estimated to be 0.4%. In contrast to familial hypercholesterolemia mutations, about 17% of such patients were predisposed by their DNA on the basis of a high polygenic score.

Reference
1. Khera AV, Chaffin M, Zekavat SM, et al. Whole-genome sequencing to characterize monogenic and polygenic contributions in patients hospitalized with early-onset myocardial infarction. Circulation. 2019;139(13):1593–602.

254. Correct Answer: D

Rationale
Although a high polygenic score confers significant inborn risk for myocardial infarction, "DNA is not destiny." Both adherence to a healthy lifestyle and statin therapy have been linked to a 40–50% reduction in risk of incident events among individuals with a high polygenic score.

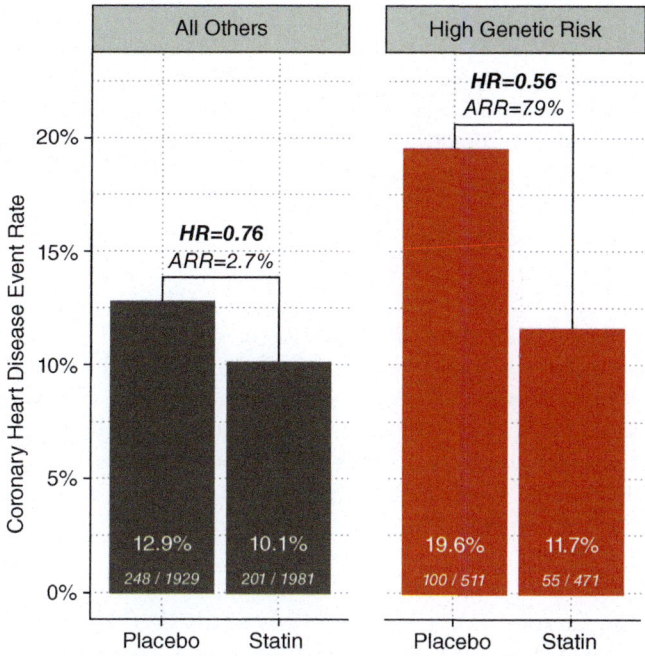

Incident coronary heart disease events by statin therapy and genetic risk group in WOSCOPS (West of Scotland Coronary Prevention Study). Nonfatal myocardial infarction or death resulting from coronary heart disease rate is shown by randomized treatment group and polygenic risk group in WOSCOPS. Absolute events (and percentage) per individual in each group are shown at the bottom of the bars. This represents 604 events over 64,031 total patient-years of follow-up. The follow-up period within the trial was 4.8 years (SD, 0.7 years) for both the placebo and statin groups and out of the trial was 8.1 years (SD, 3.4 years) for the placebo group and 8.4 years (SD, 3.0 years) for the statin-treated group. ARR indicates adjusted relative risk; and HR, hazard ratio. (Figure and legend reproduced with permission from Circulation. 2017 May 30;135(22):2091–2101)

References
1. Khera AV, Emdin CA, Drake I, et al. Genetic risk, adherence to a healthy lifestyle, and coronary disease. N Engl J Med. 2016;375(24):2349–58.
2. Natarajan P, Young R, Stitziel NO, et al. Polygenic risk score identifies subgroup with higher burden of atherosclerosis and greater relative benefit from statin therapy in the primary prevention setting. Circulation. 2017;135(22):2091–101.

255. Correct Answer: B

Rationale
ACC/AHA Guidelines recommend ticagrelor or prasugrel over clopidogrel in patients with ACS (acute coronary syndrome) undergoing revascularization. Ticagrelor, but not prasugrel, can be preferred to clopidogrel in ACS. Prior stroke or TIA (transient ischemic attack), advanced age, frailty, and high bleeding risk are contraindications to institution of prasugrel therapy.

Reference
1. Levine GN, Bates ER, Bittl JA, et al. 2016 ACC/AHA guideline focused update on duration of dual antiplatelet therapy in patients with coronary artery disease: a report of the American College of Cardiology/American Heart Association task force on clinical practice guidelines. J Thorac Cardiovasc Surg. 2016;152(5):1243–75.

256. Correct Answer: A

Rationale
While older clinical trials showed a reduction in cardiovascular events with aspirin, recent clinical trials have shown mixed results. ASCEND showed a reduction in vascular events in those with diabetes while bleeding risk was increased. ARRIVE and ASPREE failed to show a benefit of aspirin in high-risk primary prevention and older adults in primary prevention, respectively. ASA has never been studied in an RCT (randomized clinical trial) among those with elevated CAC scores.

References
1. Gaziano JM, Brotons C, Coppolecchia R, et al. ARRIVE Executive Committee. Use of aspirin to reduce risk of initial vascular events in patients at moderate risk of cardiovascular disease (ARRIVE): a randomised, double-blind, placebo-controlled trial. Lancet. 2018;392(10152):1036–46.
2. ASCEND Study Collaborative Group, Bowman L, Mafham M, Wallendszus K, et al. Effects of aspirin for primary prevention in persons with diabetes mellitus. N Engl J Med. 2018;379(16):1529–39.
3. McNeil JJ, Wolfe R, Woods RL, et al. ASPREE Investigator Group. Effect of aspirin on cardiovascular events and bleeding in the healthy elderly. N Engl J Med. 2018;379(16):1509–18.
4. US Preventive Services Task Force, Davidson KW, Barry MJ, Mangione CM, et al. Aspirin use to prevent cardiovascular disease: US preventive services task force recommendation statement. JAMA. 2022;327(16):1577–84.

257. Correct Answer: F

Rationale
Several landmark publications provide the evidence base that stenting/PCI does not reduce death or MI but only angina.

References
1. Boden WE, O'Rourke RA, Teo KK, et al. COURAGE Trial Research Group. Optimal medical therapy with or without PCI for stable coronary disease. N Engl J Med. 2007;356(15):1503–16.
2. Gersh BJ, Boden WE, Bhatt DL, et al. To stent or not to stent? Treating angina after ISCHEMIA-introduction. Eur Heart J. 2021;42(14):1387–8.

3. Brown DL, Boden WE. Impact of revascularisation on outcomes in chronic coronary syndromes: a new meta-analysis with the same old biases? Eur Heart J. 2021;42(45):4652–5.
4. Manolis AJ, Boden WE, Collins P, et al. State of the art approach to managing angina and ischemia: tailoring treatment to the evidence. Eur J Intern Med. 2021;92:40–7.

258. Correct Answer: E

Rationale
Patients with atherosclerosis in the peripheral arteries, including the legs, are at heightened risk of major adverse cardiovascular events, including myocardial infarction and stroke and are at particularly high risk if they have both coronary and peripheral atherosclerosis (i.e., polyvascular disease). Patients with peripheral artery disease are at high risk of major adverse limb events and functional decline related to impaired perfusion. Due to their heightened cardiovascular risk and the frequent existence of comorbidities, patients with peripheral artery disease are at high risk of cardiovascular and all-cause mortality.

Reference
1. Gerhard-Herman MD, Gornik HL, Barrett C, et al. 2016 AHA/ACC guideline on the management of patients with lower extremity peripheral artery disease: executive summary: a report of the American College of Cardiology/American Heart Association task force on clinical practice guidelines. Circulation. 2017;135(12):e686–725.

259. Correct Answer: E

Rationale
The Heart Protection Study demonstrated that lowering LDL-C with statins reduces major adverse cardiovascular events as well as peripheral revascularizations. Two trials of PCSK9 inhibitors (FOURIER and ODYSSEY OUTCOMES) have demonstrated that lowering LDL-C with a PCSK9 inhibitor on top of statins reduces major adverse limb events (MALE) and revascularizations as well as major acute coronary events (MACE). Multiple real-world datasets demonstrate underutilization of lipid lowering therapies in patients with atherosclerosis and in particular in patients with peripheral artery disease.

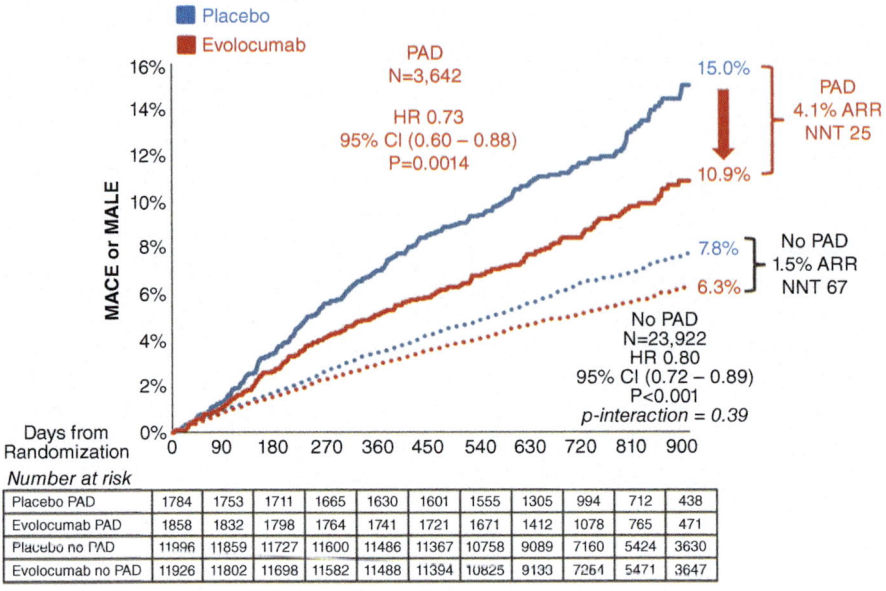

Major adverse cardiovascular and limb events in patients with and without peripheral artery disease. The composite of major adverse cardiovascular events (MACE; cardiovascular death, myocardial infarction, or stroke) and major adverse limb events (MALE; acute limb ischemia, major amputation, or urgent revascularization) by treatment (evolocumab in red, placebo in blue) in patients with (solid lines) and without (dashed lines) symptomatic PAD. *ARR* absolute risk reduction, *CI* confidence interval, *HR* hazard ratio, *MACE* major adverse cardiovascular event, *MALE* major adverse limb event, *NNT* number needed to treat, *PAD* peripheral artery disease. (Figure and legend reproduced with permission from Bonaca et al. Circulation. 2018 Jan 23;137(4):338–350)

References

1. Heart Protection Study Collaborative Group. Randomized trial of the effects of cholesterol-lowering with simvastatin on peripheral vascular and other major vascular outcomes in 20,536 people with peripheral arterial disease and other high-risk conditions. J Vasc Surg. 2007;45(4):645–54.
2. Bonaca MP, Nault P, Giugliano RP, et al. Low-density lipoprotein cholesterol lowering with evolocumab and outcomes in patients with peripheral artery disease: insights from the FOURIER Trial (Further Cardiovascular Outcomes Research With PCSK9 Inhibition in Subjects With Elevated Risk). Circulation. 2018;137(4):338–50.
3. Schwartz GG, Steg PG, Szarek M, et al. ODYSSEY OUTCOMES Committees and Investigators. Peripheral artery disease and venous thromboembolic events after acute coronary syndrome: role of lipoprotein(a) and modification by alirocumab: prespecified analysis of the ODYSSEY OUTCOMES randomized clinical trial. Circulation. 2020;141(20):1608–17.

260. Correct Answer: B

Rationale

This patient, despite only having minimal stenosis, has extensive plaque which involves at least 5 coronary segments. Her symptoms, which are described as rare and non-exertional, are unlikely to be due to the minimal stenosis that she has. Although PET could be useful to assess for microvascular dysfunction in the right clinical context, this patient has non-exertional symptoms and a high exercise capacity, and thus this is less likely to be useful in this scenario. It is important to recognize that the amount/extent of plaque is associated with a higher future risk of CV events. The patient also has mildly elevated LDL-C. As such the most important next step would be lipid lowering therapy (in addition to lifestyle changes). Her Lp(a) is only mildly elevated and would not warrant any therapy. Genetic testing has not been shown to add much to risk prediction, especially once data on actual presence of plaque (from CAC or CCTA) is available.

Reference

1. Narula J, Chandrashekhar Y, Ahmadi A, et al. SCCT 2021 expert consensus document on coronary computed tomographic angiography: a report of the Society of Cardiovascular Computed Tomography. J Cardiovasc Comput Tomogr. 2021;15(3):192–217.

261. Correct Answer: A

Rationale

Coronary CTA is generally considered most appropriate for symptomatic patients. Thus, choices C and D would not be correct. Those patients could be evaluated with coronary artery calcium testing. Coronary CTA is less useful in patients who have undergone prior PCI or CABG as it is difficult to visualize the lumen of the stent (if prior PCI) and patients with prior CABG often have severe amount of coronary calcifications. Patients with very extensive coronary calcifications are also not good candidates for coronary CTA.

Reference

1. Narula J, Chandrashekhar Y, Ahmadi A, et al. SCCT 2021 expert consensus document on coronary computed tomographic angiography: a report of the Society of Cardiovascular Computed Tomography. J Cardiovasc Comput Tomogr. 2021;15(3):192–217.

262. Correct Answer: A

Rationale

More than 30 million people in the United States have some form of chronic venous disease (CVD). The prevalence of CVD is 10 times that of peripheral arterial disease and is underdiagnosed and undertreated. Chronic venous disease is a major source of morbidity and most admissions are for venous ulcers. The direct cost of treating venous disease in the United States is $3 billion annually. Risk factors for CVD vary, but they tend to be related to conditions that lead to venous dilation or other disruption of basic vein structure. These include older age, family history, female sex, pregnancy, obesity, occupations performed while standing, high-impact physical activity, and comorbid conditions such as deep vein thrombosis (DVT), superficial thrombophlebitis, and obstructive sleep apnea. Prevention is aimed at reducing risk factors and focused on management of obesity, increasing physical activity and reducing venous pressure by treating sleep apnea, elevation of legs and modifying activities that predispose to these.

Reference
1. McArdle M, Hernandez-Vila EA. Management of chronic venous disease. Tex Heart Inst J. 2017;44(5):347–9.

263. Correct Answer: E

Rationale
All of the answers support the accurate pathogenesis, prevalence and clinical benefit of CAC in CVD risk discrimination.

Using 10-year ASCVD risk estimate plus coronary artery calcium (CAC) score to guide statin therapy				
Patient's 10-year atherosclerotic cardiovascular disease (ASCVD) risk estimate:	<5%	5-7.5%	>7.5-20%	>20%
Consulting ASCVD risk estimate alone	Statin not recommended	Consider for statin	Recommend statin	Recommend statin
Consulting ASCVD risk estimate + CAC				
If CAC score =0	Statin not recommended	Statin not recommended	Statin not recommended	Recommend statin
If CAC score >0	Statin not recommended	Consider for statin	Recommend statin	Recommend statin
Does CAC score modify treatment plan?	✗ CAC not effective for this population	✓ CAC can reclassify risk up or down	✓ CAC can reclassify risk up or down	✗ CAC not effective for this population

Reference
1. Greenland P, Blaha MJ, Budoff MJ, et al. Coronary calcium score and cardiovascular risk: JACC state of the art review. J Am Coll Cardiol. 2018;72:434–47.

264. Correct Answer: E

Rationale

In this woman with traditional risk factors for ASCVD and an anginal equivalent symptom who is found to have a large defect on nuclear perfusion imaging, the presumed diagnosis is chronic coronary syndrome. In the setting of chronic coronary syndromes, many large-scale randomized trials including the ISCHEMIA and COURAGE trials have not shown a marked difference in survival or composite cardiovascular events between an invasive revascularization strategy or optimal medical therapy.

The correct answer is to obtain a coronary CT angiogram, as the presence of left main disease or three-vessel disease with a reduced ejection fraction has not been ruled out. In this subset of patients, revascularization is recommended so further anatomical evaluation is warranted.

In this patient, it is not currently recommended to add a second antiplatelet agent, such as clopidogrel or initiate a low-dose anticoagulant (COMPASS trial) in the context of primary prevention. Recall, the COMPASS trial only included secondary prevention individuals. Although improving the patient's antianginal regimen is desired, her heart rate of 52 beats per minute makes further titration of metoprolol challenging. Lastly, CAC testing is not indicated in symptomatic patients and would not be recommended.

References
1. Maron DJ, Hochman JS, Reynolds HR, et al. ISCHEMIA Research Group. Initial invasive or conservative strategy for stable coronary disease. N Engl J Med. 2020;382(15):1395–407.
2. Eikelboom JW, Connolly SJ, Bosch J, et al. COMPASS Investigators. Rivaroxaban with or without aspirin in stable cardiovascular disease. N Engl J Med. 2017;377(14):1319–30.

265. Correct Answer: C

Rationale

This patient presents to clinic with refractory anginal symptoms in the setting of known obstructive CAD based on recent coronary angiogram. She is already on an effective antianginal regimen, which includes beta blocker therapy, nitrate therapy, and calcium channel blocker therapy. Although additional antianginal therapy may be considered, this patient should be offered consideration of revascularization for improvement in her quality of life. The ISCHEMIA trial reported that patients with persistent symptom burden despite optimal medical therapy had improvement in angina-related quality of life in an invasive treatment arm.

References
1. Spertus JA, Jones PG, Maron DJ, et al. ISCHEMIA Research Group. Health-status outcomes with invasive or conservative care in coronary disease. N Engl J Med. 2020;382(15):1408–19.
2. Maron DJ, Hochman JS, Reynolds HR, et al. ISCHEMIA Research Group. Initial invasive or conservative strategy for stable coronary disease. N Engl J Med. 2020;382(15):1395–407.

266. Correct Answer: D

Rationale

This patient has a history of multiple cardiovascular risk factors and is found to have a markedly elevated coronary artery calcium score, which would place her at a significantly elevated risk of incident ASCVD event. As such, she warrants an aggressive prevention regimen, which should include initiation of diabetes medications with proven cardiovascular outcomes benefit as well as targeting an LDL-C less than 70 mg/dL. The initiation of ezetimibe 10 mg daily should achieve an LDL-C <70 mg/dL as this has roughly a 10–20% expected decrease. It is not necessary to initiate PCSK9 inhibitor therapy at this time as adjunctive lowering with ezetimibe should be tried first. Regarding the patient's diabetes, empagliflozin should be added as this showed a significant cardiovascular death improvement in the EMPA-REG study. Thus, the correct answer is D—start ezetimibe 10 mg daily and empagliflozin 10 mg daily.

References
1. ElSayed NA, Aleppo G, Aroda VR, et al, on behalf of the American Diabetes Association. 10. Cardiovascular disease and risk management: standards of care in diabetes-2023. Diabetes Care. 2023;46(Suppl 1):S158–90.
2. Arnett DK, Blumenthal RS, Albert MA, et al. 2019 ACC/AHA guideline on the primary prevention of cardiovascular disease: a report of the American College of Cardiology/American Heart Association task force on clinical practice guidelines. Circulation. 2019;140(11):e596–646.

267. Correct Answer: D

Rationale

This patient has a history of multiple cardiovascular risk factors and is found to have a markedly elevated coronary artery calcium score, which would place her at a significantly elevated risk of incident ASCVD event. As such, she warrants an aggressive prevention regimen, which should include initiation of diabetes medications with proven cardiovascular outcomes benefit as well as targeting an LDL-C less than 70 mg/dL. The initiation of ezetimibe 10 mg daily should achieve an

LDL-C <70 mg/dL as this has roughly a 10–20% expected decrease. It is not necessary to initiate PCSK9 inhibitor therapy at this time as adjunctive lowering with ezetimibe should be tried first. Regarding the patient's diabetes as well as her obesity, she meets criteria for the addition of GLP1 receptor agonist and would benefit from the combined improvement in glycemic control, weight loss, and cardiovascular benefit. Thus, the correct answer is D—start ezetimibe 10 mg daily and tirzepatide 2.5 mg weekly. Moreover, the 2022 ACC Expert Consensus Decision Pathway on non-statin therapy considers the addition of ezetimibe beyond statin therapy in those with a CAC score ≥100 if the LDL-C is still 70 mg/dL or higher.

References
1. ElSayed NA, Aleppo G, Aroda VR, et al. on behalf of the American Diabetes Association. 10. Cardiovascular disease and risk management: standards of care in diabetes-2023. Diabetes Care. 2023;46(Suppl 1):S158–90.
2. Frías JP, Davies MJ, Rosenstock J, et al. SURPASS-2 Investigators. Tirzepatide versus semaglutide once weekly in patients with type 2 diabetes. N Engl J Med. 2021;385(6):503–15.
3. Lloyd-Jones DM, Morris PB, Ballantyne CM, et al. 2022 ACC expert consensus decision pathway on the role of nonstatin therapies for LDL-cholesterol lowering in the management of atherosclerotic cardiovascular disease risk: a report of the American College of Cardiology Solution Set Oversight Committee. J Am Coll Cardiol. 2022;80(14):1366–418.

Index

A
2022 AACE guidelines for the diagnosis and management of NAFLD, 52
ABCG1, 219
2018 ACC/AHA cholesterol guidelines, 28, 48, 96, 176
ACC/AHA guidelines, 140, 225, 245
2018 ACC/AHA guidelines for the management of blood cholesterol, 50, 182, 205
2020 ACC/AHA guideline for the management of patients with Valvular heart disease, 127
2019 ACC/AHA guideline on primary prevention, 124
2017 ACC/AHA hypertension guideline, 236
ACC/AHA primary prevention guidelines, 140
2018 ACC/AHA/Multi-society cholesterol management guidelines, 8, 112, 113
2018 ACC/AHA Multisociety guidelines, 101, 108, 155, 188
2021 ACC/AHA/SCAI guideline for coronary artery revascularization, dual antiplatelet therapy, 127
2014 ACC/AHA stable ischemic angina guidelines, 106
2020 ACC Expert Consensus Decision Pathway on Management of Bleeding in Patients on Oral Anticoagulants, 128
2017 ACC Expert Consensus Decision Pathway for Periprocedural Management of Anticoagulation, 128
ACE inhibitor, 46
Acupuncture, 32, 137
Acute myocardial infarction (AMI), 68, 229
Acute pancreatitis, 56
Aerobic and resistance training, 175
Agatston coronary artery calcium score, 59, 200
Agatston score, 77
Aggrastsat to Zocor trial (A to Z), 213
Agatston units, 25
Aggressive lipid-lowering, 69
AHA/ACC 2018 Cholesterol Guidelines, 69
AHA/ACC 2018 Cholesterol Practice Guidelines, 231
AHA/ACC Guideline on the Management of Blood Cholesterol, 139
AHA/ACC hypertension guideline, 147
2018 AHA/ACC/multisociety guideline on primary prevention, 14, 101, 104, 105
2019 AHA/ACC/multisociety guideline on primary prevention of cardiovascular disease, 149
2019 AHA/ACC Prevention Guidelines, 122
2013 AHA/ACC/TOS Obesity Treatment guidelines, 222
AHA/American College of Cardiology pooled cohort equation, 173
Alcohol-containing beverages, 4
Alcoholic cardiomyopathy, 30
Alcohol ingestion, 31
American Association for the Study of Liver Diseases (AASLD), 51
American Association of Clinical Endocrinology (AACE), 51
2022 American College of Cardiology Expert Consensus Decision Pathway (ACC ECDP), 55, 188, 189
American Heart Association, 8, 193
Androgen deficiency, 195
Anemia of kidney disease, 62
Ankle brachial index (ABI), 3, 83, 96

Antihypertensive drug therapy with stage 2 hypertension, 71
Anti-obesity medication, 4, 87
Antiplatelet agents, 180
Antiplatelet drug therapy, 49, 181
Anti-sense non-coding RNA (ANRIL), 165
Appendectomy, 47
Arachidonic acid (AA), 180
Aromatase inhibitor therapy, 4
ARRIVE, 246
Arteriosclerotic cardiovascular disease (ASCVD), 10, 13, 15, 55, 84, 85, 100
  biomarkers, 31
  CAC, 60
  cardiovascular risk assessment, 50
  pooled cohort risk calculator, 44, 168
  primary and secondary prevention of, 13, 14, 24
  related events, 2, 16, 19, 112
  risk category, 55, 101, 103–105
  risk estimator or borderline, 82
  risk reduction therapy, 20
  risk score, 56
  traditional risk factors, 251
  treatment of lipid disorders, 119
  treatment approach, 44
ASCEND, 246
ASPC clinical practice statement, 79
Aspirin resistance, 179
Aspirin's antiplatelet therapy, 179
Aspirin therapy, 38, 74, 115
ASPREE, 246
Astrocytes, 231
Atherosclerosis in peripheral arteries, 247
Atherosclerosis risk in communities (ARIC) study, 200
Atherosclerotic cardiovascular disease
  female-specific risk enhancing factors, 28
  risk, 20
  treatment of lipid disorders, 22
Atorvastatin, 104
Atrial fibrillation, 44, 166, 167
  occurrence, in Blacks, 21, 117

B
BARI-2D, 223
Behavior therapy, 65
Blood brain barrier, 69, 231
Blood cholesterol, management, 205
Blood pressure
  dietary sodium intake, 160
  lifestyle management, 160
  management, 41, 159
  non-pharmacologic treatments, 130
  patient centered recommendations, 42
  pharmacologic therapy, 42
  stages, 41
  treatment and follow-up, 160
Blood pressure control, 41, 43
Body mass index (BMI), 5, 43
Borderline dyslipidemia, 73
BP-lowering medication, 235
BP reduction with continuous positive airway pressure, 241
Bupropion, 125

C
Canadian Cardiovascular Society (CCS) Class 1-2 angina, 15
Canakinumab Anti-inflammatory Thrombosis Outcome Study (CANTOS), 63, 69
Canakinumab for Atherosclerotic Disease (CANTOS) trial, 39, 152, 214, 233
Canakinumab for Atherosclerotic Disease Study (CANTOS) study, 39, 154
Cardiac apex, 11, 12
Cardiac chest pain, 223
Cardiac computed tomography, 109
Cardiac imaging, 29, 54, 132
Cardiac microvascular dysfunction, 29
Cardiac performance of long-distance runners, 122
Cardiac rehabilitation (CR), 8, 97
Cardiac valve surgery, 97
CARDIA study, 23, 121
Cardiology practice, 57
Cardiometabolic health, 5
Cardioprotective dietary patterns, 24
Cardiorespiratory fitness, 121
Cardiovascular clinical trials, 1, 36, 79, 144, 145
Cardiovascular disease (CVD)
  antiplatelet therapy, 49
  mortality rates, 72, 240
  pretest and posttest, 116
  reproductive risk factors, 36, 143
  risk discrimination, 250
  risk factors, 43, 59
  subclinical measures, 45
  in symptomatic or asymptomatic women and men, 89, 90
Cardiovascular health
  optimization, 4
  psychological factors, 58
Cardiovascular manifestations, 24

Cardiovascular medications, 20
Cardiovascular medicines, 77
Cardiovascular mortality, 4
Cardiovascular risk, 38
    assessment, 35, 46, 173
    factors, 99
    management, 2
    optimization, 5
Cardiovascular screening evaluation, 59
Chest discomfort, 75
2021 Chest Pain guidelines, 223
Cholesterol management guideline, 74, 243
Chronic kidney disease (CKD), 26, 62, 206
Chronic venous disease (CVD), 1, 76, 79, 81
    first line therapy, 82
    prevalence, 249
    treatment, 2
Cilostazol, 86
Clinical-etiology-anatomy-pathophysiology (CEAP) classification system, 81
Clopidogrel, 38
Clopidogrel or initiate a low-dose anticoagulant (COMPASS trial), 251
Cognitive behavioral intervention on depression, 58
Comprehensive cardiac rehabilitation, 8
Congestive heart failure, 26
Continuous positive airway pressure (CPAP), 234
CORAL trial, 241
Corona phlebectatica, 81
Coronary anatomy, 131, 187
Coronary angiography, 242
Coronary artery calcification, 17, 240
Coronary artery calcium (CAC), 169
    scan, 17, 110
    score, 2, 16, 18, 34, 49, 61, 66, 77, 101, 111, 142, 169, 182, 204, 252
        assessment-guided strategy for statin therapy, 111
        asymptomatic primary prevention, 60
        burden, 60, 202
        clinical benefit, 250
        evidence-based guidance, 202
        pathogenesis, 250
        prevalence, 250
        radiation exposure in single computed tomography scan, 56, 191
        testing, 108, 109, 114, 115, 223, 251
Coronary artery disease (CAD), 15, 73, 127
    pre-and post-menopausal women, 28
    prevalence, 126
    by stress testing, 90
    therapeutic lifestyle intervention, 75

Coronary bypass graft (CABG) surgery plus medical therapy in the STICH trial, 16
Coronary computed tomography angiography (CCTA), 15, 33, 50, 76, 132, 184, 188, 249
Coronary flow reserve (CFR)/myocardial flow reserve (MFR), 193
Coronary plaques with positive remodeling, 184
C-reactive protein (CRP), 213

D

Dept of Health and Human services, 141, 227
Diabetes, cardiovascular complications, 45
Diabetes mellitus (DM), 84
Diabetes support and education (DSE), 86
Dietary Approaches to Stop Hypertension (DASH) diet, 24, 32, 123, 138, 162, 163, 178
Dietary Guidelines for Americans 2020–2025, 135
Dilated veins around the ankle, 81
Direct-acting oral anticoagulants (DOACs), 27, 127
Dual antiplatelet therapy (DAPT), 27, 38, 147
Duke treadmill score (DTS), 7, 242
Duplex scanning, 81
Dutch Criteria, 191
Dyslipidemia, 3

E

Early lipid screening, 190
Early-onset myocardial infarction, 74
ECG exercise testing, 88
Ejection fraction with exercise, 73
Elevated LDL-C, 41
Elevated Lipoprotein (a) [Lp(a)], 135
Emerging risk factors collaboration, 168
Endocrine Society Clinical Practice Guideline, 196
Enhancing Recovery in Coronary Heart Disease (ENRICHD) study, 194
Erectile dysfunction, 59, 198
2019 ESC chronic coronary syndromes guidelines, 106
Estimated glomerular filtration rate (eGFR), 41
Evidence-based care, 23, 120
Exercise, 137
Exercise testing, 7, 94, 95
Exercise treadmill test, 93
Ezetimibe, 113

F

Familial hypercholesterolemia (FH), 31, 71, 136, 244
Fasting triglycerides, 37
Fatal/nonfatal MI/stroke, 91
FDA approved pharmacotherapies, 104
Fertility therapy, 129
FIB-4, 184
Finland Cardiovascular Risk Study (FINRISK) risk calculator, 173
Framingham Risk Score, 173

G

Gene polymorphism, 43
Generalized anxiety disorder questionnaire-2, 194
Genetic polymorphism, 43
Glucagon-like peptide-1 receptor agonist (GLP1-RA), 67, 98, 227
Glycemic control in T2D, 24
Goals and Metrics Committee of the Strategic Planning Task Force of the American Heart Association, 96
Guideline directed medical therapy (GDMT), 229
Gut microbiome, 63

H

HbA1c, 10
Heart failure and preserved ejection fraction (HFpEF), 71, 97
Heart failure and reduced ejection fraction (HFrEF), 235
Heart Protection Study, 232, 247
Heart rate index equation, 23, 121
Heart rate recovery, 90
Hemoglobin A1c, 9
Heterozygous familial hypercholesterolemia (HeFH), 18, 110
HgbA1c, 62
High sensitivity C-reactive protein, 63
High sensitivity troponin I, 68
High sensitivity troponins, 229
Holiday heart syndrome, 30, 133
Hormone replacement therapy, 129
Human bacterial microbiome, 209
Humor, 67
Hypercholesterolemia
   evaluation, 61
   management, 61, 62
Hypertension, 28, 120
   large randomized controlled clinical trials, 42
   management, 33

non-pharmacologic therapy, 33, 139
randomized controlled clinical trials, 164
staging and risk of heart failure, 164
treatment, 53, 186
Hypertriglyceridemia, 2
Hypothyroidism, 18

I

IDEAL trial, 178
IMProved Reduction of Outcomes: Vytorin Efficacy International Trial (IMPROVE-IT), 213
Incident coronary heart disease events by statin therapy, 245
Inflammasomes, 152
Inflammation, 211
Intensive lifestyle intervention (ILI), 86
International normalized ratio (INR) goal, 27
Invasive coronary angiography, 15
ISCHEMIA trial, 33, 138, 251
Ischemic heart disease, 46
Ischemic stroke, 37

J

Justification for the Use of Statins in Prevention: an Intervention Trial Evaluating Rosuvastatin (JUPITER), 39, 70, 154, 233

K

Kaplan–Meier analysis of time to incident heart failure, 161
Kaplan-Meier curves, 119
Ketogenic diet, 47, 175
Kidney Disease Improving Global Outcomes (KDIGO), 155, 156

L

Lactic acidosis, 67
L-arginine, beetroot and cocoa flavonoids, 136
Laughter, 67
Lipid management, 36
Lipopolysaccharide (LPS), 210
Lipoprotein (a) [Lp(a)], 31, 44, 57, 113, 114, 135, 168, 193
Lipoprotein-associated phospholipase A2, 64
Liver stiffness measure (LSM) test, 52
Liver stiffness measurement (LSM) based on Fibroscan, 185
Look AHEAD Research Group, 87
Look AHEAD trial, 86
Low-carbohydrate diets, 200

Low density lipoprotein cholesterol (LDL-C), 25, 40, 55, 56, 61, 62, 172, 204
Lower extremity peripheral artery disease, 75
Lower extremity revascularization procedure, 86
Low-salt and Mediterranean diets, 148
LpPLA2, 215

M

Macrophages scavenge lipoproteins in the extracellular milieu, 219
Major acute coronary events (MACE), 247
Major adverse cardiovascular events (MACE), 86, 155, 248
Major adverse limb events (MALE), 247, 248
Major associated cardiac events, 57
Major depression disorder in the United States, 57, 194
Mechanical aortic valve replacement (AVR), 27
Mediterranean diet, 137, 178, 199
Metabolic syndrome, 65, 176, 222
Metformin, 9, 228
Metformin monotherapy, 87
METS, 35
Monofilament test, 10
MRI proton density fat fraction (MRI-PDFF), 184
Multi-ethnic study of atherosclerosis (MESA) cohort follow-up, 161, 182, 191
  participant, 116
Multivariable-adjusted hazard ratios, 204
Myocardial infarction (MI), 19, 21, 40, 74, 149, 244
Myocardial flow reserve (MFR), 193

N

National Center for Health Statistics (CDC), 117
National Institute of Alcohol Abuse and Alcoholism (NIAAA), 135
National Lipid Association (NLA), 100, 113, 123
National Lipid Association expert opinion guidelines, 191
National Lipid Association Scientific Statement, 147
Neurocognitive impairment, 69
Neutrophils, 64, 220, 221
NHANES data, 240
NHIS data, 95
NIH-sponsored CV clinical trials, 145
NLRP3 inflammasome, 152, 153
Non-alcoholic fatty liver disease (NAFLD)
  prevalence, 51
  simple steatosis, 51
Nonalcoholic steatohepatitis (NASH), 185
Nonfatal myocardial infarction/death, 245
Non-imaging exercise treadmill test, 6
Non-pharmacologic therapy plus BP-lowering medications, 105
NSAID therapy, 151
Nuclear perfusion scan, 76

O

Obesity, 29, 53, 186, 187
Obstructive coronary artery disease, 17
Obstructive sleep apnea (OSA), 73
  in hypertensive sleep apneic patients, 72
  increased neck circumference, 222
Olive oil, 70
Optimal medical therapy (OMT), 75
Optimism, 195

P

Patient Health Questionnaire-2 for depression, 194
Pericytes, 231
Perineal infections, 67
Peripheral arterial disease (PAD), 4, 86
  asymptomatic and uncomplicated, 3
  prevalence, 3, 85
  risk factors, 3, 85
Periprocedural bridging
  of anticoagulation, 27
Physical activity (PA), 35, 66, 141
Pitavastatin, 22, 117
Prevention of Decline in Cognition After Stroke Trial (PODCAST), 148
Polycystic ovary syndrome (PCOS), 35
Polyvascular disease, 247
Pooled cohort equations (PCE), 48, 101, 142
9p21 polymorphism, 165
Pravastatin or Atorvastatin Evaluation and Infection Therapy trial (PROVE-IT), 213
Preeclampsia, 101
Prevention After Stroke-Blood Pressure (PAST-BP) trial, 148
Preventive cardiology, 67
Primary care physician (PCP), 40
Progressive claudication symptoms, 1
Proprotein convertase subtilisin/kexin type 9 (PCSK9) inhibitor, 34, 71, 113, 115, 147, 238, 239, 247, 252, 253
Prospective Cardiovascular Munster Score, 173

Prospective Urban Rural Epidemiology (PURE) cohort studies, 200
PROSPER trials, 232
Psoriasis, 155

R
Randomized clinical trial with lipid-lowering agents, 232
Randomized control trial, 175
Recreational drug use, 47
Recurrent Stroke Prevention Clinical Outcome (RESPECT) trial, 148
REDUCE-IT trial, 192
REDUCE-IT. A PCSK9 inhibitor, 172
REGARDS study, 168
Renal-artery stenting, 72
Renin angiotensin system inhibition (RASi), 62, 126, 206
Resident macrophages within atherosclerotic plaques, 64
Risk assessment tools, 16

S
SCOT-HEART trial, 140
Secondary prevention of small subcortical strokes (SPS3) trial, 148
Semaglutide, 227
Severe hypertriglyceridemia, 191
Sex-specific Kaplan-Meir failure, 167
SGLT-2 inhibitors, 98, 158, 162, 206
SGLT2 therapy, 228
SHARP trial, 156
Short chain fatty acids (SCFAs), 210
Simone Broom Criteria, 191
Single-photon emission computed tomography (SPECT), 188
Smoking, 175
Smoking cessation, 25, 125
Social determinants of health, 23, 120
Sodium-glucose co-transport in the proximal tubule of the kidneys, 126
Sodium glucose transport protein inhibitor (SGLT2i), 62, 155, 207, 208
SPARCL trial, 178
Specialized pro-resolving molecules, 63
Stable ischemic heart disease (SIHD), 27, 242
Stage 1 hypertension medical therapy, 41, 71
Standup comics, 228
Statin therapy, 12, 13, 44, 54, 145
Stimulus (cue) control, 223
STITCH trial with ischemic cardiomyopathy, 107
STOP-ACEi trial, 206

Stroke, risk assessment, 20
Supervised exercise therapy (SET), 8
SUSTAIN-6 trial, 87
Supraventricular tachycardia (SVT), 18
Symptomatic coronary artery disease, 27
Symptomatic lower extremity peripheral artery disease, 75
Symptomatic peripheral arterial disease (SET), 97
Synergistic toxicity, 133
SYNTAX score, 66, 223
Systemic coronary risk evaluation, 173

T
Testosterone, 196, 198
  deficiency, 230
  supplementation, 196
Testosterone replacement therapy (TRT), 68, 230
Ticagrelor, 151
Tirzepatide, 5, 29, 53, 88, 97, 131
TNT trial, 178
Treadmill exercise testing, 6, 16, 107
Triglycerides, 166
Triglyceride (TG) profile, 56
Trimethylamine-N-oxide (TMAO), 210
Type 2 diabetes mellitus
  management, 42
  on metformin monotherapy, 87

U
Uncontrolled HTN (hypertension) among US historically marginalized populations, 22
Underreporting of alcohol intake, 30, 134
UK QRISK2 risk assessment tool, 173
Urinary albumin to creatinine ratio values, 125
US Preventive Services Task Force (USPSTF), 48, 115, 178

V
Vegan/vegetarian diets, 178
VIRGO study, 229
Visceral adipose tissue, 64, 217, 218
Vitamin E, 185

W
West of Scotland Coronary Prevention Study (WOSCOPS), 245
Women's Health Study, 43, 165

SPRINGER NATURE

GPSR Compliance

The European Union's (EU) General Product Safety Regulation (GPSR) is a set of rules that requires consumer products to be safe and our obligations to ensure this.

If you have any concerns about our products, you can contact us on ProductSafety@springernature.com

In case Publisher is established outside the EU, the EU authorized representative is:

Springer Nature Customer Service Center GmbH
Europaplatz 3
69115 Heidelberg, Germany

The manufacturer's authorised representative in the EU is Springer Nature Customer Service Centre GmbH, Europaplatz 3, 69115 Heidelberg, Germany. If you have any concerns regarding our products, please contact ProductSafety@springernature.com

Printed and bound by CPI Group (UK) Ltd, Croydon, CR0 4YY
25/03/2026
02078177-0005